OPTIONS FOR HEALTH
AND HEALTH CARE

Options for Health
and Health Care
THE COMING OF
POST-CLINICAL MEDICINE

Alfred E. Miller

Maria G. Miller

Foreword by Wilbur J. Cohen
Former Secretary
Department of Health, Education and Welfare

A WILEY-INTERSCIENCE PUBLICATION

JOHN WILEY & SONS   New York • Chichester • Brisbane • Toronto

Library of Congress Cataloging in Publication Data

Miller, Alfred E   1930-
  Options for Health and Health Care
  (Health, medicine, and society)
  "A Wiley-Interscience publication."
  Includes index.
  1. Medical care—United States.   2. Social medicine
—United States.   3. Medical economics—United States.
4. Medical policy—United States.   I. Miller, Maria G.,
joint author.   II. Title.   [DNLM: 1. Costs and cost
analysis.   2. Delivery of health care—United States.
3. Health services—Economics—United States.   W 84
AA1 M58c]

RA395.A3M477   362.1′0973   80-27755
ISBN 0-471-60409-7

Printed in the United States of America

10 9 8 7 6 5 4 3 2 1

TO PEGGY, ERIC, AND PETER

Foreword

Health and medical care services in the United States constitute a vast and growing business. Science and technology have radically changed the services provided during this century. The extension of the insurance concept to the financing of health services has had an important impact on the access to and the delivery of medical care. Both the public and private sectors are heavily involved in health and medical care programs, as well as Federal, state, and local governmental agencies, voluntary associations, and the educational system at all levels.

Although it may be difficult to understand such a complex and changing system, it is even more difficult to guide and direct its future course. For instance, efforts to constrain cost increases, expand early access to preventive and primary care, provide services to underserved areas, reduce unnecessary hospital and nursing home care, to judge and improve the quality of care, extend home health services, or to provide appropriate care to the mentally ill or mentally retarded—all involve substantial organizational as well as economic resources that tax the administrative and creative talent of a wide range of personnel. The establishment of priorities in the medical care area is fraught with difficult moral issues. Questions of life and death, pain and suffering do not easily fit within cost-benefit and cost-effective evaluations.

Those who attempt to analyze and propose constructive and controversial changes in the health delivery system thus must approach their task with both a sense of humility and a respect for the challenge. It is possible to understand and describe how we arrived where we are. It is even possible to try to surmise where we are likely to be in the near future on the basis of present trends. But to choose new lines of action, to encourage innovative institutional changes, to disturb the status quo, all take both understanding and conviction with recognition of the possibility of error, defeat, and sometimes even success.

In the late 1970s, the United States was utilizing some 30 percent of all health and medical expenditures for the approximately 10 percent of the population age 65 and over. As the older population continues to increase, medical expenditures are bound to increase to meet the needs of this group.

vii

The provision of nursing home care and alternatives to institutional care have become persistent, continuing issues. Questions concerning the extent of medical care for terminal illness confront not only physicians but also philosophers, families, the courts, and the legal system.

The role of health maintenance organizations and nation-wide health planning during the 1980s will provide many opportunities for cooperative efforts between providers and consumers and for a wide range of professional competencies in the management of these enterprises. A changing balance of power within the health and medical care decision-making system may have extensive ramifications that cannot be clearly and completely foreseen. It may be said with some certainty that unexpected developments in the future will affect the system, just as they have in the past. The ability to turn such unexpected developments into constructive and beneficial improvements will be important. The leaders in the health professions in the future will have to be more sensitive than the leaders in earlier years to the consideration of options, priorities, tradeoffs, the attitudes of the consumer, and the objectives and goals of national economic, political, and social policy.

This book gives the reader the opportunity to understand and comprehend the challenge ahead for the health and medical care system and the providers and consumers who enable the system to function. I look back on the 1940s and 1950s when the number of courageous and insightful students of the system as a whole were few and far between. It was neither safe nor sound to present a comprehensive diagnosis of the system's difficulties or possible future lines of change. Such a comprehensive approach was subject to attack as being radical, impractical, or visionary. Today, the situation is markedly different. There are innumerable diagnoses publicly available and a wide variety of proposed changes. There are more facts and descriptions to study and more panaceas to choose from. The student, provider, consumer, or legislator who tackles the medical care system must absorb huge quantities of information and be prepared to evaluate what is offered within some framework that helps toward an effective decision-making process.

I think *Options for Health and Health Care* will help in that difficult political and intellectual effort. It is worth trying and worth doing. The health of every individual, of the family, and of the community is a precious resource beyond the capacity of economists to price. Each effort to understand our health and medical system and to improve it is a contribution toward maximizing and perfecting the human condition.

The present system of medical care delivery is probably not as good as its most avid defenders say it is, but, at the same time, it is probably not as bad as its severest critics claim. There is no perfect health delivery system nor is one in sight within our lifetime, or possibly ever. Physicians and consumers must learn to live with an imperfect, complex, and controversial system.

But it is clear as we look back over time that our health and medical care system has changed, is continuing to change, and that it is capable and able to change. Consider this optimistic note when reading this book.

WILBUR J. COHEN

Former Secretary of Health,Education and Welfare, 1968–1969
Professor of Public Affairs
Lyndon Baines Johnson School of Public Affairs
The University of Texas at Austin

Preface

Medicine since the 1930s has made tremendous strides in its ability to prevent disease and to intervene successfully once illness has struck. Yet, despite this continued improvement, we hear increasing dissatisfaction with the health care system. Hardly a year goes by without several new books describing the "crisis in health care." Frustrations created by the discrepancy between public expectation and what actually occurs in the health sector have led to a growing incidence of malpractice suits and denunciations of the medical profession, hospitals, and other providers of care as well as repeated legislative attempts aimed at reforming various aspects of the health system.

The purpose of this book is not to add another voice decrying the failures of health care to fulfill its apparent promise. The goal instead is to provide an understanding of why the system functions as it does—both its strengths and its weaknesses—and where it is going. Health problems and health care inadequacies are discussed at length, but not in order to deprecate the accomplishments of medicine or impune the integrity of the dedicated men and women working in the field. Consideration of the problems is intended primarily as a tool to gain sharper insight into the nature of health and disease in society and the operation of our health system. The objective is to learn how we can bring medicine's advances to bear most effectively on the health needs of the nation.

Most policy-oriented analyses of the health system focus on individual problems of immediate concern to policy makers, such as infant morality, prevalence of chronic diseases, maldistribution of health care workers, overutilization of services, cost escalation, and quality of care. It is a central thesis of this book that the major problems of health and health care are not isolated phenomena to be "solved" one by one—let alone something to be blamed on identifiable individuals or groups. Instead they are primarily results of the structure of society and of the health care system as a whole. The life style of post-industrial society is largely responsible both for the improvements in health and for the ascendancy of the chronic diseases prevalent today. The fundamental orientation of the health system is responsible for many of the triumphs of medicine, but at the same time it entails certain inherent disjunctions making it ill-fitted in important ways to deal with the new needs of society for care.

Our aim is to look at this larger picture, to provide an integrated analysis of the overall structure and behavior of the American health system. The book is meant to offer informed citizens, health policy makers, administrators, health services researchers, and other students of the health sector with an overview of the system, an understanding of why it behaves as it does, the problems it faces, and the options for dealing with them. This goal has necessitated an analytic perspective different from that usually found in books on health care.

This new methodological approach involves three elements. The first is structural analysis. While individual problems and issues confronting policy makers represent serious concerns that call for resolution, in many instances they are merely symptoms of deeper incongruencies of the system. An examination of its structure as a functional whole, and of its basic tensions, is necessary to understand the true nature of the immediate problems. Only then will the most effective strategies to overcome the individual problems become obvious. Otherwise, attempted solutions are likely to remain little more than temporizing or cosmetic patchup undertakings.

The second element is analytic history. The features of organizational, social, and professional structures that are significant for understanding the system and its key problems are not always immediately evident. A major methodological aid in identifying them is reexamination of the historical development of those structures and patterns of behavior from the vantage point of today's problems—a process we think of as analytic history. The history of institutions lives on in their inner dynamics and basic orientation, which determine their responses to everyday concerns and to attempts at restructuring them. Thus analysis of institutional evolution provides a special insight into the underlying forces influencing current structure and behavior, which may not be accessible from contemporary analysis alone.

The third element is the social dynamics of institutions. Having identified the key structural features of institutions and their basic orientations, we are still faced with the question of why these characteristics persist in the face of the dysfunction they often entail. We therefore attempt to discern the constellation of social interactions that sustain the institutions and create the incentives, norms, and other social influences on the behavior of individuals involved in them. These interactions are neither random nor static. They create a dynamic but stable pattern of mutually reinforcing social forces that perpetuate the structure of the institutions and the behavior of individuals involved. This pattern imparts momentum to an institution, making it highly resistant to outside functional needs or attempts to influence institutional behavior. Analysis of institutional social dynamics attempts to discover these self-sustaining patterns of interaction and to identify leverage points for influencing them.

The tightening limitations on resources for social programs and the growing burden of disease faced by post-industrial society will increasingly force policy makers to choose between difficult social tradeoffs in the coming years. We believe the holistic structural approach employed here will become more important in attempting to reach rational decisions about those tradeoffs and avoid the temptation to hide from them through self-deception and budgetary gimmickry.

A number of conclusions that grow out of our analysis must, we believe, become essential starting points for making these difficult decisions and for restructuring the health system to meet the new needs of society more effectively and efficiently. For example, health and disease are social phenomena. The health of the population is more a product of socioeconomic living standards and general technological development than the effectiveness of medical care. The marked reduction in the incidence and mortality of infectious diseases during this century was due primarily to improved living conditions, nutrition, sanitation, and to some extent immunization. Little of the decrease can be attributed to the improved clinical care that emerged during the same period. Similarly, the increased mortality and morbidity today from chronic illnesses, such as heart disease, strokes, and cancer, as well as from accidents and violence, result primarily from the life styles of post-industrial society.

Moreover, the revolution in medical science at the end of the last century created the potential for effective medical intervention for the first time in history. This success transformed the prestige and role of the medical profession and reoriented the organization of medical care to emphasize sophisticated technological methods based on the new scientific discoveries. The resulting social dynamic of the health system and its technology makes it more a product of its own objectives and its special technologies and less of the needs of society than was previously the case. This organization and its orientation toward care are increasingly less appropriate for the predominant chronic disease problems of today—creating a growing mismatch between the health care system and patients' needs.

Consider the system of financing medical care, which evolved from the growth of employment-derived health insurance and then tax-supported government insurance programs. This has created an incongruent mixture of elements from free-market, public-service, and regulated-utility types of economies. This mixture distorts the usual economic mechanisms necessary to control costs, allocate resources and utilization in accord with need, and provide leverage to force the health system to adjust to the new needs of patients and society. Instead the financing and reimbursement system reinforces the inappropriate emphasis on intensive technology rather than preventive and supportive care.

Strategies for reforming the health care delivery and financing system, for containing costs, and for establishing national health insurance are usually based on ideological commitment to one or another of the three economic structural types (free market, public service and regulated utility) as the ideal or only legitimate one. Each strategy seeks to correct the deficiencies of the one economic type by eliminating the distortions caused by admixture of the other types—using tactics such as increasing competition, public budgeting, or rate and investment regulation. The competing ideologies

about the proper nature of the health economy are politically at logger-
heads so that legislative initiatives often come to an impasse.

Finally, major structural reforms are necessary to bring the function of
the health system into better match with the new needs for care and to re-
introduce effective economic mechanisms for controlling cost and allocating
resources. Nevertheless, we do not have the option of starting from scratch
and building up an ideal system—even if agreement could be reached as to
how such a system should look. The health system has an existing structure
that cannot be radically or suddenly reorganized. For example, to believe
that the economic organization of the health sector, which now is financed
largely like a public service, could be transformed into an effective competitive market simply by reforming the tax laws fails to recognize the powerful
momentum of existing institutions and social structures. The same fallacy
underlies the belief that professionally (provider) dominated decision making
could be converted into control by consumers simply by making patients
directly responsible for a larger component of the payment. On the other
hand, it is equally naïve to think that significant improvement can be
achieved by trying to solve isolated symptomatic problems in a piecemeal
fashion. Continuing efforts are needed to deal with urgent immediate problems, but it is also necessary to look for leverage points that can be used to
gradually influence the basic structural problems in a direction more congruent with today's health needs. No single change in the system can accomplish this, but a coordinated strategy of such changes may be able to do
so over time.

Although this book is foremost an original treatise on the health system,
it can serve as a primary textbook for courses in medical sociology or survey
courses on the health system for students of health administration or health
policy. The first half of the manuscript grew out of lectures in medical
sociology given by one author at the City University of New York from
1972 to 1977. The second half evolved from experience in health policy and
health politics at the Department of Health, Education and Welfare (now
the Department of Health and Human Services) from 1977 to 1980. The
book is not intended to give a detailed description or complete review of
the standard knowledge about the health system, but it provides a unified
overview and analysis of the underlying forces for understanding the dynamics of the system and its components. It can also be used as supplemental reading for courses in medical economics or health politics.

Besides direct relevance for the health field, we believe that the new
methodological approach to the study of institutions used here is applicable
in other areas. This perspective may be of general interest to sociologists,
economists, political scientists, and public administrators for application in
many sectors besides health. For sociologists the approach merges structural–
functional with interactionist analysis in a complementary fashion. Each of
these traditional approaches alone was found wanting as a means of explaining the institutional momentum and yet dynamic evolution of the
medical profession, hospitals, and the financing system—in the face of grow-

ing dysfunction vis-à-vis the larger society. For economists, the analysis of
the structure and mechanisms of the health care market raises questions
about the limitations of standard economic interpretations of the health sector. The examination of the link among economics, ideology, and politics
in relation to health care offers a potentially useful method for extending
the context of political economy in other sectors. For political scientists, the
history of political forces in health policy and the investigation of the ideological foundations for diverging political strategies to contain costs, reform
the delivery system, or establish national health insurance affords new insights into the political alignments of the Congress and interest groups in
regard to health issues. It serves as a case study in the interrelationships of
social, technological, economic, and professional forces within the political
process.

Finally, for public administrators, policy makers, and informed citizens,
we believe the health sector may present a microcosm illustrating many features beginning to appear in the larger economy—perhaps with lessons in
regard to certain problems confronting post-industrial society in general as
we move further into the 1980s. Attempts to draw these analogies explicitly
would be beyond the scope of this book. However, the nature of institutional momentum driven by technology, as found in health care, brings to
mind parallels in the energy field. The politics of special interests and the
impact of budgetary self-deception recall attempts to control inflation in
many sectors. The role played by changes of social structure and by the
revolution of life styles in influencing disease patterns makes one think of
our energy, environmental, and urban problems. It is conceivable that the
more encompassable health care sector could be a prototype laboratory
for learning about and perhaps developing methods for dealing with some
of the challenges that advanced industrial society will have to cope with in
the coming years.

Many friends and colleagues have patiently read parts of the manuscript
at various stages in its genesis and have given us valuable comments and
advice. We would particularly like to thank Wilbur Cohen, David Mechnic,
Arnold Weinberg, Joseph Eichenholz, Reginald Fitz, Steven Jonas, Richard
Warden, David Banta, William Weissert, Lester Breslow, Milton Roemer,
and Odin Anderson for their helpful contributions. The early preparation
of the manuscript was supported by a generous grant from the Commonwealth Fund of New York. The opinions expressed in this book are our
own, in our capacity as private citizens, and are not intended nor should
they be construed to represent official positions of the Department of Health
and Human Services or the Administration.

ALFRED E. MILLER
MARIA G. MILLER

Washington, D.C.
February 1981

Contents

OPTIONS FOR HEALTH
AND HEALTH CARE

CHAPTER ONE

Introduction:
An Overview of the Arguments

THE MISMATCH BETWEEN THE HEALTH CARE
SYSTEM AND TODAY'S HEALTH PROBLEMS

During the last 50 years there has been a growing mismatch between the health problems of the nation and the system of services intended to treat them. Since 1900 the kinds of diseases responsible for the most mortality and morbidity in our society have shifted markedly. Previously the important illnesses were predominantly acute infectious diseases. Today they are primarily chronic debilitating disorders, requiring modes of prevention and care very different from those that were common before. The structure of the health care system has also changed radically since 1900 but not in a way that would make it most effective for dealing with the newly prevalent illnesses. A new organization of health care emerged during the period when the infectious diseases were coming under control. This organization took on a momentum of its own as a result of the enhanced prestige of medical science, the vested interests in medical institutions, and the financing system that evolved parallel to the development of medical technology. Unfortunately, this momentum has carried the system of care in a direction that is not well suited to the kinds of diseases that are most prevalent today. The dysfunction created by this mismatch between health needs and health care is a major cause underlying many of the more obvious difficulties of the health system—including serious misallocations of resources, failure to prevent needless disability and suffering, inappropriate care for many illnesses, overuse of expensive medical services and technologies, excessive costs, and general dissatisfaction with the responsiveness of health care to patients' needs. Correcting this basic mismatch must be a primary concern of health policy makers in devising strategies to overcome the more commonly recognized specific problems.

THE NEW PATTERN OF DISEASES

In 1900 a third of all deaths in this country were caused by infectious diseases. Today only 3% of deaths fall into this category, nearly all from the pneumonia-influenza disease group. These occur almost exclusively among the elderly, premature infants, or other individuals weakened in some way. This decline in infectious diseases was partly due to changes in the structure of society, and partly to the breakthrough in the knowledge about disease that occurred after 1880 (Chapters 2 and 3). A major element of the decrease was simply a continuation of the improvements already underway throughout the nineteenth century as a result of better living standards and working conditions. The epidemics from diseases like typhoid largely ceased after the turn of the century because of better sanitation, food inspection, and water purification. Diphtheria almost disappeared after 1925 because of immunization. Tuberculosis and scarlet fever had virtually come under control because of better nutrition, better housing, and isolation of contagious cases, long before the antibiotics became available (around 1950) that made effective treatment possible. Antibiotics did make a major difference in the mortality and morbidity from pneumonia, ear infections in children, and streptococcal throat infections, which can lead to heart damage from rheumatic fever or chronic kidney damage (glomerulonephritis). Yet, only a small fraction of the reduction in morbidity and mortality from infectious diseases can be attributed to clinical intervention (i.e., treatment once an illness is in progress). Today except for viral upper respiratory infections, where medical intervention seldom makes any difference, only a tiny fraction of medical practice deals with infectious diseases. They account for only 2% of health care costs.

Currently 70% of all deaths result from heart disease, strokes, and cancer, compared to 18% in 1900. The next most frequent cause of death is violence: accidents, homicide, and suicide. In the 1 to 35 age group, violence is the most common cause of mortality and disability. Accidents alone account for 7% of health care costs and 15% of the productivity lost due to health disability. Diabetes, cirrhosis of the liver, and chronic lung disease together account for another 5% of total mortality. Thus chronic diseases and disabilities now make up the overwhelming portion of social loss due to health impairment and are responsible for the major share of health care costs.

Chronic disabling conditions are quite different in their causes, prevention, treatment, and effects from the infectious diseases of previous times (Chapters 4 and 5). The increased prevalence of chronic diseases is as much a product of the changes in society as was the decrease in infectious diseases (Chapter 5). In part chronic diseases are merely an unfortunate but predictable and largely unpreventable consequence of aging. As the age distribution of the population shifts with the increasing life expectancy and as acute infectious episodes, even among the aged, can be controlled, chronic illnesses are bound to be more prevalent. This creates the paradox that the healthier a society is in terms of longevity, the more disease is present at any time. Yet, chronic diseases are not just something left over after the acute infectious disease has been eliminated. Modern, affluent post-industrial life styles, including overeating, stress, and lack of exercise, as well as cigarette smoking, have contributed to heart disease. It is estimated that between 75 and 95% of all cancers are consequences of exposure to factors in the workplace, in the environment, or of social behavior like smoking, eating, and drinking habits (Chapters 4 and 5). Given the massive increases in environmental pollutants and food additives in recent years and the lag of 30 to 40 years from exposure until appearance of tumors, the incidence of these diseases will undoubtedly continue to increase in years ahead. Similarly, auto accidents and violence are largely a result of social structure and personal life style; most cirrhosis is the product of alcoholism; chronic lung disease is mainly a consequence of smoking or occupational and environmental exposure to pollutants.

These chronic conditions with their slow, diffusely caused onsets require approaches to prevention and treatment very different from the infectious diseases of the past. Rather than single specific disease agents, like bacteria, against which specific prevention and/or treatment can be targeted, today's diseases and disabilities have multiple causes that are difficult to interrupt at any one point. Prevention would require modifying patterns of personal, economic, and social behavior. Effective treatment for these disorders requires early detection, long-term surveillance, dependable patient management, maintenance and social support that provides for many diverse aspects of a patient's life needs (Chapter 5). The disabling and usually incurable nature of today's diseases makes improving the quality of life while suffering from them as important as increases in longevity. Consequently, the support that physicians give patients to increase their functional capacity and comfort or to help them cope with continuing illness and disability becomes as crucial as the purely technical therapy. To facilitate this, a very different organization of health care would be necessary than individually practicing physicians can provide. Ideal care for chronic diseases would call for coordinated teams of professionals to supply the diverse array of necessary services as well as supervision and information systems to ensure the integration and continuity of such care.

The medical situation (and health care needs) created by today's illnesses might be called "post-clinical" medicine to distinguish it from the structure of classic clinical medicine aimed so predominantly at curative intervention in acute limited episodes of illness. The term "post-clinical medicine" is meant in the same sense as "post-industrial society"—which does *not* imply that industry now plays a less essential role. Post-industrial society entails a continuing central role for industry, but one modified by the massive expansion of the service sector. Similarly post-clinical medicine implies the continuing importance of clinical medicine, but with major expansion of the supportive maintenance, patient management, and new preventive elements of care. To fulfill its new and growing role in the post-clinical era without creating intolerable costs, clinical medicine must become more efficient and better organized. It must become more responsive to the changing health needs and social context if it is to provide solutions to the health problems of society rather than adding to the burden.

An additional factor in changing health needs is the transition from extended families and close-knit supportive communities to isolated nuclear families, which has accompanied urbanization and increasing social mobility (Chapter 9). This restructuring of society adds to health care needs and costs by transferring demand for supportive care (particularly of the aged) to the health system instead of providing it within the family setting. These same changes in social structure also intensify the demand for physicians as personal counselors and sources of general social support not easily obtained elsewhere in our depersonalized society. Further need for the supportive and maintenance aspects of health care arises from the growing tendency to redefine many essentially social or behavioral problems as "diseases," for example, drug abuse and learning disabilities. These personal and social functions of medical care tend to be at odds with the highly specialized technical role of the physician—something equally desired by patients.

THE NEW STRUCTURE OF HEALTH CARE

The medical profession and the health care system built around it have changed radically since the 1930s—but not in a way that best fits the new needs for care. Until very recently in history medicine had little to offer in a technical sense that could make such difference in the outcome of disease (Chapter 3). A few exceptions were bone setting, some simple surgical procedures, obstetrics in certain circumstances, and a few drugs like quinine and digitalis discovered by folk medicine that happened to have specific therapeutic effects. The bloodletting, purging, and use of ineffective but toxic drugs, still standardly practiced until the late nineteenth century, undoubtedly sped more patients toward their demise in the course of history than were ever helped by medical techniques. The major positive role of the healing professions was allaying the anxiety of illness by reassuring patients and maintaining social order in the face of the disruption created by disease. As the guardians of the mysterious knowledge about death and disease, physicians have served as a kind of priesthood. Using this priestly mandate to define a "proper" controlled response to illness, they made it possible to carry on workable, if modified, social roles when the terror of disease struck.

Today the situation is almost reversed. Physicians command a technology that clearly can make a difference in the outcome of many illnesses—although it probably contributes much less to the improvement of health than is often believed. The application of this powerful technology has become the primary concern of medical practice at the expense of the social and personal supportive role of the past (Chapter 6). Almost every aspect of the profession and of the present health system emphasizes the specialized, high-technology elements of practice—medical education, the professional prestige system, financial incentives, the organization of the health system increasingly centered around hospital practice, the reimbursement system, and the expectations of the public generated by the apparent success of the new medical technology. Because of the predominant need for longer-term supportive and maintenance services, however, this sophisticated technological approach to medical care is increasingly less appropriate for the kinds of chronic illness to be dealt with today.

Ironically, a major factor in the internal dynamic that carries the health system in a direction so poorly matched to the needs of society derives from the very success achieved by medicine during the past hundred years. From 1850 to 1900 a new and remarkably successful theory of disease emerged, often referred to as the "germ theory" but actually much broader. It provided a framework for understanding diseases as disturbances of the newly understood normal physiological mechanisms of the body. These disturbances resulted from interference by particular disease agents or specific defects of other kinds. Based on this new theory, medical research discovered many of the most important bacterial, parasitic, and nutritional-deficiency disease agents from 1880 to 1900 (Chapter 3). This enabled public health professionals to devise measures for interrupting their transmission, in many cases almost immediately. It soon made immunization techniques possible for preventing other important diseases, such as diphtheria and tetanus. The development of anesthesia, knowledge of bacteriology, and better organization of hospitals and nursing allowed the rapid advancement of surgery.

After 1900 infant mortality, life expectancy, and other indicators of the health of Americans began to improve rapidly. In part this was simply a continuation of the improvement that had been going on during the nineteenth century as a result of better standards of living, housing, nutrition, sanitation, and working conditions. But it suddenly became much more visible as a nationwide system of vital statistics was established, and as health reform groups became more vocal. The rapid successes of public health in eliminating the epidemic scourges like cholera, typhoid, and diphtheria were clearly aided by the new technology of medicine. These accomplishments, together with the dramatic achievements of the new surgical capabilities, brought the medical profession rising prestige, which seemed primarily attributable to the new technology—whether or not this was actually justified (Chapter 4). Clinical medicine shared in this new technology-centered prestige from the beginning—despite the fact that it contributed very little to the improvement in health until after 1945. In fact, clinicians often received most of the credit because their visibility was greater than public health physicians and because of their traditional social status as overseers of health and disease in the community.

Discovery of antibiotics, hormones, and other drugs allowed physicians to intervene effectively in the course of many types of illnesses already in progress for the first time in history. These successes were responsible for a revolution in the role of physicians, in the structure of the health care system, its cost and financing, and in public expectations about medical care. The technical role of the physician using specialized methods to deal with specific disorders has become the major source of prestige. The growth in prestige and the concomitant financial incentives, which largely stemmed from these technological accomplishments, have been the driving forces in reshaping the structure of the profession and the health care system. They continue to carry it in the direction of its past success—despite the decrease in appropriateness for today's problems. The successful technological method oriented the profession almost entirely toward the use of specialized techniques for counteracting the specific organic defects rather than toward dealing with the patient's personal problems or the behavior leading to the organic pathology. Many developments in the organization of the profession also stemmed from this technological prestige. Medical education, for example, was completely reorganized to emphasize the scientific basis of the new technology, leading to increasing technical specialization of practice (Chapter 6).

To be sure, there are acute episodes within chronic illnesses when high-technology care is called for. Certain stages of some cancers are appropriately treated with complicated surgery, chemotherapy, or radiation. Acute episodes in heart disease often require intensive specialized treatment. Diagnosis of certain disorders can be assisted by complex procedures to determine the nature of the illness. But because of the single-minded orientation toward these approaches to medical care, costly and often questionably effective technology tends to be markedly overused and inappropriately used. More *"care*-oriented," supportive, and maintenance treatment is needed rather than *"cure*-oriented," episodic, high-intensity intervention (Chapters 5 and 10). High-technology care is directed toward particular physiological defects or episodes with the intent of overcoming them. It fosters a physician perspective and organization of practice that concentrates primarily on the episode. It leads to neglect of the means for dealing with the long-term problems—the social and personal context where a patient needs assistance in coping with the disabilities and adjusting to limitations. It also detracts attention from efforts toward individual and environmental preventive measures. The personal counseling and social expediting (and social control) functions that dominated the former physician role have fallen victim to the technological revolution in medicine. Yet, the prevalent chronic disease problems and social structure of post-industrial society increasingly require a health care system that fulfills these functions.

CONSEQUENCES OF THE MISMATCH

This mismatch between the structure of the health system and the pattern of diseases affects virtually every aspect of health care. It lies at the root of many of the more obvious problems facing health policy makers—overspecialization, maldistribution of manpower and resources, fragmentation of care, overuse of hospital care, unnecessary utilization of services, and runaway costs. The large percentage of physicians trained as specialists in order to master a portion of the complex technology is a direct result of the emphasis on the technical aspects of medical care. The abundance of specialists, in turn, increases the utilization of the technology that they are trained to employ—in many cases beyond the proven efficacy or real need for its use (Chapter 8). Almost no regard is given to the cost/benefit relationship in considering potential tradeoffs with other modes of care. The profession largely abides by the ideology that whatever *can* be done technically in a given situation, *must* be done—the so-called technological imperative (Chapters 6 and 10). The technological approach derives from a philosophy aimed at *cure* of specific physiological defects. This goal dominates treatment strategies—even when alternative approaches to care might be more appropriate—at the expense of other goals such as disability reduction, limitation of suffering, or prevention of less immediate but potentially more serious problems. The focus on diseases rather than patients, which goes with the technology-oriented, specialist-dominated approach to medicine, also adds to the depersonalization of health care—an important element in current patient dissatisfaction.

The increasing complexity of technology and the cost of the new equipment and facilities has forced its centralization into hospitals and encouraged physicians to concentrate on hospital practice. The new role of hospitals has also brought about profound changes in their organization and function. Hospitals began as custodial institutions established to provide asylums of last resort for the indigent sick. With the development of effective surgery and complicated medical interventions, hospitals became essential for good medical practice and were rapidly transformed to meet the demands of the middle class for such care (Chapter 7). At first the new hospitals were simply workshops where physicians could apply the products of the new scientific medicine in their practices. The growing complexity of technology and the open-ended financing made available by the new insurance system of payment further transformed hospitals into complex, highly departmentalized organizations. They developed their own goals and vested interests. The spawning of new semi-independent professions to operate the increasingly sophisticated technology made it more difficult to coordinate the various departments into an efficiently functioning whole—let alone to make the organization responsive to the needs of the communities they serve.

Specialization and growth of hospital-based practice contribute to the geographic maldistribution of physicians, since specialists and hospitals tend to concentrate in large urban areas. Large populations are needed to assure enough of the problems that specialists' technologies are designed to treat (Chapter 8). Since providers largely determine the utilization of their own services, and since the insurance method of payment allows almost unrestricted revenues, providers compete in regard to prestige rather than price. Consequently, higher concentrations of physicians or hospital beds tend to drive up unit costs rather than holding them down through price competition. The misallocation of health manpower and resources contributes significantly to the soaring cost of health care while leaving major gaps in availability of services. As a net result of the misallocation and the payment system, resources are overutilized for health care in relation to other sectors of the economy where they might actually do more to improve the health of the population (Chapters 5 and 7).

The growth in complexity and cost of medical technology has also fragmented the health care system into many specialized subsystems. The medical profession is fractionated into many specialty subdivisions and increasingly separated into hospital-based and office-based practitioners. Hospitals have become conglomerates of many semi-independent departments. Nursing homes, the drug industry, medical suppliers, the health insurance industry, health planning agencies, the public health system, all became specialized organizations built around the use of a particular part of the technology of health care. Each of these subsystems has taken on a life of its own—to some extent independent of the other components—with its own goals, its own organization, its own financing methods, and a vested interest in its own specialized technology. There is no longer an overall means of coordinating these components into a unified system responsive to the health needs of the population—as physicians once did (Chapters 7 and 8). Patients with little guidance have difficulties in negotiating their way through the maze of services. In many instances the independent objectives and directions of the various subsystems work at cross-purposes leading to inefficiency, inappropriate utilization, and waste.

As American society moves further into the era of post-clinical medicine, the present trends in the pattern of chronic diseases and in the structure of the health care system will most likely continue. This will intensify the functional mismatch unless vigorous measures are taken to change the present trends. Health policy makers must deal with these deep-seated roots of the more apparent problems if they hope to succeed in improving the function of the system through the major health reforms presently being considered. Given the mismatch between illnesses, the organization of the health care system, and the expectations of patients, pouring additional resources into the present system will accomplish little except to increase costs even further. New funds will simply be absorbed without significant improvement unless something is done to bring the components into a better fit and to solve their structural problems.

THE CAUSES OF THE MISMATCH

In the face of the major need for care of chronic illnesses, it seems paradoxical that the medical profession and health care system have changed in a direction so poorly matched to these health problems. The reasons lie in the self-propelling momentum of the medical profession and the institutions (especially hospitals) developed to implement the new technology. The semi-independent subsystems within the health care sector have acquired vested interests in their particular segments of the technology. Such an interest, together with the social organization built around the employment of the technology, creates an institutional momentum that carries the system in a direction largely independent of the actual needs for the services it provides.

The insurance system of payment, which developed in response to the costs of high-technology medical care, also became a superstructure reinforcing the structure and dynamic of other parts of the system. The stepwise emergence of the health financing system produced its own set of dysfunctional incongruencies among the economic mechanisms that would appropriately control costs and allocation of budgets in accord with consumer needs in most economic sectors. The perverse incentives of the resulting payment system are responsible for much of the inordinate cost increases for health care—and the inappropriate allocation of expenditures. As a result, cost escalation for some services are far out of proportion to benefits while other medical services suffer from inadequate resources. These dysfunctional economic incentives fuel the trend toward overutilization of inappropriate sophisticated technology. As a result of its unique financing methods, the health care system is largely freed from the usual market constraints or public accountability that force most economic sectors to conform their activities more nearly to the demands of society. Instead, it is left to be driven by its own internal priorities (Chapters 11 and 13).

The health insurance system of financing medical care began as a means of protecting patients against the highest unpredictable costs of illness. The growing expectations in regard to the accomplishments of medical science and technology brought a growing demand for guaranteed access to medical services. Meaningful access requires protection from the possible financial impact associated with the complex new technology, particularly in hospital care. As a response to this demand (and the concern on the part of hospitals for assured payment of the large bills generated by their services) health insurance was developed (Chapter 11). Its expansion was accelerated by becoming a major demand of collective bargaining as a fringe benefit of employment. Because of the preoccupation with the technological aspects of care and the high cost associated with it, health insurance benefit packages first emphasized hospital care, then surgery and other technology-intensive care, while neglecting primary (ambulatory) care and prevention. The availability of guaranteed payment through insurance coverage reinforces the emphasis on technological elements of care at the expense of supportive modes of caring for and preventing disability from today's prevalent diseases.

The rapid expansion of health insurance as a fringe benefit of employment soon made it the principal means of financing health care. In 1965 the largest remaining groups without health insurance, the elderly and the very poor, were given entitlement to government paid health insurance through the Medicare and Medicaid legislation. As a consequence of public and private insurance, the health care economy became an incongruent mixture of economic mechanisms derived partly from the free market, partly from public service, and partly from regulated-utility economies—without the usual checks and balances built into any of these economic systems when they exist in their pure forms (Chapter 13). Today health care is largely collectively financed as if it were a public service either directly through tax dollars or indirectly through fringe benefits of employment. Such employer costs are passed along as a burden to the general economy in the form of higher prices on goods and services produced as if they were a payroll tax. Yet, in contrast to overt public services, there is little opportunity for public decision making about health budgets. The insurance system of payment disperses the budgeting process into a myriad of individual utilization decisions. These are made mostly by providers unencumbered by the obligation to pay—in fact gaining financially. Overall budgeting and allocation take place only retrospectively and under no control from those who actually bear the burden of payment. Open-ended insurance payment methods and physician control of decisions for over 80% of their own utilization allow providers to determine their own budgets almost independently of consumer demand (Chapter 12).

With similar inconsistency, market entry is strictly limited by licensure and expertise requirements, as in a natural monopoly utility. Yet, distribution of supply is neither controlled by franchising nor by pressure of competition. Supply and service distribution decisions are left to providers as if health care were a free-market commodity (or with minimal constraints imposed by planning agencies). The price mechanism, necessary for provider competition, has been largely eliminated as a means to allocate services in accord with consumer demand. Thus, the internal incongruencies of the economic mechanisms in the health sector have made the financing system into an uncontrolled superstructure to the health system that frees it from the normal economic constraints existing in most parts of the economy. This perverse economic structure accounts for much of the cost escalation, inefficiency, and misallocation of resources in the health care system.

POSSIBLE STRATEGIES FOR ALLEVIATING
THE MISMATCH PROBLEMS

There are two sides to the health care mismatch equation: the new pattern of diseases and the structure of the health care system. Either can potentially be the focus of strategies to bring them into better congruence. The ideal strategy would be to prevent the chronic diseases by removing the original causes, but the easy strategies of prevention have largely been implemented already. These new disorders are primarily products of personal, social, and economic life style. Their prevention would require changing important features of personal or social behavior and environmental conditions. Besides curtailing cigarette smoking, this might include decreasing use of the automobile, rich diets, food additives, and industrial products that are carcinogenic—or even restructuring our metropolitan areas to make the quality of social life healthier for large segments of the population. Even if there were agreement about how to accomplish such social engineering, it would probably require actions and restraints that are incompatible with our political and ethical beliefs about personal freedom and privacy (Chapter 5).

The economic and social upheavals and tradeoffs in social priorities required by such behavior modification and social engineering strategies would have to be carefully weighed if any major long-term improvements in health are to be sought by this route. In order to make the difficult choices in the political arena, either at the national or local level, much better information would be needed concerning the relative effect on health and welfare produced by different options. For example, the costs in disruption to the economy, social structure, or personal freedom required by some methods of decreasing morbidity and social loss from accidents, homicide, coronary heart disease, or alcoholism might be unacceptable. On the other hand, it is conceivable that investing in mass transit or housing or schools, or even subsidizing healthful personal life styles would do more for health (even in the narrower sense) than the same investment in improved medical care. These are the kinds of alternatives that future preventive health policy decisions will have to deal with. The difficulties in making adequate evaluations for such choices are immense because we still know so little about the social factors determining the health status of a population. Major efforts toward developing such "health impact statements" will have to be made by health policy analysts who attempt to deal with the mismatch by changing the disease side of the equation (Chapter 5).

Even if many of these difficulties are overcome and major progress in prevention is achieved, there are inherent limits to strategies for disease prevention. Increased longevity is not immortality, and there is no way to arrange that all body systems reach their mortal limit at the same time. Short of morally unacceptable decisions not to treat failure of certain body systems after specified ages, we will be faced with increasing numbers of chronically ill patients requiring long-term maintenance and support. Thus, aside from any strategies to improve prevention of chronic diseases, it will be necessary to restructure the health care system to provide better and more efficient care for chronically ill patients. Measures to control the unnecessary cost of high-technology care will be essential so that resources remain to deal with the inevitably growing maintenance needs.

A number of strategies are already being attempted for reforming certain aspects of the health system (Chapter 10). The health planning approach seeks to direct new investment into facilities and services most needed by the population. The HMO (Health Maintenance Organization) strategy brings provider incentives into more efficient accord with patients' needs for care by eliminating the utilization-inducing influence of fee-for-service payment. Technology assessment evaluates the potential benefits (in comparison to cost) of new and existing medical technologies and procedures. As a mechanism of system reform, assessors would make technology utilization recommendations to providers or even employ economic incentives to encourage valuable and discourage less effective methods of diagnosis and treatment. Each of these strategies has some promise of improving certain elements of the system, but all are very limited in their leverage on the overall system priorities as long as the present financing system is left intact. Any realistic reform of the health care delivery system will have to be combined with restructuring the system of payment.

Some of the alternatives being put forward as national health insurance proposals would establish health care economies that are more internally consistent (Chapter 14). Two plans propose bringing expenditures and allocation more into line with consumer needs by reinstituting one or another of the traditional economic models for doing this. One plan would recreate a competitive market between complete packages of care so that consumers would have clear alternatives for comparison shopping. The Federal subsidy to premiums for each plan would be equal and restricted without further tax deductibility so that consumers would feel the difference in price among plans. By informed purchase (shopping) consumers would have economic leverage to force providers to offer plans more in accord with their actual health needs. Another type of plan acknowledges the present largely collective (public service) financing of health care and would institute corresponding public control of expenditures and allocation of services by negotiated prospective regional budgets within overall authorized limits. The National and State Health Boards established by the plan could use the economic leverage of budgeting to achieve system reform.

Either of these two economically consistent approaches would, in the long run, probably be more effective than current law or compromise plans in limiting costs and increasing the leverage to make the health system more responsive to the needs of the nation. Yet, political realities probably make it impossible to enact either of them. Creating the new internally consistent economic structures would require major departures from the present system of organization and financing. Congress will be more likely to embrace some plan instead that patches up the major gaps in coverage and seeks to deal with the cost and organizational problems by using the less effective but politically time-honored method of increasing regulation. The most pressing coverage problem in the eyes of the middle class is the danger of catastrophic expenses from an illness that exceeds one's insurance benefits. One type of plan targeted at filling gaps would simply mandate catastrophic coverage for all employees using whatever minimum government subsidies are necessary to make it feasible and equitable. This could be combined with some as yet undetermined improvements in entitlement for persons presently without adequate insurance. The Carter administration's National Health Plan would link such a catastrophic insurance approach with a set of measures to achieve certain reforms in the health system and enfranchise groups still without coverage. It would federalize Medicaid and combine it with Medicare. Cost control and system reform would be attempted through separate provisions without attempting fundamental change in the financing system.

Legislating reform of the health care system will be an interesting test case of how the democratic process in this country can come to grips with social policy in the new political and economic context of the 1980s. The coming decade promises unprecedented political dilemmas created by the growing limitations of resources, more effective political power of vested interests, and increasing complexity of organizational relationships in all major economic sectors. Today in the face of runaway inflation, limited economic growth, and increasing need for services, failure to grapple with long-range, total-system problems may force us to cut back on other equally needed services because of budgetary limitations. As in the case of the energy problem—with which there are many political parallels—failure to act decisively on health system reform is a decision in itself, with its own consequences imposed through the unavoidable impact on the economy of the forces already in motion.

Political decision making in this country has traditionally taken place through so-called incrementalism—solutions of major problems in many steps, each tested by its effects before going on to the next. Incrementalism tends to compromises that simply add on new components as a system grows, rather than by restructuring the system within existing parameters or facing difficult tradeoffs between competing demands for resources. When interrelationships between the various parts of an economic sector are relatively simple, it is possible to deal with one part at a time. With today's health system, however, a more comprehensive legislative package may be necessary to establish a congruent, efficient system of providing and financing care that is responsive to the needs of the nation.

The question is whether we will be able to face the real implications and tradeoffs of allocating limited budgets and resources in the face of strong opposition from powerful vested interests. Our political system is at the mercy of short-range pressures. The broad reform and long-term vision necessary to create a more rational health care system for the era we are entering is particularly difficult in today's political climate—the payoff for the nation is years ahead while the political process must face the always impending next election. If we cannot reach a consensus about long-range goals and act decisively to attain them, it seems unlikely that we will be able to redirect the present inappropriate direction of development of the health system or appreciably slow the escalation of its costs.

PART ONE

THE MISMATCH BETWEEN HEALTH CARE AND TODAY'S HEALTH PROBLEMS

Part 1 describes the origin and character of the mismatch, which has arisen during this century, between the predominant types of diseases affecting the population and the nature of the health care system for dealing with them.

Chapter 2 begins by tracing the history of disease in societies until the turn of this century. This not only serves as a baseline for appreciating the changes that have occurred since then, but it also demonstrates the underlying relations between the patterns of diseases in populations and their characteristic social structures. Social forces are the major determinants of nutrition, life style, and other factors that influence the incidence and impact of various diseases. These relations are more easily understood in past societies. Today the preoccupation with medical care tends to obscure the more fundamental dependence of health and disease on social factors. Yet societal characteristics and related personal behavior are still the primary determiners of mortality and morbidity—and the necessary point of intervention if significant improvements are to be achieved.

Chapter 3 traces the historical development of the medical profession that took place parallel to the trends described in Chapter 2. Again, the analysis not only provides background for understanding the transition during this century, but also illuminates the basic social role of the medical profession and its relation to society. These social forces underlying the healing role continue to influence physician and patient behavior today despite their overshadowing by the emphasis on the technical role of medicine.

Chapter 4 examines the interplay between the medical profession, society, and ideas during the emergence of scientific medicine in the nineteenth century. A revolution in the conception of disease and in methods for combatting it occurred late in the century. The technological success based on this new theory of disease markedly changed the orientation of physicians to their patients, the organization of medical care, and the expectations of patients. These new attitudes and structural professional changes have acquired a momentum of their own—to a large extent independent of the functional needs of patients and society for care. Yet enough of the old attitudes and social relationships remain to cause serious ambivalence and tensions between the parties involved. The relationships of the old healing role persist because the underlying social needs and forces that evoked them continue to exist and are even intensifying again today in the face of increased chronic disease.

Chapter 5 analyzes the emergence during the twentieth century of the new pattern of illnesses characteristic of post-industrial society. This pattern is marked by the decline of infectious diseases and the rise of chronic illnesses, presenting problems of prevention, treatment, and social support quite different from before. We have designated this new situation and its needs as "post-clinical" medicine. Instead of adapting to meet the new needs, however, the health care system has continued to develop in the direction set by its technological success early in this century. This has eventuated in a serious incongruence between the type of care provided and the needs of society arising from the new pattern of diseases.

CHAPTER TWO

Changing Patterns of Disease:
The Relations Between
Technology, Society, and Health*

The major shifts in the pattern of diseases from predominantly acute infectious disorders to primarily chronic degenerative ones has produced one side of the mismatch between the health problems of our society and our health care system (Chapter 1). One strategy suggested for improving this situation is to find ways of preventing the chronic disorders—as we did for the acute diseases. To assess the potential success of various strategies for influencing the incidence and outcomes of different diseases, we must understand the factors that determine the pattern of diseases occurring in a society and the factors that change it. A first step is to analyze what brought us to our present situation of health and disease.

Because the decline of acute infectious diseases took place parallel to the revolution in medical science, it is often assumed that improved medical technology was the *cause* of the change in the disease pattern. In small part, medical intervention has been a factor, but most of the positive and negative trends in morbidity and mortality from various diseases in this century represent almost straight-line continuations of trends already established in the nineteenth century, long before the medical technological revolution was underway. The principal causes of the beneficial trends were actually improved nutrition, living standards, and sanitation. The negative trends were largely caused by increasing exposure to environmental carcinogens, improper diet, and other features of post-industrial life styles. In the course of the century improved public health measures, such as water purification and food inspection; preventive measures, such as immunization or control of contagion; and finally clinical intervention were also superimposed on these trends modifying them to some degree.

It is difficult to separate the various factors influencing the changing pat-

* Where not otherwise attributed, standard historical data used in this chapter are taken from Rosen, 1958; Singer and Underwood, 1962; or Shryock, 1968.

17

tern of diseases if we look only at the process during this century. But this transition is not the only major shift in the pattern that has occurred in the course of history. Equally profound changes in disease incidence and out-comes have taken place parallel to every major transition in the structure of society. Examining some of the important historical changes in societies and their diseases lends useful insights into the factors and relations at work in the present century. This analysis helps assess the relative impact of factors influencing health and disease and the potential of various strate-gies for dealing with the health problems we now face.

Much the same types of diseases that we know today seem to have afflicted societies since the beginning of human existence. Pathologists who investi-gate residues of diseases left in archaeological remains have found evidence of most kinds of diseases known today (Sigerist, 1951). Description of dis-eases by ancient physicians and other chroniclers of human affliction are sometimes recognizable by modern clinicians as characteristic of diseases fa-miliar now. In this way historians of disease conclude that the great ma-jority of human diseases occurring today have occurred throughout most of mankind's existence—presumably always caused by agents or factors similar to those that cause them now (Ackerknecht, 1972).*

Yet, despite this persistence and universality of most disease types, the patterns of incidence and effects of diseases in different societies are remark-ably varied. In Asia and Africa the major causes of death are still epidemic and endemic infectious and parasitic diseases, while in the United States and other advanced industrial countries this ceased to be the case early in the present century. Even between social groups at the same time in the same city, marked differences in incidence and effects are found. For exam-ple, the infant mortality rate in Harlem, a poverty area of New York City,

---

* To be sure, there are diseases that seem to have suddenly appeared *de novo* in human societies, or disappeared. A famous case is the so-called English sweating sickness, which decimated Tudor armies and cities in several waves between 1485 and 1551, apparently surpassing even bubonic plague in its fearsome effects. Then, as mysteriously as it came, the strange contagion disappeared from sight, never to return. Clinical descriptions of the disease do not allow us to recognize it as any known today or previously (Dubos, 1965). Genetically determined diseases arise spontaneously by mutation (at least once, though often repeatedly) and can then be transmitted by inheritance. Likewise, exposure of populations directly or by way of environmental pollution to new agents that are results of industry and new technology has sometimes led to toxic diseases, to genetic or birth defects, and even to new tumors not previously known. For example, a characteristic pattern of congenital abnormalities arose from the unfortunate use of thalidomide as a sedative during pregnancies. Similarly, nearly all cases of mesothelioma (a rare type of cancer of the lung) are traceable to inhalation of asbestos dust produced in industrial processes (Kilbourne & Smillie, 1971), an occurrence that only goes back a few decades. In these ways new diseases can emerge in a population. In addition, certain diseases like tuberculosis and syphilis have apparently changed their virulence and other characteristics over time. However, these instances of newly arising or changed disease types and of dis-eases that have apparently disappeared only underscore the basic persistence of most disease categories.

was still 26 per 1000 live births in 1976, while the rate in Forest Hills, an affluent middle-class area of the same city, was 9 per 1000 in the same year (New York City Health Department, 1978). Such differences in mortality are only gross indications of many subtler variations in the patterns of morbidity.

As striking as the *differences* are, the *persistence* of the characteristic patterns of diseases in any population of a society is just as remarkable. Actuaries and epidemiologists can usually predict with disturbing accuracy how many cases and deaths from each disease type will occur in a given population on the basis of trends from the past. The patterns of disease incidence in populations are clearly not arbitrary. While disease patterns result from a host of factors, they are just as typical of each society as other distinctive features of its social life. There must be causes embedded in the nature of societies that determine the particular patterns of diseases found. The question is what these causes are and how they account for the radical change in incidence of disease types in our society since the turn of this century.

Geographic differences account for some of the variation and persistence of disease patterns. Trypanosomiasis (African sleeping sickness) occurs only in Africa because it can be transmitted only by the tse-tse fly, which thrives nowhere else. Yet, while many parasitic diseases are found only in tropical countries today, some like malaria and yellow fever, which we now think of as tropical diseases, were common in the Mississippi Valley and along the Atlantic coast during the nineteenth century (May, 1958). Massive cholera epidemics occurred in New York, London, and other major industrial cities until almost the turn of the present century, just as they do today in underdeveloped countries (Duffy, 1974). As recently as 1920, fifty of every 1000 live-born infants in the United States succumbed to so-called "weanling diarrhea" of the same sort that causes much of the high infant mortality in poor nations today (Kilbourne & Smillie, 1971). Clearly, geographic idiosyncrasies alone cannot account for the gross differences in patterns of mortality and morbidity found in different countries, different subcultures of the same country, and at different times of history among the same peoples. We must look elsewhere to explain differences in the incidence and outcomes of the diseases that are responsible for the bulk of mortality and morbidity in populations—and thus understand the significance of the changes in disease patterns that have occurred in this country since 1900 (McKeown, 1965).

Examination of the overall historical development of societies shows that the major, characteristic differences in the incidence, morbidity, and mortality from various disease groups is most clearly correlated with the state of technological development and social organization. It has come to be widely recognized that the health status or disease pattern* of a society is

---

* Incidences of diseases and mortality rates are, of course, not strictly a measure of "health," at least not in the positive and encompassing sense of the World Health Organization's definition of health as "a state of complete physical, mental and social well-

a product of its overall life style, economic affluence, cultural habits, and social structure—not just a result of the specialized activity of its medical care system (McKeown & Lowe, 1974).

To clarify the forces responsible for the patterns of diseases in societies, we analyze societies at various stages of technological development—first, in regard to the general societal technology determining overall economic structure and then the more specialized technology of the health care system within industrial societies. The developmental stage of technology is commonly used for classifying societies. The level of technology commanded by a society is a primary determinant of its economy, style of life, demography, and social structure. Technology also has great influence on the other features of society that impact on health, such as socioeconomic organization, living standards (nutrition, housing, personal hygiene, sanitation, and general affluence), and the health care system. In the course of history these elements, along with the environment, have been increasingly modified by technological developments.

PREAGRARIAN SOCIETIES

The technology of preagrarian societies is very limited, leaving the population essentially at the mercy of the environmental forces surrounding it. Demography, socioeconomic organization, and health care adapt passively to the requirements of that environment. Archeological evidence and studies of tribal societies and nomadic shepherd groups today suggest that preagrarian societies are in a kind of ecological balance with their food supply and with parasites or other disease processes. The food supply is limited by the plants and wild life that occur naturally in the area, so it is impossible to sustain a high population density. Food and disease crises are kept within tolerable limits by passive adaption to the environmental situation through culturally transmitted customs and social behavior. Social methods of birth control seem to have been established in most preagrarian societies. According to Dubos (1965):

Prolonged breast-feeding, prohibition of sexual intercourse during the period of nursing, the use of various contraceptive techniques, abortion and infanticide are among the many methods used by primitive people in the past and still used by them today.

The high death rate in such tribal societies also constrains the growth of population. Thus, disease itself is a major factor in maintaining population

---

being and not just the absence of disease" (World Health Organization, 1944). However, the pattern of diseases comprises a major component of the state called the "health of a population"—and the part that health policy (in the strict sense) can deal with.

balance. Infant mortality alone often approaches 50% because the babies are subject to intermittent malnutrition (to which infants are very sensitive), serious respiratory infections in cold climates, and intestinal infection with diarrhea in hot climates.

Infant mortality from pneumonia and diarrheal disease is itself a complex affair, as shown today by studies of underdeveloped countries with marginal food supplies. Death from diarrhea usually occurs during the period of weaning, and is therefore referred to as "weanling diarrhea." Although clearly infectious in nature, it is neither epidemic (as it would be if carried by a common water or food supply) nor are ordinary pathogens (such as dysentery or salmonella food poisoning that cause gastroenteritis in adults) usually identifiable in the infants. When the mother's milk is withdrawn and before adult foods are taken, the low-protein, low-calorie infant diet often yields poor resistance to the ordinary bacteria carried harmlessly in the gut of adults (Scrimshaw & Behar, 1971). The personal hygienic habits of these cultures—such as prechewing of food for children, not washing hands, eating on the ground—and the prevalence of flies and vermin expose the infant to the body flora of adults before its antibody system is able to cope with it. Infants depleted by malnutrition have poor antibody (protein) synthesis.

A similar phenomenon occurs with pneumonia. Childhood fevers, like measles, mumps, and rubella, have very low mortality rates in societies with well-nourished children. In marginally nourished populations, childhood viral infections are frequently complicated by pneumonia and ear infections, raising the case mortality rate to several hundred times that of similar illnesses in the United States (Kilbourne & Smillie, 1971).*

In tropical climates the food problem is usually less severe, but there is a high incidence of parasitic diseases, such as malaria, schistosomiasis (blood flukes), or trypanosomiasis (sleeping sickness), which are carried by the surrounding insect and animal population. Accidents and hardships of hunting and food gathering also take a high toll.

Even where the choice of food supply is quite limited, tribal societies have usually developed abilities to select and obtain a balanced diet. Dubos (1959) reports:

Primitive cultures manage to derive fairly adequate nourishment from even the most desolate areas if the ecological conditions under which they live are stable. Thus, the Otomi Indians have found sufficient sustenance to survive for many generations in the Mesquital Valley of Mexico, a semidesert with many months of drought yearly. They exhibit little, if any, clinical evidence of malnourishment

---

* It seems likely that infant mortality from these problems is actually higher today in tribal societies that have been forced onto reservations or that live as squatters in crowded unsanitary conditions on the edge of urban societies. These groups participate only marginally in the new culture, retain many of the habits of the original tribal settings, and often have even worse weanling nutrition.

even though they consume few of the foods usually considered essential for a balanced diet. Their consumption of meat, dairy produce, fruit, and the conventional
vegetables is extremely low. Along with their tortillas, they eat purslane, cactus
fruit, pigweed, and sow thistle for greenstuffs, and drink pulque. Yet their diet
when tested a decade ago was found to supply a better nutritional combination
than eaten by certain city dwellers in the United States examined at the same
time. It is probable that every component of the Otomi diet provides some essential nutrient. The alcoholic beverage, pulque, which is used unfiltered, contains
all the factors of the agave juice from which it is made, as well as those generated
by the microorganisms involved in the fermentation process.

Besides the cultural behavior of tribal societies limiting the birth rates
and selecting adequate diets to achieve equilibrium with the natural habi-
tat, considerable biological adaptation to prevalent disease agents also
seems to occur. The low population density and relatively infrequent cross-
contact between tribal groups limits the types of infectious and parasitic
diseases to which a particular group is exposed. Over the generations the
group builds up a so-called herd immunity* to some of these diseases, which
allows the group to live in a state of endemic equilibrium with the common disease agents of its environment. Contact with the outside world,
however, can easily upset this delicate balance. A tragic example is the way
that American Indian societies were decimated in early colonial times by
smallpox, measles, and other contagious diseases brought by Europeans—
among whom they had a relatively mild effect because of the long history
of endemic accommodation. A similar situation occurred later with tuberculosis when Indians and Eskimos were exposed more closely to Whites.

Thus in preagrarian societies man is at the mercy of his environment,
and population remains in a balance determined by a survival equation in
which population density is constrained between the forces of the food
supply and endemic diseases. This situation is little modified by human activity except through sociocultural adaptation to the constraints, such as
diet selection from available food more adequate than random gathering
would produce, and cultural mores that achieve a birth rate regulation appropriate for the food supply. Avoidance of disease through "preventive
medicine" or "public health" (sanitation, etc.) may occur by way of mores
concerning care of food, sources of water, and, perhaps, infant feeding habits. These adaptations have little effect on the major sources of adult contagion from the surrounding animal parasitic reservoir. High adult mor-

* "Herd immunity" is the biological explanation given for the marked differences in susceptibility to the same disease agents exhibited by various inbred groups. The phenomenon
is still poorly understood, but it is believed to be due to genetically transmitted variations
in the antibody producing mechanisms or other factors that determine the ability to
resist the effects of particular disease agents. One striking example of nonantibody mediated herd immunity is the resistance of certain African populations to malaria as a
result of the genetic modification of the hemoglobin that leads to sickle cell disease if
they are exposed to colder climates.

tality occurs from these endemic parasitic and other infectious diseases, accidents, and high maternal death rates, leaving few persons surviving to old age.

AGRARIAN SOCIETIES

The first major impact that human culture and technology had on the natural equilibrium of populations with their environments was in regard to the availability of food. The agricultural revolution, which first occurred in neolithic societies, produced the great agrarian civilizations of the ancient and medieval world and those that continue to characterize much of Asia today. The greater availability of food and the changed social structure necessary to accommodate to the landed economy weakened the social checks on birth rates. The incentives shifted toward larger families to work the land and provide "social security" for parents in their old age. Civilizations with the greatest populations could support the largest armies and survive best in the large-scale warfare that developed over the possession of the richest farming lands. Because of the greater food production much higher population densities were possible, and a marked change in the pattern of diseases occurred.

Infant mortality fell as a result of improved nutrition. On the other hand, the population density and contact between groups increased sufficiently so that many new respiratory and enteric infections became endemic and took a high toll of each new generation. Nevertheless, the higher birth rates and improved nutrition more than overbalanced any increases in childhood mortality from contagion. Death from certain parasitic diseases decreased in all age groups as the carrier animal population was pushed away from the centers of human population. On the other hand, drainage canals and rice paddies, in which men, snails, mosquitos, and other disease agents or vectors came to coexist, intensified such other endemic parasitic diseases as malaria and schistosomiasis (still so prevalent and debilitating in the Near and Far East).

The rapid population growth and higher densities would have been more than the land could support for long, had it not been for the frequent intervention of major disasters such as famines, wars, and plagues. Tied to the land and no longer able to move to other areas if the food supply failed, agrarian societies were subject to widespread starvation when drought or other natural disaster brought on crop failure. Most characteristic of the disease pattern of the great agrarian civilizations, and perhaps more important than even the wars in shaping the tide of history, were the great plagues (Zinsser, 1934). Throughout antiquity and the Middle Ages, societies were swept periodically by pestilences of acute infectious diseases with high mortality rates (especially smallpox in early times, but later bubonic plague) as the combination of high population densities and increased world trade made certain epidemics possible. Population groups were adapted to their own endemic pathogens so that mortality from them was relatively low and often limited to childhood. A new disease agent introduced to the susceptible adult population from outside, however, led to rapid epidemic spread and high mortality within the dense pool of potential victims. The infection would sweep through the entire population until most were either dead or had recovered from the disease, thereby developing an immunity that prevented reinfection (McNeill, 1976). Those few susceptible individuals who somehow escaped infection were then too sparsely scattered to sustain the further spread of contagion, and the epidemic burned itself out. Another epidemic of the same disease would not recur until a new generation of susceptibles had grown up and the disease was reintroduced from outside (or by asymptomatic carriers of the pathogen, as with typhoid).

As population density increased and trade intensified, the frequency of contact between groups multiplied so that epidemics of certain diseases, such as smallpox, became increasingly common but also less virulent. They began to occur primarily among the younger members of the population (the older members already being immune from the last epidemic), and "herd immunity" was gradually built up. Thus many of the diseases that were once epidemic plagues gradually took their place among the endemic infections of the population. On the other hand, still higher levels of population density eventuated in new diseases that reached epidemic and pandemic proportions. The louse-borne typhus, for example, often became epidemic in particularly crowded and dirty conditions, such as those sustained by armies in the field or cities under siege (Zinsser, 1934). Where common water supplies could be contaminated by sewage, enteric epidemics such as cholera and typhoid fever took their toll. Bubonic plague ravaged Europe periodically during several centuries of the Middle Ages then stopped because of changes in exposure to the rat and flea population that carried the bacteria between human epidemics. This occurred partly because of an improvement in housing construction, which kept out the rats, and partly because of the migration of a new species of rat into Europe from Russia around 1750 that was less susceptible to plague (Dubos, 1959). Other epidemic diseases seem to have waxed and waned because of modification of the disease agent itself.*

The changes in disease incidence in agrarian societies were largely inadvertent consequences of changes in technology and population distribution that either facilitated or hindered transmissions of infectious processes. However, some degree of conscious public health activity (sanitation) oc-

---

* The exact relationship between disease agents, herd immunity, and other environmental and social conditions in regard to each type of epidemic disease is a fascinating study, but we must limit ourselves here to illustrating the general principles involved as a background for the sociology of health care. Interested readers are referred to the works of Zinsser (1934), McKeown (1971), Rosen (1958), and Dubos (1965, 1959).

curred in the few great cities that flourished in each major agrarian civilization. Cities can grow beyond a small critical size only if certain arrangements are made for water supply and waste disposal. Therefore some sanitary engineering was necessarily a part of the technology in every agrarian civilization successful enough to produce great cities. Beyond this there was little that would qualify as preventive medicine or public health. To be sure, as far back as we have historical record, there was apparently some belief in "contagion," with attempts to isolate lepers, quarantine ships coming from known areas of plague, and so forth, but this was usually sporadic, unsuccessful, and often ill-advised. Because of inadequate knowledge of contagious processes, persons were often quarantined or avoided when the true carrier was the rat, insect, or contaminated water supply that easily slipped through the assumed barrier (Rosen, 1958).

Thus the more adequate and dependable food supply in agrarian societies radically modified the population equilibrium by increasing the birth rate and decreasing infant mortality. Yet, it also led to new problems on the disease side of the survival equation. In becoming masters of their fate in regard to nutrition, societies lost many of the adaptive cultural mechanisms for living in equilibrium with nature that they had acquired over long periods of time. The Malthusian problem of population growth outstripping the productivity of the land was first unleashed, which still continues to plague the world with cycles of abundance, overpopulation, crop failure, and famine. The increased population density also introduced a whole new set of epidemic disease problems that preagrarian societies had not experienced. The first in a series of cycles was initiated in which technological advancement solved one set of health problems only to create a new set—an enigma that we continue to face today.

EARLY INDUSTRIAL URBAN SOCIETY

With the coming of the Industrial Revolution in Europe in the eighteenth and nineteenth centuries, there arose a new urban structure of society well chronicled by sociologists and social historians. It was accompanied by a new pattern of diseases which is less commonly discussed. The transition to urban industrial society brought another order-of-magnitude shift in population concentration as a result of massive migration from farms to city factories. Large-scale urban living created a new set of social customs and living situations which produced quite different health problems. In agrarian societies the problems were those of not producing enough food for the growing population and of contagions, partly endemic and partly epidemics from outside. In industrial societies the health problems began to stem from the ill effects of man's own products and living conditions in the urban settings necessary for the factory system of production.

The initial health impact of the new urban industrial social structure was

a result of residential crowding, filth, factory accidents, and pollution—
problems with which the previously tiny Renaissance cities simply were not
equipped to cope. The epidemic plagues that had swept across the conti-
nents of Europe and Asia in the Middle Ages and in early modern times
were replaced by more concentrated epidemics and endemics of diseases
spreading within the dense population of cities. Because of the poor sanitation and contaminated food and water supplies, cholera and typhoid epidemics became almost annual summer events in one city or another. Tuberculosis was a great killer, especially among the working classes crowded
together in dark factories and slum housing. Birth rates began to drop
again. Even though child labor was common, children were less of an economic asset in the city than on the farm, and the social mobility and growing affluence of urban life shifted values away from families to material
goods. Children died of infections common to crowding, such as diphtheria
and scarlet fever. Many grew up stunted and crippled physically or mentally from the living and working conditions and from diseases such as rickets, caused by lack of sunshine and by dietary deficiency (Rosen, 1958).
Women died of childbed fever spread by the poor hygiene of the midwives
and obstetricians. Workers died from industrial accidents and toxins. Industrial environmental pollution also came to be a danger of the new urban living, with an increasing incidence of chronic bronchitis from smoke
and dust inhalation and occupational malignancies, such as scrotal cancer
frequently occurring in chimney sweeps exposed to coal tars. The conditions of living in the early industrial cities were such that the death rate
actually exceeded the birth rate (Singer & Underwood, 1962). Yet, despite
all the drawbacks, the potential economic opportunity and glamour of city
living continued to attract migration from the growing surplus of agricultural labor. Urban industrial centers grew at an unprecedented speed, leading to further crowding and unsanitary conditions in the slums and
factories.

The worst of this situation was relatively short-lived as social history
goes. For example, infant mortality rates in London are estimated to have
been between 400 and 500 per 1000 live births from 1730 to 1750 (Singer &
Underwood, 1962). Yet by 1800 the rate had dropped to 240 per 1000 and
continued to fall throughout the next century, reaching about 140 per 1000
by 1900. This drop occurred despite the fact that population density continued to grow rapidly and that very limited formal public health measures
were undertaken before 1900.

The explanation for this improvement in health probably lies in the nature of the changes wrought by industrialization itself. Along with the
problems of urban industrial society came the wealth, technological expertise, attitudes, and organization that also made it possible to deal with
these very problems created by urbanization, though considerable time
elapsed before any effect was evident. Not that the leaders of this society
perceived of themselves as attempting to solve health problems—such aware-

ness came only much later in the mid-nineteenth century, with the self-conscious, so-called Sanitary Movement. Rather, the actions taken were commercially, pragmatically, and to some degree humanely motivated.

Low as wages were, the joint spendable income of the working class began to represent a major factor in the economy and attracted significant investment in new housing. Poor and crowded as the new tenements were, they were a considerable improvement over the hovels in which the first generation of migrants to the cities had been forced to live, and probably constituted better living conditions than those to which infants were exposed on the equally poverty-stricken farms. With the doubling and quadrupling of population in many cities within a generation, there was no choice but to construct new water supplies and sewage disposal systems (Cole & Postgate, 1961). Even without explicit concern about the sanitary conditions of these new systems, they were much less prone to disease-producing cross-contamination—simply as a consequence of the more effective construction resulting from improved civil engineering.

Another factor that operated indirectly to mitigate the unhealthy conditions of the new urban population was the same constellation of sociocultural behavior that contributed an important element to the Industrial Revolution itself—the capitalist-puritan ethic and the philosophical "enlightenment" or humanist rationality of the eighteenth century. According to Max Weber (1958) the Protestant belief in achievement, frugality, and hard work in the service of one's calling, was an important underpinning of capitalist industrial society. Akin to this belief were the norms of cleanliness, orderliness, and civic pride that included willingness to work for effective governmental organization. Coupled with a renewed emphasis on charity to the poor, these motivating factors fostered repeated attempts to improve the welfare of the working class and clean up living conditions in the cities—if only to remove offensive eyesores. The Enlightenment philosophy of progress and belief in man's ability to improve his own lot in life through control of nature augmented the puritan ethic. It led some to take as their mission the education and "moral improvement" of the poorer classes. Methodists, Quakers, and other activist puritan sects worked to elevate the standards of living and aspirations of the downtrodden (Trevelyan, 1942). Local governments imbued with the new spirit of progress undertook to establish orphanages, hospitals, and work houses. Harsh as they were by present standards, these did provide a kind of baseline welfare.

It is difficult to estimate how much of the improvement in living standards, and hence in the level of health, was due to any one or all of these humanitarian or rationalistic attempts to correct the evils of the new urban conditions. Much of the improvement may have been merely an inadvertent trickling down of the new affluence created by industrialization. Part of the credit may also go to motivational factors insofar as rising affluence manifested by the already successful entrepreneurial class created working-class aspirations toward higher standards of living (better food and housing, cleanliness, education, etc.). Whatever the specific causal routes by which they were achieved, these changed conditions of life in the new industrial cities began to have a significant impact on the health of the population long before any conscious effective measures toward public health or preventive medicine were undertaken. As noted, various measures of quarantine and isolation were attempted, but until the particular means of transmission of specific diseases were discovered, these methods were much less significant in preventing disease than the general sociocultural improvement in the standard of living.

NINETEENTH CENTURY URBAN SOCIETY—
THE EFFECT OF PUBLIC HEALTH REFORM

The characteristic patterns of diseases associated with the three societal types discussed thus far were entirely a result of their *general* socioeconomic technologies. These technologies had their effects on health *indirectly* by way of primary influences on demography, social structure, and living standards and hence on nutrition, housing, sanitation, and hygiene. The patterns of diseases of the three remaining societal types have been at least in part the outcomes of technological developments within the health care sector proper, first public health and sanitary reform, then preventive medicine oriented to specific diseases, and finally curative clinical medicine. The fact that health technology came to have an influence on the pattern of diseases did not mean that the general socioeconomic technology of the society no longer had an impact on its health. On the contrary, the continued improvement in standards of living, nutrition, housing, and sanitation throughout the nineteenth century was a major reason for the decline in many important types of morbidity and mortality, such as infant mortality and tuberculosis. In fact these factors were probably the chief cause of improvement in health until at least 1880.

Moreover, the emergence of successful medical technologies was itself the result of advances in the more general societal technologies and of social forces such as urbanization. Public health technology was the culmination of advances in sanitary engineering, administrative systems, vital statistics analysis, and epidemiology, all of which evolved from the general intellectual progress of Western civilization (in particular from the philosophies of mercantilism and the Enlightenment; Rosen, 1958). Preventive medicine developed on the basis of pathology, which emerged in large urban teaching hospitals, and bacteriology, which was a product of nineteenth century industrial chemistry as well as pathological research. Effective clinical medicine was the result of an even more complex convergence of developments stemming from many sources in the general technological and intellectual stream of Western society as well as particular discoveries within the field of medicine proper. The emergence of effective ("scientific") preventive and clinical medicine is discussed in Chapter 4, since it is so closely intertwined with the development of the medical profession itself.

The development and implementation of public health technology and organization in Europe and the United States is of interest not only for understanding the impact they had on the pattern of diseases, but also as an object lesson in the relationship between ideology, technological evolution, and politics in bringing about change in the health and health care of a society. The problems faced in the American health sector today (with the coming of "post-clinical medicine"; Chapter 5) have many similarities to those encountered by the so-called public health movement.

Despite the faith of the Enlightenment that progress in all human affairs could be achieved through the application of scientific methods, most improvements in health and welfare during the eighteenth century had little scientific basis. Empirical methods were simply not yet available for investigating health problems of populations (or of individuals)—nor was there any administrative machinery for dealing with public health problems even if their causes had been known. After 1800 both these necessary elements for constructing a rational utilitarian approach to public health problems developed rapidly. Initially the new methods were used primarily as weapons in political battles for social and sanitary reform. In the long run, however, they provided a continuing rational basis for dealing with health problems that is essential for modern urban industrial societies.

The scientific element of public health technology consisted of using sociodemographic and vital statistics (and their analysis by means of probability calculus) to determine the correlates (and assumed causes) of diseases—part of the process we now call epidemiology. This method made it possible to plan points of intervention for preventing diseases, and to test the relative effectiveness of various modes of intervention. Vital statistics analysis was an outgrowth of the seventeenth-century mercantilist philosophy, which assumed that the welfare of society depended on the wealth and strength of the national state. It was presumed that the nation would be strengthened by having a large, healthy, well provided-for population that could be used effectively in economic production and other national objectives (Rosen, 1958). To further this policy William Petty developed "political arithmetic," the use of statistical data to estimate the impact of factors such as birth rate, illnesses, and mortality on the economy and polity. John Graunt carried out the first study of "bills of mortality" (death certificates) in London in 1662, demonstrating the relative constancy of death rates due to different causes and the excess of urban over rural mortality rates. Petty tried to calculate the economic loss due to disease, and advocated a Health Council for London to deal with public health matters, but this fell on deaf ears.

During this period mathematicians began working out the laws of probability which were essential for more sophisticated analysis of statistics. In 1693 Edmund Halley (an astronomer, mathematician, and disciple of Isaac

Newton) published the first life-expectancy tables. This enabled the calculation of annuity costs and other actuarial data needed for the sound operation of the commercial life insurance plans that came into existence in
the early eighteenth century. Such commercial uses of the data, in turn, fostered the more systematic collection of census and vital statistics records.
Throughout the eighteenth century demographic and vital statistics were
improved, and the mathematical theory of probability and statistical inference was further developed. In 1760 Daniel Bernoulli used probability theory to demonstrate that the difference in mortality of inoculated and non-
inoculated persons during a smallpox epidemic was sound evidence for the
effectiveness of inoculation. In 1786 Pierre Laplace showed how to estimate
the probable range of error of population projections made on the basis of
birth rates. In his great treatise on probability in 1812, Laplace provided
a firm foundation for the whole field of statistical inference.

The establishment of public health departments resulted from the political victories of the sanitary movement between 1800 and 1880. But the organizational theory for designing these agencies began as an outgrowth of
the mercantilist and Enlightenment philosophies of the seventeenth and
eighteenth centuries. As early as 1714 Nehemiah Grew, Samuel Hartlib,
and John Bellers argued publicly for a national health service available to
all on the grounds that "illness and untimely deaths are a waste of human
resources" (Rosen, 1958). Their proposals, however, lead to no concrete action—perhaps in part because they ran contrary to the major prevailing political and administrative trends of the times. In contrast to the mercantilist
philosophy of the seventeenth century, the dominant belief of the century
following was that the role of government should be limited to regulation
and protection in regard to the economy and that laissez faire capitalism
should be allowed to carry out the actual provision of services. Even some
traditional public services, such as municipal water supply and garbage
and sewage disposal, were moved from the public into the private sector.
Similarly today sound proposals for reform of the health care system based
on careful rational analysis may fail to be implemented because they run
counter to the current strong antigovernment philosophy of the Congress
(Chapters 13 and 14).

The Enlightenment philosophy of the eighteenth century advocated rational restructuring of society according to scientific principles to bring
about human progress (but not control of the economy). These beliefs
prompted health professionals to develop extensive schemes for systematic
reform of health conditions. The most elaborate was Johann Peter Frank's
System of a Complete Medical Police, published in six volumes from 1779
to 1817. In the spirit of the "enlightened despotism" dominant on the European continent at that time this system proposed regulation of everything
from personal hygiene, marriage, pregnancies, child health, nutrition, housing, and sanitation to vital statistics collection and hospital construction.
Similar if less elaborate systems of health surveillance and regulation by or-

ganized government bureaucracies were proposed by other physicians of the period, and feeble attempts were made to implement some of the ideas. However, the Napoleonic wars brought an end to most of the experiments, and another 50 years passed before effective public health organizations were established.

After 1800 the death rates in cities, which had been declining since 1750, again began to climb. This was due in part to the ravages of the Napoleonic wars with the disruption of food supplies, the destruction of housing, and massive epidemics of typhus, cholera, and smallpox that were carried from one region to another by the movements of armies and refugees. It was also attributable in part to the new wave of population growth, beginning about 1750, that doubled the European population by 1800, causing still further crowding into urban centers. This was accompanied by a marked rise in the incidence of tuberculosis and influenza. The rising death rates, now better documented by government-collected vital statistics and interpreted by more sophisticated professionals attuned to the significance of such data, led to the so-called Sanitary (or Public Health) Movement—a new round of attempts at reform of the public health sector.

The elements in this Sanitary Movement and the constellation of forces allied for and against sanitary reform provide interesting parallels with problems faced today in bringing about reform of the American health care system. For the success of public health reform, then as now, it was crucial that both the political climate and the scientific basis were ripe for the changes. The political and philosophical doctrines of individualism and laissez faire progress that fired the French Revolution had ended in the disaster of the Napoleonic wars. The resulting conservative political reaction of the early nineteenth century was reflected in the more collectivist philosophies of government and economics exemplified by the utilitarianism of England and the utopian socialism of the Continent. Both embodied a partial return to the paternalism of the mercantilist period. There, however, the similarity between countries ended.

France, possessing a highly centralized government bureaucracy restructured during the Revolution and Napoleonic era, was quick to respond to health professional leadership. Government directives from the top enabled rapid implementation of new technical and organizational public health innovations. French science, medicine, and technological advancement had moved into the forefront in the period just before and after the Revolution, and it is not surprising that French health professionals took the lead in applying the new statistical methods to public health research. In 1828 Louis Villermé, a physician, began the study of differential mortality rates in Paris and showed that death rates were a function of the living conditions of the working class. This demonstrated correlation between death rates and living conditions reinforced the movement already underway to regulate the factory system and other social conditions. In 1841 child labor laws were passed, and in 1848 Health Councils were established throughout France to advise the magistrates of each area on public health matters. Thus in France public health machinery was established and incorporated into the existing government bureaucracy as soon as scientific methods convincingly demonstrated its need (Rosen, 1958).

In England (and also in the United States), on the other hand, the very decentralized governmental system was only responsive to broadly based political pressure, which made it necessary to mobilize support for sanitary reform from many different groups. At this time England's medical profession was much more traditional than the French, with the less research-oriented clinicians exerting more control than the academicians. In England the public health research and reform came not from the health professionals but from lay social reform groups inspired by Jeremy Bentham's utilitarianism. In 1832 Edwin Chadwick was appointed head of a Royal commission to investigate the Poor Laws and advise reform measures. He recommended sweeping changes in these laws concerning work houses and other welfare measures. But he also seized the opportunity to investigate the "sanitary conditions of the labouring classes" in order to encourage improvement of these conditions through implementation of a governmental system for regulating health and sanitation.

Chadwick's theory, which he shared with many reform-minded Benthamite utilitarians in the Sanitary Movement, was that *filth* itself is the cause of disease. Since the Middle Ages contagion had been assumed to cause certain obvious epidemic diseases like bubonic plague and smallpox, but the mechanisms of contagion were unknown. The growing trend in clinical medicine at this time was to assume a specific cause for each disease type, so that, even if a disease seemed to be contagious, this did not imply any necessary connection to unsanitary conditions. There was little inclination among physicians to accept the sanitary-reformist ideas which appeared to reduce all disease causation to a single common denominator—filth.* Physicians also resented the sanitary movement as an attempt by laymen to invade their area of expertise and were less willing to weigh the evidence impartially than if it had come from their own camp (Shryock, 1969). The reformists, on the other hand, tended to ignore well-founded criticisms by the physicians, belittling their efforts and resorting to political or polemic weapons, which the physicians felt were unfair and inappropriate for such questions.

* In 1848 Edwin Snow studied the London cholera epidemic of that year and conclusively demonstrated the source of contagion to be the Broad Street pump by tracing the geographic clustering of cases to people who had obtained their water from that source. Thus a clear connection between poor sanitation and contagion was shown for at least one disease, but by then it was too late to mediate between opposing camps. The significance of Snow's study was only clear 20 years later, after Pasteur's and Koch's work finally demonstrated the bacterial nature of the causation and transmission of cholera and many other diseases. During this interim period the controversy raged between contagionist and anticontagionist theories of disease, as well as between miasmic (filth) and specific-cause theories.

The sanitary reformists, however, held the political initiative and were able to capitalize on it. Chadwick, taking his lead from Villermé and armed with new improved tools of statistics, clearly demonstrated in his report of 1842 that the unsanitary living conditions of the English working classes were related to their higher mortality, and that these conditions were responsible for great economic loss through disease, disability, and early deaths. Chadwick joined forces with the Chartist Movement, Owenite socialists, other liberal reform groups, and even with industrial interests looking for a better labor supply. The coalition was able to secure enactment of a series of new laws regulating public health and social welfare. Beginning with the Poor Law Amendments of 1834, they culminated in the establishment of a National Board of Health in 1848—probably urged on by the great London cholera epidemic of that year.

The lay social reform movement maintained the political initiative and dominated social action until the English Public Health Act of 1875 put physicians back in command of health policy matters. Even though based on a false (miasmic) theory, the measures taken by the new boards of health were soon effective in improving the health conditions of urban populations. By the end of the century—long before any measures based on the new bacteriology, such as immunization or water chlorination, could have a significant impact—mortality from cholera and typhoid fever was falling rapidly, as was infant mortality and the overall death rate among the working class. According to Shryock (1969):

Statisticians, engineers, and social philosophers all made their contributions to the public health movement. For one generation, about the middle of the (19th) century, it seemed indeed as though mathematicians might do more for public hygiene than could the medical men themselves. Statisticians revealed problems and engineers found solutions, at a time when the best medicine tended toward nihilism and seemed to have little to offer.

Thus again a change in technology—this time health administrative technology combined with sanitary engineering technology—and the resulting changes in social organization and behavior, led to a radical change in the pattern of diseases.

A similar series of events took place in the United States a few years later. American urban health problems were analogous to those in Europe but compounded by the rapid flow of impoverished immigrants into eastern seaboard cities. From 1804 onward New York City had a City Inspector of Health who was part of the police department (Duffy, 1974). He was primarily responsible for the quarantine of vessels arriving at the port but also was on guard for outbreaks of epidemics within the city. In 1845 and 1848 Dr. John Griscom, the New York City Health Inspector, issued reports on the unsanitary condition of the laboring population in New York similar to Chadwick's and obviously influenced by it. In addition to reviewing strictly sanitary conditions, Griscom detailed the problem of New York's crowded tenement housing.

In 1850 Lemuel Shattuck, a Boston publisher, convened a commission that produced a similar sweeping sanitary survey of Massachusetts. It made strong recommendations calling for state and local health departments to collect vital statistics; to control environmental sanitation, food, and water supplies; and to provide child health services, including vaccination for smallpox. Vaccination was still not widely practiced despite its demonstrated effectiveness. Unfortunately, no practical action was taken on the basis of Shattuck's report for another 19 years. Between 1857 and 1860 four national Quarantine and Sanitary Conventions were held. In 1864 another New York sanitary survey finally led to action, and in 1866 the New York City Municipal Board of Health was authorized by the state legislature. After a reorganization in 1870 it took the lead in sanitary reform and disease control through efficient administration, which set the standard for the nation and the world. In 1869 Massachusetts finally adopted many of Shattuck's recommendations, and other states followed suit. At the national level the United States Public Health Service came into being only with the advent of the "preventive medicine era" of health care.

Thus the development of vital statistics analysis and other techniques of social epidemiology made it possible to detect and focus public attention on the factors that were responsible for major variations in the incidence of important epidemic and endemic diseases. Political action combined this knowledge with the administrative organization and authority to take action against assumed sources of disease. As a result marked improvement in the health of urban populations occurred even before more precise knowledge about the nature of the disease agents was available. The so-called miasmic or filth model on which the reform movement was based turned out to be wrong, but it nevertheless provided the justification and political leverage needed for the establishment of health departments and sanitary engineering activity. The model succeeded because it pulled together the many findings of epidemiological research into an easily saleable package.

Given the legal mandate to carry on surveillance and act against presumed sources of disease, health departments could simply follow the lead of their epidemiological findings—which had become independently valid and no longer dependent on the underlying theory. These agencies could act directly on the basis of whatever worked. Purification of water supplies, control of garbage, and sewage disposal virtually eliminated major epidemics of cholera, typhoid, and dysentery that had killed thousands every summer in crowded urban areas during the first half of the nineteenth century. Cleaning streets, removing refuse, eradicating rats and other vermin, and improving tenements dramatically lowered the incidence of typhus outbreaks. Quarantine and isolation of cases of smallpox (and legally enforced vaccination), diphtheria, scarlet fever, and tuberculosis reduced endemic levels and interrupted many epidemics (Duffy, 1974).

Thus many of the major scourges of urban populations were well on the way to control before medical science could identify their causes. For the first time in history the pattern of diseases was significantly affected by the ability of health professionals to intervene in the process. The advent of effective public health (and later medical technologies), however, does not mean that the nutritional, living standard, and sanitary engineering factors brought to light in our analyses of earlier societal transitions are now any less important. They remain the essential basis on which the health of any society must be built. In setting health policy we must not allow concern for these fundamental factors to be overshadowed by the more dramatic impact of newer developments. Before examining the impact of effective scientific medicine, however, it is necessary to backtrack in history to trace the development of the medical profession, which had to implement this new knowledge and technology.

REFERENCES

Ackerknecht, Erwin H., *History and Geography of the Most Important Diseases,* New York: Hafner, 1972.

Cole, G. D. H., and Postgate, Raymond, *The British Common People, 1746–1946,* London: Methuen, 1961.

Dubos, Rene, *Mirage of Health,* New York: Doubleday Anchor, 1959.

Dubos, Rene, *Man Adapting,* New Haven: Yale University Press, 1965.

Duffy, John, *A History of Public Health in New York City, 1866–1966,* 2 vols., New York: Russell Sage Foundation, 1974.

Kilbourne, Edwin D., and Smillie, Wilson G., *Human Ecology and Public Health,* London: Macmillan, 1971.

May, Jacques M., *The Ecology of Human Disease,* New York: MD Publications, 1958.

McKeown, Thomas, *Medicine in Modern Society,* New York: Hafner, 1965.

McKeown, Thomas, "A Historical Appraisal of the Medical Task," in McLachlan, G., and McKeown, T., Eds., *Medical History and Medical Care,* New York: Oxford University Press, 1971.

McKeown, Thomas, and Lowe, C. R., *An Introduction to Social Medicine,* 2nd ed., Philadelphia, Pa.: Lippincott, 1974.

McNeill, William H., *Plagues and People,* New York: Doubleday Anchor, 1976.

New York City Health Department, *Vital Statistics Report,* New York: Department of Health, 1978.

Rosen, George, *A History of Public Health,* New York: MD Publications, 1958.

Scrimshaw, Nevin S., and Behar, Moises, "Malnutrition," in Kilbourne, E. and Smillie, W., *Human Ecology and Public Health,* London: Macmillan, 1971.

Shryock, Richard H., *The Development of Modern Medicine: An Interpretation of the Social and Scientific Factors Involved,* New York: Hafner, 1969.

Singer, Charles, and Underwood, E. Ashworth, *A Short History of Medicine*, Oxford: The Clarendon Press, 1962.

Sigerist, Henry E., *A History of Medicine, Volume I: Primitive and Archaic Medicine*, New York: Oxford University Press, 1951.

Trevelyan, George M., *English Social History*, London: Longmans Green, 1942.

Weber, Max, *The Protestant Ethic and the Rise of Capitalism* (translator, Talcott Parsons), New York: Scribner, 1958.

World Health Organization, "The Constitution of the World Health Organization," *WHO Chronical*, 1:29, 1944.

Zinsser, Hans, *Rats, Lice and History*, Boston: Little, Brown, 1934.

CHAPTER THREE

Development of the Medical Profession: Social Mandates, Healing Efficacy, and Divergent Professional Traditions

Chapter 2 examines the history of the social factors influencing health and disease. This chapter examines the social forces that produced and continue to influence physicians' attitudes, organization, and behavior by tracing the historical development of the medical profession. As with the social causes of diseases, the social forces influencing physician behavior are often overlooked in our overconcern with their technical role in providing medical care. Important as this technical role has become in recent times, it is always exercised within a less obvious social context of (1) cultural tradition that defines the physician's status and social mandate, (2) professional organization that maintains a system of norms, incentives, and vested interests influencing the treatment situation, and (3) ideology about the nature of health, disease, and the physician's role in dealing with them, which focuses attention on certain problems at the expense of others.

These characteristics of the medical profession shape not only physicians' attitudes and behavior but also those of patients. Patients are part of the same cultural tradition; they perceive the physicians' status and their own roles as patients in terms of the cultural norms governing these relationships. Patients are influenced by the forces of professional organization because there are no equivalent counterveiling forces on the client side. To a large extent they accept uncritically the ideological perspective of the medical profession in regard to health and disease because of the profession's high prestige and the difficulty that outsiders have in evaluating the mysterious and frightening nature of medical knowledge and practice. We return explicitly to the question of patient behavior in Chapter 9, but it should be remembered that, insofar as the patient's role has a history at all, it is largely caught up in the cultural development of the medical profession.

When we analyze their role, physicians must be understood as both technicians providing a highly regarded service over which they hold a monopoly and also as agents of society with a mandate to control the anxiety and socially disruptive impact of illnesses. The first function has become increasingly a matter of public concern and analysis. The second function, however, is usually recognized only indirectly in the nostalgic desire to have physicians play a more personal role in caring for their patients. Despite its apparent secondary nature today, this social function continues to exert a major influence on the performance of the technical function as well as on the status and authority of physicians in society and on patients' expectations in regard to medical care. Freidson (1970, 1970a) has emphasized how physicians use their social authority, including their mandate to define disease, as an instrument to maintain dominance over patients. Yet, this is only one of the many ways that the social components of the physician's role influence the behavior, attitudes, and organization of the profession. The broader context of the professional mandate to exercise social control of illness behavior can be illuminated by examining the way it operated through much of history when it was the primary determinant of physician behavior.

Until very recently virtually the only effective service physicians could provide was the relief of anxiety by means of their official social function as controllers and caretakers of the sick. This function still constitutes a major component of the physician's role—although its importance is obscured by the growth of the technological function. In fact, in many ways the social control role has become a handmaiden to the technical one. This reversal of the relationship between social and technical functions is an important root of the growing patient dissatisfaction over what is referred to as the "impersonalization of the physician-patient relationship." In tracing the history of the profession we find that this impersonal perspective is largely a product of the very effectiveness of medical technology today—in contrast to its impotence until quite recently. Such submersion of the social function of medicine by its enhanced technological capabilities has important implications for the present organization of medical care.

If the social authority of the physician indeed has continued importance for the health and welfare of society, then the overascendancy of the technological function calls for deliberate measures to shore up the social functions of medicine. The norms built into cultural institutions like medicine have been weakened by the diffuseness and specialized nature of social interaction. As a result it is unlikely that the desired behavior can be brought about simply by moral exhortation or professional socialization that attempts to inculcate the appropriate values. Continuing organizational structures are necessary that encourage the desired behavior through adequate incentives, sanctions, and continuing group pressures. In examining the history and structure of the medical profession, we will seek to learn what kind of professional organization might serve this purpose by comparing the effects of the constellations of control in the past.

The second major feature of professional organization and behavior analyzed in this chapter is the differentiation of the original priestly physician
role into several traditions that remained separate throughout much of history: the guild (artisan) tradition, the learned academic tradition, and the
public service (hospital) tradition. Though tenuously reunited around the
turn of this century, these different traditions have left their mark on
the present structure of the profession and continue to be represented in
important groupings today. In many periods of medical history these traditions have been at odds with each other. They have had different processes
for training and socialization, different organizational structure, different
technologies, and therefore divergent vested interests. This division was
partly eclipsed for a short period as a result of the revolutionary breakthrough in medical technology in the late nineteenth century, which all
the traditions wanted to share. Today, however, the divisions are reassert-
ing themselves in a new form (see Chapter 8). These divergent professional
traditions were a result of the interplay between the division of institutional responsibility in regard to the social mandates of the profession and
the development of medical technology that changed the way these mandates could be carried out.

These different historical traditions constitute more fundamental influences on physician behavior than the subdivisions of the profession by
specialty. Concerns about overspecialization, maldistribution of practice location, or inadequate quality of care have led policy makers and health
service investigators to concentrate on the effect of medical education, financial incentives, and surveillance methods in controlling physician behavior.
This assumes a uniformity within the profession that a careful historical examination of its development shows does not in fact exist. The different historical traditions have quite dissimilar incentive and organizational systems
so that measures aimed at influencing one part of the profession may be totally ineffective in reaching the rest.

Medical historians have contributed to the illusion of homogeneity by
portraying a straight-line evolution of the scientific tradition of the profession. This account of medical history is misleading because it concentrates
entirely on the learned (academic) tradition of medicine, which is better
documented through publications and lasting discoveries. It neglects the
guild tradition of the ordinary practitioner and the separate public-service
tradition represented by hospitals throughout much of history. It also fails
to recognize the revolutionary nature of the changes in the conceptual
model of disease in the late nineteenth century and the profound and sudden change in physician organization that this revolution engendered. The
new theoretical model of disease first made biology effectively applicable to
medicine and fundamentally changed physicians' attitudes and behavior toward patients. With an eye to current policy implications, we reexamine
the history of the profession with these questions in mind.

THE SOCIAL ORIGIN OF THE MEDICAL
PROFESSION IN PREAGRARIAN SOCIETY

To understand the social forces determining the organization and behavior of physicians, we must first ask a more fundamental question: Why did healing professions arise at all, and what mechanisms have sustained them in societies? Physicians or their equivalents have had positions of importance, respect, and power in every known civilization—despite the fact that, until the end of the last century, there was very little they could do to change the outcome of most diseases. Throughout most of history physicians, using bloodletting, purges, and toxic drugs, probably have hastened the demise of more patients than they helped. To be sure, folk medicine and shamans sometimes stumbled onto herbs and other remedies containing active ingredients that do in fact aid in treatment. However, with a few notable exceptions such as quinine against malaria, these usually produced only symptomatic relief. Most controlled clinical trials of such drugs today show no significant difference in the outcome of the illness when they are compared to the effect of an inert placebo.

Admittedly, people have always *believed* that physicians could help them, and this belief itself is an important factor in the effect that physicians are able to have on patients. Most illnesses get better on their own, no matter what is done for them—or even in spite of things done that actually weaken patients' resistance in fighting a disease. This obviously worked in favor of physicians who could claim credit for nature's cures, thus enhancing the faith that their patients had. This faith, in turn, was and is an important therapeutic tool. Many diseases are psychosomatic or at least have a significant psychological component that can be helped by the faith in the healer. Even where no cure occurs, belief in the potential power of the healer provides solace and socially sustaining support for patient and family. Using this belief, the physician is able to accomplish considerable good even when he can do nothing to influence the course of the disease itself.

Yet this faith in the healer is precisely the puzzle we need to understand. If it is arbitrary faith that helps, why does the physician's role take such a similar form as a social institution in every society? Why do the organizational characteristics of the healing profession persist with such tenacity? The same faith could just as well be attached to simpler less powerful institutions. Why the physician, with his mystery, prestige, and close association to the central authority of the society? The tenacious persistence of the characteristic social institution of medicine, with its prestigious professional role despite the lack of technical success, is a puzzle. This apparent paradox calls for explanation in terms of other social forces, for instance, what the sociologist, Robert Merton (1968), calls "latent functions." Such forces that have maintained and shaped the professional tradition of medicine are more easily seen by examining the healing profession in its most primitive form, where its role is most clearly social.

Medicine in preagrarian societies was and is a mixture of religious ritual, magic, and socially institutionalized responsibility for the sick. In such societies the tribal priest, the seer, and the medicine man or shaman are often one and the same person, and this combined religious and healing role represents what can be called the "priestly tradition" of medicine (Sigerist, 1955). Birth, death, and illness are mysterious, anxiety-producing phenomena in all societies (Ackerknecht, 1943). An important problem is posed by the social effects of illness, whether or not anything can be done to change the course of the disease. Each society needs some measure of social control over the sick individual's reactions to anxiety and pain, especially over behavior that may appear potentially dangerous to others. This social control is usually exercised in conjunction with means for giving comfort, solace, and psychological support to the patient (Ackerknecht, 1942, 1942a). In order to maintain necessary social activities in the face of illness, the social control and assistance often are required not only for the sick person but also family and others interacting with the patient. Here strong direction and sanctions are even more essential because the nonsick are in a less dependent position and less amenable to control. Consequently, every society needs a strong system of norms and institutionalized decision-making about social behavior in regard to illness.

These problems of social control of illness behavior make it very likely that any society will develop institutions and roles for dealing with them as part of its cultural tradition. To exercise authority in the face of anxiety and suffering, a powerful role has arisen that is vested with a cultural mandate to do this. The person in this role is authorized to make and enforce decisions about the fate of the sick, and often of the nonsick who are in some way affected by the illness. This healing role, coupled with direct service to the sick person, also requires justification for the privileged access to information and the right to examine and manipulate the body of the patient. The constellation of authority, privilege, and responsibility vested in the healing role, therefore, demands a high degree of integration into the moral and power system of the society—with special justification for the unique powers of the role. Much of the physician's power over the patient is accomplished psychologically by the air of mystery involved in the treatment and the dependency engendered in the patient by the anxiety of the illness. This is reinforced by social sanctions available to the priestly healer. The mysterious knowledge and its use in ritual or magic, are primary means of providing psychological support and solace to the patient as well as buttressing the authority needed for social control.

Since the sick in preagrarian society were often believed to be possessed by evil forces, the use of magic and ritual also reaffirmed the moral order of the society in the face of the threat posed by the illness (Ackerknecht,

1943). The potentially disruptive elements of fear, sorrow, or despair were actually converted into sources of solidarity by participation in the ritual and by the sharing in the power of the culturally sanctioned magic. Consequently the medicine man performed an important latent function (Merton, 1968) in supporting social stability. It is not surprising, therefore, that the priestly healing tradition was closely tied into the religious and moral order of society. The phenomenon of creating conformity to moral standards and social solidarity through participation in rituals in the face of threatening situations is familiar to sociologsts in many contexts (Durkheim, 1893; Coser, 1952). The mechanism is best documented and understood in regard to morally deviant behavior where collective action against it produces greater solidarity among the participants (Erikson, 1966). Condemning the deviant reaffirms the norms of society, strengthens identification with the norms, and heightens the sense of membership in the society by drawing a clear boundary between those who are excluded from the moral order, "them" (the deviants), and those who do belong, "us."

Even though in modern society sickness is no longer looked upon as caused by evil forces and therefore akin to moral deviance, it is still socially threatening and in this sense a form of deviance (Mechanic, 1968). Participation in the social processes for controlling it continues to lend a sense of heightened societal identification to those involved. The person officially empowered to label such a threat and direct social defenses against it plays a crucial normative role in the structure of society—one that will always remain very close to the central cultural authority. A high degree of this moral sanction remains in the role of physicians today. Much of the physicians' power over patients, and their status in society derives from their authority to label disease and to determine the assistance and sanctions of society to be employed in regard to patients (Freidson, 1970). The mysterious knowledge and seemingly occult power, which physicians use to treat disease and indirectly to dominate patients, are a continuation of the magical power and moral authority of the primitive priestly physician role.

Possession of this occult knowledge and command of the mysterious cultural rituals vest physicians with high prestige and power in the social hierarchy. Therefore, a strong, culturally institutionalized and socially organized system evolved for transmitting and protecting this knowledge, ritual, and skill (Sigerist, 1955). A method was established for selecting, initiating, and socializing new members of the healing group, and for training them in the secret knowledge and skills. The institutionalized system for doing this came to have a self-perpetuating social momentum of its own. This institutional self-propagation further reinforced the functional reasons for the continuation of the role—much as religious institutions do for the priesthood. The physician role and its social organization have many parallels with the role of the priest, and major elements of this priestly role have been maintained by the medical profession throughout its history.

Side-by-side with the priestly physician role in preagrarian societies, there existed a much more pragmatic, less prestigious healing activity. This was based on the store of knowledge and skills making it possible to deal with certain simple injuries, infections, common symptoms such as fever, and with childbirth. In tribal societies, and to some extent in more complex societies, these skills and knowledge are transmitted by a cultural tradition distributed widely throughout the population as "folk medicine" (Coe, 1970). In more complex societies with a greater division of labor, the knowledge and practice of the pragmatic medical skills were restricted to special members of the society such as midwives, bonesetters, barber surgeons, herbalists, and the like (Sigerist, 1960). Unlike the duties of the priestly role, these pragmatic medical tasks usually dealt with less mysterious and terrifying conditions. The problem of social control was not so central, and pragmatic healing roles were seldom shrouded in cultural mantle of mysterious knowledge, social power, and prestige. Folk medicine practitioners still had to solve the problem of patient compliance and had to justify their privileged access to information and right to manipulate the patient's body. However, this was accomplished largely by transaction, the patient granting the special privileges only as a condition necessary for receiving the particular service. Because much less mystery, authority, prestige, and cultural sanction were involved, the processes of initiation, socialization, and transmission of knowledge and skills usually took place by means of simple apprenticeship or self-instruction and experience in practice.

Thus in the beginning healing activities were divided between a priestly physician role embodying the social control aspects of the profession and other separate roles or diffuse knowledge and skills providing the more utilitarian aspects of the medical profession. The priestly (social control) role had the greatest prestige and power and the highest degree of institutionalization within the social order. It justified the privileges and special authority of physicians and prescribed their responsibilities to patients and society. The social control functions of the priestly tradition have persisted to the present. They have been modified, however, and divided among several professional traditions in the process of incorporating more sophisticated, pragmatic healing functions as medical knowledge and technology advanced. The initial division took place in Greece during the Classical Period.*

DEVELOPMENT OF THE MULTIPLE PROFESSIONAL TRADITIONS OF MEDICINE IN ANCIENT GREECE

At the beginning of Greek history the situation was as in the early societies discussed: a priestly healing group and folk medicine. By the end of the

---

* Similar developments and divisions of the profession probably took place in Egypt and other ancient civilizations, but we do not have sufficient records to know precisely what form it took. Besides, the Greek developments are those from which our own traditions have directly descended.

Greek classical period this had been replaced by three separate healing traditions: the Hippocratic artisan (guild) tradition, the academic (learned) tradition, and the hospital (public service) tradition. The groups representing the three traditions divided the old priestly mantle among themselves in the process of assuming different elements of the growing technical functions of medicine. In early Greek times the Asklepiad healing priesthood had a monopoly over the occult knowledge and social control functions of healing just as did similar priestly groups or cults in previous civilizations (Sigerist, 1961). Greek mythology included the physician demigod, Asklepios, in its pantheon. There were temples dedicated to him throughout Greece where patients came from afar in hopes of miraculous cures. The spalike setting, where patients were treated with rest, exercise, diet, meditation, and advice from the priests, seems to have been effective in improving either the physical or mental state of many. The temple remains are as filled with votive works made by grateful pilgrims as is the Grotto of Lourdes with discarded crutches. The Asklepiad priesthood and its healing tradition continued throughout Greek classical history. However, its original undisputed authority and sole institutionalized healing role were challenged by new healing traditions that arose and were also institutionalized in that period.

The first new role established was the artisan healer who provided certain straightforward but effective services to patients on a "fee-for-service" basis, with minimal privileges and duties of the social control type. Because of the typical social organization of these artisans in later times, this role can be called the "guild tradition."* This tradition of Greek medicine may have split off from the Asklepiad priesthood, as legend has it, or it may have arisen through the growth, pragmatic success, and institutionalization of folk medicine, or both (Sigerist, 1961). The individualistic and commercial culture of classical Greece saw the development of secular knowledge and learning in many areas (Farrington, 1953). The rise of independent artisan groups organized into guilds allowed the transmission of this knowledge from one generation to the next by the apprenticeship system. Artisan physicians had already established themselves in pre-Socratic times, developing a tradition that accumulated practical knowledge about health and disease based on theories in terms of natural rather than supernatural causes. A number of early Greek natural philosophers were artisan physicians (Clagett, 1955).

As the craft tradition of medicine developed and a growing corpus of practical and theoretical knowledge became available, guilds established organized schools as an adjunct to the apprenticeship system in transmitting the knowledge. The most famous was the school of Hippocrates on the Island of Cos (Sigerist, 1958). When they had finished their schooling and

* There were important cultural and organizational differences between the Greek "techne" (crafts) and the medieval "guilds," but their social functions were similar and for our analysis of the medical professional traditions, these differences were not as crucial as the similarities.

apprenticeship, Greek artisan physicians practiced by traveling from town to town selling their services as they could. A few cities employed physicians, but unlike the well-established healing priesthood, whose members lived from charitable donations and from the production of their temple land holdings, most guild physicians had to support themselves from their professional activities alone. Financial support, and patient compliance, entailed a commercial relationship that required client satisfaction because there were no strong social sanctions and cultural norms to back these physicians. As a result, artisan physicians had to be very pragmatic and prudent in their craft. They limited active intervention to the few conditions where they could achieve satisfactory effects such as lancing boils and setting broken bones. They employed only a few drugs derived from mild herbs, and relied mostly on diet and natural regimens.

Their reputations were built on the judicious selection of patients with good outlooks for recovery rather than attempts at dramatic cures or intervention in hopeless cases. Consequently they developed the art of prognosis to a high degree, establishing the practice of systematic clinical description necessary to recognize the crucial signs, symptoms, and clinical courses of illness that would allow them to foresee the probable outcome. They used this clinical prognostic ability to "secure a good reputation when visiting a new town by being able to tell a patient right away what his trouble was without having to ask questions" (Marti-Ibanez, 1960). Thus, commercial necessity led to an improved empirical approach to clinical medicine that proved to be a lasting contribution. This empirical attitude encouraged the accumulation of systematic observations and transformed the approach to practice even though it gave no satisfactory causal understanding of diseases.*

Their vulnerable position as commercial private practitioners also led artisan physicians to organize guilds for mutual protection and professional solidarity. Protection of professional interests was not guaranteed by culturally mandated institutions as with the priestly role. It was necessary to develop organizational forms to strengthen the rights of practitioners, control competition, and present a united front to society in regard to guild interests. By setting ethical standards, such as the Hippocratic oath still taken by physicians today, the guilds protected the reputation of the profession as a whole, making it easier for each member to practice (Sigerist, 1961). Such ethical codes also served to prevent unfair competitive practices

---

* The humoral balance theory of Hippocratic medicine was apparently useful in guiding treatment (or alleviation) of symptoms in the hands of Greek physicians trained in moderation and restraint in therapy. However, its use by later generations of physicians who were less astute clinicians often led to senseless bleeding and purging of patients that undoubtedly caused many needless deaths. Moreover, entrenched in dogma as it was from Greek times through the eighteenth century, it blinded most physicians to the observation of other possible causal relationships in the clinical patterns of disease. Thus it probably played a role in delaying the emergence of effective methods of prevention and treatment based on intervention against causes of pathology rather than on symptoms.

among guild members. No doubt many abuses and conflicts still occurred, but the organization and attitudes that developed in response to guild physicians' vested interests did produce a new mode for practice of the healing arts. Thus, the priestly and the guild traditions of the healing profession came to exist side by side dealing with quite different problems, using very different techniques of diagnosis and treatment, and educating, organizing, and supporting their members in quite different ways.

The second new professional tradition of Greek medicine was the academic or learned profession. This developed as part of the general evolution of Greek cultural life in which a speculative but empirically and logically based philosophy, rational criticism of traditional beliefs, and the pragmatic search for solutions to technological problems, all joined to produce a great period of intellectual flowering (Snell, 1953; Farrington, 1953). Institutionalization of these achievements included the development of the medical learned profession, which has retained its own tradition throughout the subsequent history of medicine. The Greek intellectual heritage contained a new element of social organization that made the preservation and extension of the new knowledge possible—a learned class, whose fulltime role was maintenance, transmission, and enlargement of the learned tradition. To be sure, every great civilization had a learned tradition of some kind, and the transmission of any culture involves an intellectual heritage. Before Greek classical civilization, however, this tradition had always been inextricably mixed with the religious and moral system of the culture. Such traditions had been transmitted primarily by the priesthood and the political bureaucracy, as for example in ancient Egyptian and Mesopotamian civilizations. In Greece, for the first time, a separate "pure" intellectual tradition came into being with an existence independent of the religious and political order, entrusted to a group whose sole role was to maintain and improve knowledge (Jaeger, 1945).

Hippocratic medicine combined with Aristotelian biology became the central content of the medical knowledge that was taken up, transmitted, and gradually enlarged by this learned tradition. Asklepiad priestly medicine was not transmitted and disseminated in the same way, although it had probably played as important a role in Greek society as had guild medicine. There were several reasons for this. Hippocratic medicine was written down and therefore more available for transmission as part of the Greek intellectual influence than was the mysterious knowledge of the priestly healing cult. It was less tied to the parochial Greek moral and religious order and therefore more easily adapted to the cultural orders of the new societies that took it up, together with the rest of the Greek philosophical and scientific heritage. Finally, limited though it was in changing the course of most diseases, it offered some definite advancements over folk medicine and shamanism in dealing with illnesses. Hippocratic medicine was widely accepted as part of the successful empirical tradition of Greek technology that succeeding civilizations were eager to adopt and emulate. Even when the learned professional tradition reverted to the priesthood, as it did for long stretches of European history, there was a content clearly distinct from the theological and moral aspects of religion. This made it possible to maintain a separate medical learned tradition, and eventually provided the basis for the re-uniting of an improved, medical-biological science with the clinical guild tradition.

Before disappearing the Asklepiad tradition spun off one other new institution that became the third healing tradition, the hospital or public service component of medical care. As a primarily commercial society, ancient Greece had a large urban population including many indigent, homeless, or sick who had no place to turn for help. In tribal and early agrarian societies, the sick and the indigent had been cared for by families or in some other informal way. In the teeming commercial cities of the late ancient world, however, this informal system was no longer adequate. There was often no one to take personal responsibility for these homeless social undesirables. To deal with the problem in Greek cities, hospitals were established. The first were outgrowths of Asklepian temples where there had always been facilities to house the sick seeking cures (Sigerist, 1961). These hospitals were supported as a charitable public service by the temples, which were generally well-endowed by contributions from grateful patrons and those who made donations as a religious act. Later, out of responsibility for their citizens and fear of unrest or contagion among the growing indigent population, city governments took it upon themselves to support Asklepian temple hospitals or similar nonreligious institutions. Thus the final medical tradition was established—public service care for the indigent. From the beginning a pattern of support developed that combined charitable donations with church and government responsibility for the poor. This pattern of financing has continued to the present day.

These early hospitals were far from the image we have of hospitals today. Not only did they provide a place for the indigent sick, but also for the needy in general, who had no other place to go. They often served as guest houses for travelers, and during the European Middle Ages this became their primary function. In fact, the modern word "hospital" stems from "hospice," the word for guest house. Over the years the organization of hospital care for the indigent became as strongly institutionalized as the guild and learned professional traditions of medicine, spreading throughout the late ancient and medieval worlds. Rome established an efficient system of hospitals, beginning with an Asklepian temple on the Island of St. Bartholemew in the Tiber River where "sick and worn-out slaves were sent to avoid trouble" (Singer & Underwood, 1962). Military hospitals were built on the frontiers of the Roman Empire. Beginning with the Council of Nicaea in A.D. 325, the Christian Church took up the work of the Asklepiads by instructing its bishops to establish a hospital in every city with a cathedral (Rosen, 1963).

Thus at the end of the Greek classical period the development of medical knowledge and the increasing complexity of society had resulted in the birth and institutionalization of three new healing traditions. Each took up part of the social control function of the old priestly healing role and became responsible for carrying out a corresponding technical function in regard to the sick. Although it did not evolve directly out of the Asklepiad priesthood, the new medical learned profession was in many ways the clearest heir to the cultural mantle of the old priestly tradition. It was institutionalized within the universities in association with the religious faculties and in many periods of history with close links to government bureaucracies for enforcing social values and norms. This prestigious learned profession retained the mandate of defining "diseases" and the "proper" patient, physician, and social response to illness. Thus it remained responsible for the moral order of medicine, having the social mandate to set norms and values in regard to health and disease in close relationship to the general moral order of society. The learned profession accomplished this within its technical role of preserving, transmitting, and enlarging the cultural heritage of medical knowledge and skills. Even though the guilds transmitted some medical techniques and knowledge by apprenticeship, the learned profession controlled the only organized basis for doing this.

The healing guilds provided the society-wide extension of the social authority of medicine by enforcing it at the one-to-one physician-patient interface. By invoking the norms and values of the learned profession in regard to disease, the guild physicians carried out the social mandate of anxiety control and prevention of public disruption from disturbed patients and families. In part this was accomplished by sharing in the cultural authority of the learned profession, possessing some of its mysterious knowledge, and enacting the awe-inspiring rituals of medicine. However, this authority was also supplemented by offering solace, psychological support, and whatever technical services were possible in exchange for patient compliance. This service-authority relationship had been directly enforced by priestly healers in earlier societies but henceforth was largely mediated by the guilds.

The hospitals, embodying the public service tradition of medicine, were the inheritors of the more coercive aspects of the social control role. The shaman could mobilize general societal reaction against sick or deviant members of the tribe who were reluctant or dangerous. In the more complex differentiated societies after the classical period this was no longer possible. Hospitals provided an organized base for exercising the same social control, offering a refuge where the impoverished sick, the homeless, many kinds of deviants, and other social "undesirables" could be confined and regimented. Thus, hospitals provided the technical service of institutional care in exchange for patient compliance. To do this, they needed external financial support and the social license to enforce the moral order in regard to these affairs. To gain these mandates and resources they invoked the cultural mantle of the learned healing tradition to some extent, sharing in its prestige as the guild healers did. However, neither financial support nor patient compliance could be obtained by this route alone. Therefore, hospitals were forced to rely more on the church and/or state, which in turn required them to be less purely medical in their approach than the guild or learned traditions of medicine.

THE INTERPLAY BETWEEN LEARNED PROFESSION AND GUILD TRADITIONS THROUGH THE MIDDLE AGES

As late antiquity began, then, the three traditions of the healing profession were established and separately institutionalized in essentially their modern roles. This historical division of the medical profession and its evolution as three distinct traditions, however, implies neither independence of the traditions from each other, nor straight-line development. The relationship between the traditions was characterized by interdependencies and struggles for dominance usually centering around major changes in knowledge, theory, or practice during the evolution of the profession. This strife between traditions is of interest because it has left imprints on professional organization, ideology, and attitudes about the practice of medicine.

During late antiquity Greece declined as the primary academic center of the world. The Greek learned tradition, however, including Hippocratic medicine (combined with Aristotelian biology) was carried on in the new Hellenistic centers of the Near East created by the conquest of Alexander the Great: Pergamum, Antioch, Alexandria, and later Bagdad (Singer & Underwood, 1962). The Greek works were enlarged through commentary and translated first into Persian, then into Arabic, as the Moslem Empire swept over the area and assimilated Hellenistic culture. After the fall of Rome in the fifth century, the Greek medical tradition gradually disappeared in the West during the early Middle Ages. Fortunately it was preserved in these translations and in the Hellinistic-Arabic professional tradition so that it could be rediscovered by the West 500 years later (Crombie, 1959).

After the hiatus of the learned tradition in Europe during the early Middle Ages, the redevelopment of the medical profession in Western Civilization began with the establishment of universities and medical faculties at Salerno, Bologna, Montpellier, and Paris in the eleventh and twelfth centuries and with the translation of Arabic medical texts into Latin (Gordon, 1959). Since the secular learned tradition had been destroyed in the West, the new universities first grew up under the domination of the Church. The clergy was the only major group that had remained literate during this period. They were the natural ones to make use of the medical texts and manuscripts that began pouring in from the East as a result of the crusades and the reopening of trade with the Arabic world (Crombie, 1959).

Yet, the new medical faculties of the West did not automatically have undisputed control over cultural norms about disease, professional tradition, and practice. A well-established independent guild tradition predated the growth of universities (Scarborough, 1969). These guilds played an important role in providing care and social control and in molding the modern medical profession. A struggle of several centuries ensued before the new medical faculties attained hegemony over the profession. Many of the tensions and the stratification of the medical profession today had their origins in the centuries of struggle between learned and guild traditions for professional dominance. This struggle came to a certain equilibrium with the introduction of the dual licensure system (university degree and civil or medical society license) in the sixteenth century.

The guild tradition of the late Middle Ages consisted of diffusely organized physicians, barber surgeons, bonesetters, midwives, and so forth, who were trained simply by apprenticeship or by studying any available medical writings and then simply plying their trade (Riesman, 1935). There was some self-regulation of practitioners by guilds, but independent wandering entrepreneurial healers were also common, and regulation or "licensure" seems to have been nonexistent. The early universities had no control and little relationship to this heterogeneous group of practitioners, but stepwise they attained a position of dominance in medical affairs (Bullough, 1966). University faculty members became the court physicians or developed other aristocratic ties and began to have their influence on the growing, increasingly centralized governments of the later Middle Ages. First bishops and then rising secular princes of Italy, Spain, and France issued edicts restricting the practice of medicine to those who had studied and passed qualifying examinations in a faculty of medicine. Since it was very difficult to define the practice of medicine at that time, this merely meant that only those who had so qualified could call themselves "physicians" and belong to the guild of that name—which soon obtained the highest status. Practitioners such as midwives, apothecaries, and surgeons were untouched by these edicts and continued to practice in competing guilds. Thus regulation divided the healing profession more clearly into segments of different status. Nonetheless, this "professionalized" (Bullough, 1966) the university-trained physician group and placed the learned tradition again in the position of officially defining the nature of disease and the norms of medical practice. Yet, guild physicans remained an essential link as the actual mediators of the social control mandate.

The influence of the university faculties over the practicing guilds by way of official edicts was only part of the process of professional control. Even where no such legal regulation existed, the most prestigious healing guilds developed codes of ethics and self-regulation that subjected themselves to much the same standards as those set by the university faculties. In order to legitimize their authority over patients, guild physicians were dependent on sharing the prestige of the university physicians, who had the primary cultural mandate to define the norms in regard to disease, health, and healing

practices. This mandate provided the necessary authority for exercising social control of illness. The borrowed prestige was reinforced for the guilds
of university-trained physicians by acquiring many of the trappings of the
learned profession, such as knowing the mysterious knowledge of medicine
(anatomy, chemistry, pharmacy, botany). Though it had little practical
value, this knowledge was important in the defense of their domain against
encroachment from other less prestigious healing guilds. The esoteric knowledge of medicine and clinical lore became their common stock in trade, and
they had a vested interest in monopolizing its use and protecting its dissemination (Bullough, 1966). This protection depended on the university faculties. Consequently, with each new major increment of knowledge, the
learned profession gained authority, only to have it diluted again as the
knowledge was gradually diffused and became the common possession of
members of the practicing profession.

Although guild physicians needed to identify themselves with the prestigious learned profession, they also wanted independence from the academicians in order to protect their separate interests. Guild physicians provided
professional healing services to the rising middle class and to some extent
to the working classes—though the latter tended to turn to barber-surgeons,
apothecaries, or nonprofessional folk healers. Being dependent on the exchange relationship with patients for their professional survival, the guild
physicians had to make more effort to please their patients. They resorted
to more ritual, "bedside manner," and mysterious hocus-pocus to present a
professional image than did either the university physicians, who had un-
questioned prestige, or the surgeons, who merely sold a limited practical
skill.

To protect their interests guild physicians had their own professional
organizations. Yet, unlike the situation in most guilds, outsiders (university
faculties) controlled entry into the medical profession. Therefore, guild
physicians began to press for stronger protection of their professional status
by seeking a hand in the licensure process. Surgeons, usually not trained at
the universities, had long controlled entry into their own guilds, and in
Italy and France this was officially recognized as licensure. In London, far
enough removed from the influence of Oxford and Cambridge medical
faculties, guild physicians first attained control over licensure to practice.
Thomas Linacre persuaded Henry VIII to charter the Royal College of
Physicians of London in 1518 as the examining body to qualify physicians
for practice in that city (Berlant, 1975). This was soon extended to the entire country, and the principle of "dual licensure" was established (a university doctoral degree followed by guild or state examination to be allowed
to practice). This system continues to the present day in the United States
and in many countries of the world.

HOSPITALS DURING THE MEDIEVAL AND
EARLY MODERN PERIODS

Since its first founding in ancient Greece, the hospital tradition has continued essentially unbroken. In Europe during the Middle Ages the Roman
military hospitals were allowed to disappear, but monasteries usually maintained small facilities to care for the sick and indigent as well as for travelers. During the Crusades the number and size of the monastic hospitals
increased rapidly, and special orders of monks (and later knights) were
established to operate them. From the twelfth to fifteenth centuries, more
than 750 hospitals were established in England alone, and by 1350 Florence
had 30 hospitals and Paris had 40 (Rosen, 1963). As the monastic hospitals
grew, they came to have many benefactors besides the church, including
kings, nobles, rich merchants, guilds, fraternities, and municipalities. Beyond caring for the sick they sheltered the poor, the infirm, the aged, lepers,
orphans, invalids, and strangers, providing medical care, philanthropy, and
spiritual guidance. Thus hospitals were as much religious and spiritual institutions as organizations for medical care (Rosen, 1963; Kane, 1973).

By manifold religious observances, the staff sought to elevate and discipline character. They endeavored, as the body decayed, to strengthen the soul and prepare
it for the future life. Faith and love were more predominant features in hospital
life than were skill and science . . . (Clay, 1909)

Monastic orders had a religious incentive to carry on the healing work
among the poor that neither the learned profession nor the medical guild
members were willing to undertake as a responsibility. The learned profession did have an alliance with church and aristocracy, both of whom supported the hospitals, but not with the level of churchmen who operated
them. For the guild members of the medical profession there was no prestige
associated with hospital practice until much later (mid-eighteenth century)
and no financial incentive to work in the hospitals, since middle-class patients avoided them as pest houses (Churchill, 1949). As the world became
more secularized in the Renaissance it was necessary to provide more medical care and less religion within the hospitals to maintain custodial control
over indigents and social outcasts. Incentives were needed to attract guild
physicians to provide this care. This required changes in the nature of hospitals, in the medical profession, and in the prevailing ethic of society.

During the Renaissance many functions of the hospitals changed, and
financially they fell on hard times. As a result of the dissolution of the
monasteries by Henry VIII in 1536–1539 the hospital system of England
disappeared, leaving the country essentially without hospitals for 200 years
until voluntary and municipal hospitals were established in the eighteenth
century. In France flagrant abuses by patrons and wardens led to a state

assumption of authority over hospital administration, but only after the French Revolution in 1794.

Freed of religious sponsorship and domination, the hospitals gradually entered a new era. There was a rising need for professional medical care as a result of the decreasing tendency of the monastic clergy to practice medicine, and because of the epidemics that swept across Europe in the wake of wars of the Reformation. Increasing migration of peasants off the land into the new commercial centers created a growing urban poor. Because of the rising prestige of medicine during the sixteenth and seventeenth centuries and the philosophy of nationalistic mercantilism, which advocated government measures to improve the health and welfare of their populations, cities began to take steps to make physicians available in the hospitals. As early as 1377 a municipal surgeon was appointed in Frankfurt-am-Main; but in England such public provision of physician services occurred only after the Elizabethan Poor Law of 1601 required local authorities to take responsibility for the maintenance of the poor. In many cases physicians were employed by municipalities under the assumption that providing professional medical care would shorten stays and reduce the number of persons who were feigning illness and "should be in work houses instead of the hospitals" (Rosen, 1963).

REFERENCES

Ackerknecht, Erwin H., "Problems in Primitive Medicine," *Bulletin of the History of Medicine*, 11:503–521, 1942.

Ackerknecht, Erwin H., "Primitive Medicine and Culture Pattern," *Bulletin of the History of Medicine*, 12:545–574, 1942a.

Ackerknecht, Erwin H., "Psychopathology, Primitive Medicine and Primitive Culture," *Bulletin of the History of Medicine*, 14:30–67, 1943.

Berlant, Jeffrey L., *Profession and Monopoly: A Study of Medicine in the United States and Great Britain*, Berkeley: University of California Press, 1975.

Bullough, Vern L., *The Development of Medicine as a Profession*, New York: Hafner, 1966.

Churchill, Edward D., "The Development of the Hospital," in Faxon, Nathaniel W., Ed., *The Hospital in Contemporary Life*, Cambridge: Harvard University Press, 1949.

Claggett, Marshall, *Greek Science in Antiquity*, New York: Collier-Macmillan, 1955.

Clay, Rotha M., *The Medieval Hospitals of England*, London, Methuen, 1909.

Coe, Rodney M., *Sociology of Medicine*, New York: McGraw-Hill, 1970.

Coser, Lewis, *The Function of Social Conflict*, New York: Free Press, 1952.

Crombie, Alistair C., *Medieval and Early Modern Science*, 2 vols., New York: Doubleday Anchor, 1959.

Duffy, John, *A History of Public Health in New York City, 1866–1966*, 2 vols., New York: Russell Sage Foundation, 1974.

Durkheim, Emile (1893), *The Division of Labor in Society* (translator, George Simpson), Glencoe, Ill.: Free Press, 1960.

Erikson, Kai T., *Wayward Puritans*, New York: Wiley, 1966.

Farrington, Benjamin, *Greek Science: Its Meaning for Us,* Baltimore: Penguin, 1953.

Freidson, Eliot, *Profession of Medicine,* New York: Dodd, Mead, 1970.

Freidson, Eliot, *Professional Dominance: The Social Structure of Medical Care,* New York: Atherton Press, 1970a.

Gordon, Benjamin Lee, *Medieval and Renaissance Medicine,* New York: Philosophical Library, 1959.

Jaeger, Werner, *Paideia: The Ideals of Greek Culture,* 3 vols. (translator, Gilbert Highet), New York: Oxford University Press, 1945.

Kane, Daniel A., "The Organization of Hospitals in Medieval England," *Hospital Administration,* **18** (1, Winter): 44–52, 1973.

Lilienfeld, Abraham M., *Foundations of Epidemiology,* New York: Oxford University Press, 1976.

Marti-Ibanez, Felix, *Centaur—Essays on the History of Medical Ideas,* New York: MD Publications, 1960.

Mechanic, David, *Medical Sociology,* New York: Free Press, 1968 (2nd ed., 1978).

Merton, Robert K., *Social Theory and Social Structure,* rev. ed., New York: Free Press, 1968.

Riesman, David, *The Story of Medicine in the Middle Ages,* New York: Hoeber, 1935.

Rosen, George, *A History of Public Health,* New York: MD Publications, 1958.

Rosen, George, "The Hospital: Historical Sociology of a Community Institution," in Freidson, Eliot, Ed., *The Hospital in Modern Society,* New York: Free Press, 1963, pp. 1–36.

Scarborough, John, *Roman Medicine,* Ithaca: Cornell University Press, 1969.

Singer, Charles, and Underwood, E. Ashworth, *A Short History of Medicine,* Oxford: Clarendon Press, 1962.

Sigerist, Henry E., *A History of Medicine, Volume I: Primitive and Archaic Medicine,* New York: Oxford University Press, 1955.

Sigerist, Henry E., *The Great Doctors,* Garden City, N.Y.: Doubleday Anchor, 1958.

Sigerist, Henry E., *On the History of Medicine,* New York: MD Publications, 1960.

Sigerist, Henry E., *A History of Medicine, Vol. II: Early Greek, Hindu, and Persian Medicine,* New York: Oxford University Press, 1961.

Snell, Bruno, *The Discovery of the Mind* (translator, T. G. Rosenmeyer), Cambridge: Harvard University Press, 1953.

CHAPTER FOUR

The Development of
Effective Scientific Medicine

Until the late nineteenth or early twentieth century the structure of the profession and the behavior of physicians were determined primarily by the social mandate to control anxiety and potentially disruptive patient behavior resulting from illness. These functions were accomplished by using the mystery, prestige, and social sanctions embodied in the authority of the physician's role and by providing solace, psychological support, and certain (minimal) pragmatic services to patients. For all practical purposes the state of medical knowledge remained unimportant for practice until almost the end of the nineteenth century. In spite of the rebirth of empirical science including anatomy and physiology during the Renaissance, and the continued accumulation of new medical knowledge, this had little practical importance for the improvement of clinical medicine in the 300 years from Vesalius' refutation of Galen's anatomy (1543) and Harvey's discovery of the circulation of the blood (1628) until Pasteur and Koch's demonstration of the bacterial nature of certain infectious diseases (1840–1880).* The ancient humoral balance theory, which Galen had perpetuated, remained the standard justification for the continued ineffective and dangerous bloodletting, purging, and blistering that had characterized medical practice since antiquity. This symptom-oriented approach also left clinical medicine at the mercy of many fads, which were introduced as the result of each new scientific interest, such as chemistry and electrophysics (Shryock, 1969).

Nevertheless, the developments in medicine during the eighteenth and nineteenth centuries had important effects on the medical profession that

---

* This continued impotence of medicine has been obscured by most histories, which give the false impression that the growth of medical knowledge during this period was accompanied by gradual improvement of clinical practice. This misleading picture arises because these histories are in fact accounts of only the medical learned tradition and its contribution to biology, which had no significant effect on clinical treatment until the revolutions in the theory of disease and physiology took place in the late nineteenth century.

laid the basis for our present clinical approach to diseases. The evolution of medical knowledge during this period was not simply an accretion of new information gradually building the store of scientific and clinical knowledge for immediate application. Rather, it was a complex intellectual and organizational struggle with little influence on medical practice until it culminated in a revolution in the theoretical model of disease, which from then on guided thinking in medical research and practice—a "scientific paradigm revolution" (Kuhn, 1962). This new causal model attributes diseases to specific defects producing disturbances of the normal (homeostatic) physiological systems of the body.* (1) It required conceptualizing diseases as recurring, recognizable entities that are separable as objects of study from the patients suffering them. (2) It built on the discovery of self-propagating organisms ("germs") that could be physically isolated from the sick and could then produce the same disease in another animal or person. (3) It required understanding the normally functional mechanisms of human physiology and how specific disease agents or defects of other kinds interfere with its normal balance creating patterns of dysfunction, recognizable as particular diseases.

The model crystallized rather suddenly in its full-blown form out of several components that had been built up gradually (but separately) within the academic tradition. This quantum jump phenomenon in knowledge is typical of scientific paradigm revolutions (Kuhn, 1962). The components alone were only of academic or biological interest and without practical application. The completed model, on the contrary, had almost immediate sweeping practical consequences that revolutionized the nature of medical practice in a single generation. It provided a framework within which much of the older knowledge could then be put to practical use and made it easier to look for new information to fill gaps in knowledge. The discoveries that grew out of using the model made effective intervention by the medical profession possible for the first time in history—because it became possible to intervene on a causal level rather than only treating symptoms. The logic embodied in this model, the technology that developed in conjunction with it, and its clinical successes had profound impacts on the attitudes, behavior, and organization of the medical profession. These professional effects of the new model are to this day fundamental determinants of the way medicine is practiced. They also underlie many current problems of the health care system.

The logic implicit in the new model was in part a product of the development of scientific methods within the academic tradition. The components of the model built up during this period were shaped in significant ways by the context in which they developed, the organization, attitudes,

---

* It is often thought of simplistically as the "germ theory"; but in its final, broader form it is able to conceptualize more than just infectious diseases.

and incentive system of the learned profession. The earlier Hippocratic humoral balance paradigm of medicine emerged under conditions where practical considerations of patient care in its full social context played a crucial role. The evolution of the modern model of diseases, on the contrary, took place almost entirely within the academic setting where these considerations were remote. Here scientific ideology, the academic prestige system, and the hospital- and laboratory-based organization exercised major influences on the form that the final model took. For example, the development of the new model required an objectivizing and experimental approach to patients and diseases. This was only possible in the teaching hospital situation where physicians were not directly dependent on their patients for remuneration. The fee-for-service relationships of the guild physicians demanded a more empathetic attitude and did not easily allow an experimental approach to the treatment of diseases. One does not pay a physician to allow him to experiment. Patients in teaching hospitals were not in a position to be so demanding. Once established, however, the logic of the new model tended to imbue these objectivizing attitudes in all physicians using it, no matter what the financial relationship to their patients. To understand the logic inherent in the model and its effects, we trace its development in the academic tradition.*

Four major threads of development can be identified leading up to the coalescence of the final model: (1) The reinstitution of careful clinical description and study of the natural history of diseases crystallized around the disease entity theory. This made it possible to accumulate a store of systematic clinical knowledge that was passed from one generation to the next by bedside teaching: (2) The development of anatomic pathology correlated with clinical descriptions created a sound scientific basis for studying diseases objectively: (3) The development of bacteriology led to the discovery of specific causal agents, the potential for aseptic surgery, and effective preventive medicine: (4) The development of physiology and pharmacology around the functional homeostatic paradigm of biological systems, together with controlled clinical trials, led to the development of effective diagnostic and therapeutic methods for clinical intervention in diseases.

---

* Although the form of treatment by the guild practitioners was little changed during the eighteenth and nineteenth centuries, the developmental process of scientific medicine within the academic tradition did have important influences on the organization and behavior of the practicing profession. Interdependency and tensions between the traditions continued during this period, and the three traditions of the profession were consolidated into essentially their modern relationships to each other by the resurgent importance of hospitals. The struggle over hospital control between the guild and learned traditions led to the division of responsibility for patient care by the hospitals. In Europe the modern relationship of learned and guild traditions to the different kinds of hospitals was well established by the mid-nineteenth century. In America this relationship was only solidified with the widespread development of residency training programs from 1945 to 1960 (see Chapter 6).

REVIVAL OF CLINICAL DESCRIPTION, BEDSIDE
TEACHING, AND THE DISEASE ENTITY THEORY

The first component eventually leading to the new model of disease came from the work of Thomas Sydenham in the second half of the seventeenth century introducing the basic concepts necessary for a specific entity theory of disease causation. Sydenham came out of the early English empirical tradition that included Robert Boyle, Isaac Newton, and John Locke, as well as William Petty and John Graunt (Chapter 2) whose work was one of the primary roots of public health (Bronowski & Mazlish, 1960). He began to observe and record the natural history of diseases and to classify recurring patterns of symptoms and outcomes. This art had been largely neglected since ancient times, and the accomplishment earned Sydenham the appellation "the English Hippocrates" (Payne, 1900). Immersed in the experience of medical practice, he noted that recurring sets of symptoms (syndromes) were often accompanied by characteristic clinical developments. These symptom patterns became "disease species" to his eyes with characteristic behavior just as observed for particular animal species. In this way, Sydenham initiated diagnosis in the modern sense (Newman, 1924).

Certain diseases, such as smallpox and bubonic plague, had been recognized as specific entities since the Middle Ages. Before Sydenham, however, most illnesses were characterized by laymen and medical professionals only in terms of their symptoms, for example, as "fevers" or "dropsy"* (Shryock, 1969). Such symptoms had been explained as imbalances between "humors" in Galen's sense. Sydenham assumed instead that there was some entity (disease species) underlying the characteristic pattern that was the same in each patient with the same disease. This way of thinking distinguishes the diseases conceptually from the patient, thereby making the disease a possible object of empirical investigation. Sydenham hoped that identification of specific disease entities could be used as a basis for determining specific treatments. His belief in this approach was probably an outgrowth of his early success in the treatment of malaria with cinchona ("Peruvian bark" containing quinine) brought back by explorers because of its reputation among the natives for curing fevers. Sydenham found that cinchona was effective in curing the particular pattern of fever that was characteristic of malaria but not other fevers that he recognized as different diseases. Unfortunately, his success in finding specific cures for specific diseases was not repeated for a hundred years. In the late eighteenth century James Lind discovered that lime juice could cure or prevent scurvy, and Edward Jenner demonstrated the effectiveness of vaccination against smallpox. More than 200 years passed before specific pathological agents (e.g., bacteria) were identified and therapeutic methods were found to combat them.

---

* Swelling of the ankles due to fluid retention, which can be a result of heart disease, kidney failure, liver dysfunction, or a number of more obscure causes.

During these two centuries the debate raged within the medical profession whether disease species were "real" (each due to a specific entity), or whether there was only one (or perhaps a few) universal cause of all diseases, such as "humoral imbalance," "inflammation," or "nerve irritation" (Shryock, 1969). Nevertheless, the tradition of clinical observation stemming from Sydenham's work created a wealth of empirical knowledge about the symptom patterns and natural histories of diseases, which could later be matched with autopsy examinations. Although Sydenham had no direct students, his writings became known throughout Europe and inspired the great clinicians of succeeding generations. Hermann Boerhaave of Leiden, an indirect disciple, institutionalized Sydenham's art of diagnosis and clinical description in his bedside teaching. His pupils in turn spread the system to all the major universities of Europe and later of America. Boerhaave was so eminent in teaching and attracting students, it is said, that "half the doctors of Europe were trained beside these twelve beds" (Sigerist, 1958). Many of them became the leading university faculty members of the next generation as well as practicing clinicians. As a result clinical teaching soon came to have a respected position in academic medicine as well as among practicing guild physicians.

As cities grew during the eighteenth and nineteenth centuries, the concentration of patients available for teaching and research also increased. The poor who crowded into the new urban industrial centers were largely dependent on the hospitals and clinics for charity medical care. Thus it became likely that enough cases of a given disease would be seen in one place to enable clinicians to compare them in Sydenham's style and determine what was typical. Previously this had been possible only with epidemic diseases.

The trends toward bedside teaching and hospital-based research were strengthened in the eighteenth century by the voluntary hospital movement. The philosophy of the Enlightenment, worldly humanitarianism, and the public spirit of the new middle class encouraged the endowment of hospitals intended to allow the sick to regain their health and provide for themselves again without burdening the state. Guy's Hospital, the first voluntary hospital in London, was opened in 1728. It was specified that the hospital was "for the relief and maintenance of *curable* poor people" (my italics) (Churchill, 1964).* Because of their more appealing mission and their favored position as charities of the growing upper middle class, voluntary hospitals quickly gained a great deal more prestige than the public hospitals. They were able to attract the best physicians as so-called visiting staff. Bedside teaching and clinical research were institutionalized pri-

---

* The hopelessly indigent, blind, or aged, were looked upon as the only fit responsibility for the public coffers and publicly supported hospitals. Thus the tradition of separation of responsibility, short-term care of the curables in the voluntary hospitals and long-term care for the incurables in the public (municipal, county, or state) hospitals, was established from inception of the new voluntary hospitals.

marily in the voluntary hospitals and became the route to recognition and advancement within the medical profession. Any physician who aspired to greatness within the practicing profession tried to emulate Sydenham's accomplishments. Such achievements were recognized by fellow physicians through designation of a disease by the name of the clinician who first described it—the route to medical immortality.

THE DEVELOPMENT OF PATHOLOGY
AND CONTROLLED CLINICAL TRIALS

The new urban hospitals also enabled the collection of postmortem pathological studies necessary to move ahead in understanding diseases. Anatomy, as a basic biological science, had been part of the medical curriculum in Europe since the founding of medical schools in the Middle Ages. Each new generation of physicians learned its Galen—or after the Renaissance its Vesalius—as part of the lore considered necessary to call oneself a physician. Yet this training made little connection between anatomy and the theory of disease or the practice of clinical description and diagnosis. During the seventeenth and eighteenth centuries anatomists teaching in medical faculties had essentially exhausted research on the normal gross structure of the body. With the more abundant case material available for autopsy in the urban hospitals, they began to turn their attention to so-called morbid anatomy, the pathological changes found in the organs of persons who had died of a particular disease. Although anatomists had noted pathological changes since antiquity, Giovanni Morgagni of Padua (1682–1771) was the first to systematically relate autopsy findings to the symptoms and diagnoses of the patients prior to their deaths (Singer & Underwood, 1962). On the basis of his studies he put forth the theory that characteristic pathological changes in the organs were the causes of the symptoms. They were, he asserted, the true disease entities that Sydenham had postulated underlying the typical pattern of symptoms and clinical course.

After Morgagni's work (1761) the tradition of clinical-pathological correlation advanced rapidly in the new urban centers of the north. A new generation of clinician-scientist professors emerged in Paris, London, Vienna, and Berlin. Their careers combined painstaking bedside observation of disease and careful pathological investigation of autopsy material (Shryock, 1969). Within 70 years these researchers mapped out the entire spectrum of diseases and their anatomic pathology essentially as we know it today. Important as it was for the diagnosis and classification of diseases, gross pathology gave little clue to the causal nature of the changes observed in organ—or what could be done about them during life. In certain cases the gross pathological changes gave indications of the way the disease process had caused the symptoms in life. A lung filled with fluid and pus at autopsy in a case of pneumonia could be intuitively related to the patient's cough and breathing difficulty. A tumor of the colon or stomach could account for the obstruction and vomiting experienced during life. But without the aid of achromatic microscopes (giving much higher resolution and magnification) and effective tissue-staining techniques, it was impossible to relate more diffuse or subtle pathological changes to symptoms and clinical manifestations of disease or to discover causal agents such as bacteria. These techniques only became available around 1840, delaying until then the links between clinical pattern, pathological finding, and causal process. Discovery of these linkages was necessary for the new disease model to emerge.

The impact of pathology on clinical treatment was virtually nil during the first half of the nineteenth century. The specific pathological agents or causes of disease that could be attacked clinically or preventively were not yet detectable. Consequently, the sanitarians attacking "filth" could produce more concrete results than the clinicians (Chapter 2). The major advancement of clinical therapeutics (the study of treatment techniques) in this period was the development of statistically evaluated clinical trials. This research led primarily to the negative finding that nothing being done for patients significantly changed the outcome of their diseases. In the long run this method became the firm foundation of therapeutics, but initially it led to nihilism and disillusionment with the medical profession.

In 1828 Louis Villermé had used the new statistical methods based on probability theory to demonstrate the public health effects of unsanitary conditions on the working class (Rosen, 1958). In 1835 Pierre Louis turned the same method to the investigation of clinical treatment—with devastating results. He studied the therapeutic effects of bloodletting for a number of diseases by matching control populations of similar cases that had not been bled with those that had been. Statistical analysis of the outcomes demonstrated that there was no significant difference between the rates of survival or improvement in the two groups (Shryock, 1969). This technique for testing the clinical effectiveness of treatment modalities became the accepted standard of research and remains the mainstay of clinical investigation to this day. Using it, Louis attacked much of the contemporary therapeutic system, most of which consisted of the time-honored treatments handed down from the past. The rest was comprised of various fads based on sweeping, unfounded systems and theories of physiology and medicine, or simply of favorite remedies based solely on individual intuitive analysis of clinical experience. Louis found them all wanting and demonstrated that almost no treatment employed by physicians at that time accomplished any apparent good for the patient, and many times actually did significant harm.

Clinical medicine was shaken to its foundations for the next 50 years. Many of the more critical physicians turned to a therapeutic nihilism, waiting "until methods of treatment could be found that produced demonstrable positive results" (Shryock, 1969). Bitter fights ensued within the profession between the old guard and the "young Turks," while charges of charlatanism were heard from the public. This was exacerbated by the Public Health Movement, which seemed to be attacking the clinical profession for doing nothing to correct the "real health problem" (the unsanitary living conditions) while using treatments for disease that accomplished nothing. But patients wanted cures and began turning in desperation to quacks, faith healers, and nonphysician practitioners of new theories of medicine like osteopathy and chiropractics. Quackery and healing "cults" developed rapidly in the early nineteenth century just as medicine was laying the groundwork for the sound scientific and therapeutic achievements of the latter part of the century by becoming more critical of its own effectiveness. This illustrates the continuing necessity for solace and reassurance as a means of social control of the anxiety generated by illness. Wherever the officially sanctioned medical profession withdraws hope and confidence-instilling care, patients seek to replace that loss by something that promises help, however irrational it may be. We still find the same phenomenon appearing today. Magical cures are pursued for cases of cancer declared hopeless by physicians. Medicaid clinics of questionable quality are patronized in poor neighborhoods where the only other sources of treatment are hospital outpatient departments, which usually offer only impersonal, fragmented care with little feeling of concern for the patient—even though the technical quality of outpatient care may be excellent (see Chapters 8 and 9).

The different segments of the medical profession underwent changes in organization and status during the mid-nineteenth century as a result of the developments in academic research, pathology, and therapeutics. These changes had a lasting influence on the practice of medicine and the attitudes of the profession. Because of the increased sophistication of research and the need for large numbers of patients to conduct it, the prestige of medicine passed back to the university and teaching hospital faculties who could fully devote their time to the study of the new developments. The old guilds, like the Royal Colleges, had fallen under the control of the elite members of the profession. As the practicing profession divided into two groups (general practitioners and consultants associated with voluntary hospitals), the less prestigious (general) practitioners found it necessary to organize new guilds to protect their interests (Berlant, 1975). The British Medical Association was founded in 1853 and quickly became the spokesman for this group. The American Medical Association (AMA) was founded in 1847.*

* The AMA had a more ambiguous role because there was no equivalent in this country to the Royal College of Physicians and because academic medicine was still so poorly institutionalized in the United States. Consequently, the AMA represented to some extent both the learned part of the profession and the practicing clinicians until about 1915, when it became more the voice of the guild (general practitioner) interests in medicine (see Chapter 8).

THE DEVELOPMENT OF BACTERIOLOGY
AND SUCCESSFUL PREVENTIVE MEDICINE

Medicine seemed on the way to succumbing to a storm of self-criticism, internal dissension, and failure to fulfill the promise of healing. Then two new developments occurred that provided dramatic successes and bolstered the profession's sense of value. Both were unexpected because they were not outgrowths of the main clinical-pathological tradition that dominated medical faculties at the time. Yet their value was quickly recognized by both the practicing and the academic members of the profession, who quickly embraced and used them as their own.

The first development was modern bacteriology, which grew out of Louis Pasteur's work on fermentation and on livestock diseases (and parallel work by others). Microorganisms had been known since Anton van Leeuwenhoek (1632–1723) invented the microscope. His speculation that they might be involved in contagion had never been completely given up. Yet the lack of adequate techniques to study the problem, together with the enthusiasm for the anatomic organ-pathology approach to diseases, had pushed contagion theory into the fringes of medical research during the early nineteenth century. Nevertheless, between 1800 and 1840, even before the advent of the achromatic microscope, renewed interest in microorganisms was growing among biologists. Theodor Schwann, co-originator of the cellular hypothesis, had discovered that microscopic yeasts are involved in the fermentation process and postulated that they were its cause. Lucas Schoenlein proved that certain scalp infections are caused by similar organisms, while Agostino Bassi showed that a specific silkworm disease was due to microorganisms. In 1840 Jacob Henle restated the hypothesis that diseases in general are caused by living agents (parasites) and also gave the criteria to verify this in regard to any given disease: "the supposed cause must always be associated with the disease and not with others, and the supposed parasite must be isolated and then proved capable of producing the disease once more" (Shryock, 1969).

Almost 35 years were required, however, to develop the techniques and carry out the programs Henle had proposed. A series of brilliant experiments by Louis Pasteur from 1850 to 1865 finally convinced the scientific world of the role of living matter, microorganisms, in fermentation and putrefaction (Singer & Underwood, 1962). Pasteur established conclusively that these "germs" are never generated spontaneously in a sterile culture medium, but always come from other microorganisms of the same kind. Other investigators found bacteria (as they came to be called) associated with certain animal diseases and produced evidence that diseases could be transmitted by material containing the bacteria. Anthrax, an infection of sheep and cattle sometimes transmitted to man, was one such disease studied by Pasteur. In 1876 Robert Koch, a student of Henle's, isolated the bacteria of anthrax and demonstrated their role as the causal agent of the disease.

This was the first unambiguous demonstration that a specific agent was the cause of a particular disease. Following Koch's example, some of the best minds in medicine turned their attention to the identification and study of contagious pathogens. Within a decade the causal agents for many of the scourges of mankind had been tracked down: gonorrhea (1879), leprosy (1880), typhoid fever (1884), malaria and diphtheria (1884), cholera and tuberculosis (1886)—the latter two by Koch himself. By the early years of the twentieth century bacteriological researchers, together with public health epidemiologists, had succeeded in discovering the agents and means of transmission for virtually the entire range of infectious diseases—bacterial, fungal, rickettsial (an important group of subcellular but microscopically visible infectious organisms including typhus), and parasitic. Many of these agents, particularly those of tropical diseases, depend on complex life cycles involving one or more intermediate hosts. The discovery of these organisms and the unraveling of the mechanisms of transmission was an exciting detective story that captured the public's imagination for more than a generation (see deKruif, 1926). These successes did much to strengthen the reputation of the medical profession in the early twentieth century. Only the submicroscopic "filterable viruses" remained elusive until the electron microscope was invented and tissue-culture methods for growing viruses were developed many years later. Even for most viral diseases the mechanisms of transmission were worked out by epidemiological methods, despite the impossibility of isolating and identifying the causal agent (Lilienfeld, 1976).

As researchers isolated the agents of infectious diseases, hope was rekindled of finding specific means for combating the organisms infecting patients (Rosen, 1958). Besides the public health approaches, such as purifying water, pasteurizing milk, and inspecting foods to interrupt the transmission of pathogenic microorganisms, two additional lines of attack were pursued, immunization and development of drugs to kill bacteria already infecting patients. Immunization methods were the first to bring success. Vaccination against smallpox was the only such technique available in Koch's time. Beginning in 1721, the pus (containing the live virus) from patients with smallpox had been used to inoculate persons superficially with the disease, usually producing a mild case while preventing the dangerous systemic form of the disease later. However, inoculation was not widely practiced because it had an appreciable risk itself. In 1796 Edward Jenner markedly diminished this risk by introducing vaccination with cowpox (Vaccinia, an attenuated form of smallpox virus) to prevent smallpox. Despite its effectiveness, vaccination still was not widely used until health departments and other governmental organizations began to promote its use. After its use in the German army had markedly reduced mortality from smallpox, it was made mandatory in Germany in 1880. Other nations were slower in adopting this practice, but by 1920 smallpox was almost eradicated in Western industrial nations and today throughout the world.

Once the agents of other infectious diseases were isolated, attempts were soon made to emulate the success of vaccination against smallpox. Pasteur discovered by chance that a culture of chicken cholera lost its virulence with aging, but still produced immunity in chickens infected with it. In a similar way he was able to attenuate other infectious agents including those of anthrax and, finally, rabies (hydrophobia), for which he received world acclaim. Prior to Pasteur's treatment, rabies infections contracted from animal carriers, which were quite common at that time, almost uniformly led to painful, hideous deaths.

Seeking to understand the mechanisms by which the body is able to maintain immunity after recovery from a disease or vaccination, Emil von Behring discovered that something in the serum of the blood (antibodies) protects the individual, and that a passive immunity for diphtheria could be created by injecting the serum of horses that had recovered from the disease. The clinical use of this diphtheria antitoxin reduced the case mortality by 50% or more. Preventive (active) immunization soon came to be much more effective in decreasing total death rates from this disease and many other infectious diseases (Rosen, 1975). Where antisera could be developed immunization was usually possible, since both depended on the same antibody process, and the greatest effect came from prevention.* With the use of immunological techniques, methods of protection against many important diseases were developed and employed by public health departments to reduce the incidence and mortality of epidemic and endemic disease. For many infectious diseases, however, neither active nor passive immunological protection seemed to be possible.

Other investigators turned their attention to the problem of finding drugs that would affect the disease agent without harming the human host. Paul Ehrlich, another student of Koch's, was impressed by his early success in staining bacteria with analine dyes for identification under the microscope and hoped that such dyes could be used as "magic bullets" to carry toxic compounds (primarily those containing arsenic) to the bacteria without injuring the tissue or physiology of the patient. One such compound had been found effective against trypanosomiasis (sleeping sickness), and Ehrlich worked four years synthesizing one organic arsenic compound after another in the search for similar curative agents. Finally his six hundred and sixth attempt, arsphenamine, was relatively successful against syphilis. Yet, for the great majority of infectious diseases, public health or preventive immunization remained the only effective mode of intervention until sulfonamides (mid-1930s), penicillin (early 1940s), and then other antibiotics became available.

* Nevertheless, passive antisera are still used even today with moderate success against a few diseases such as infectious hepatitis and botulism, where active methods of immunization are still impossible or impractical because of rarity of incidence.

DEVELOPMENT OF SURGICAL TECHNOLOGY
AND METHODS

The second successful development that grew out of the new bacteriology was the establishment of surgery as a safe, reliable method for treating a wide range of disorders. The art of surgery is as old as medicine itself, and modern surgeons have to marvel at what their predecessors were able to accomplish before the benefits of anesthesia, infection control, and adequate preoperative diagnostic techniques. Bone setting, draining abscesses, "cutting" for bladder stones and hernia repairs had all been undertaken since antiquity with enough success to permit their continuation. Wound surgery (including amputations), particularly for battle injuries, has been a necessity throughout human history. Much of the development of surgical technique has been associated with it. Certain externally obvious tumors, such as those of the breast and thyroid and large ovarian tumors, were occasionally excised successfully before the modern era of surgery. On the other hand, attempts at abdominal surgery were almost uniformly fatal, as were abdominal wounds, until the introduction of sterile operating techniques. Few statistics are available on survival rates from surgery in earlier times, but as recently as during the American Civil War 14,000 amputations were reported, with only 3000 survivals (Singer & Underwood, 1962). Lister himself reported a 50% mortality rate for amputations before introducing his antiseptic method which reduced the death rate to 15% (still very high by today's standards where mortality rates for wounds requiring amputation, even under battle conditions, are less than 1%).

The great enemies of the surgeon have always been pain, infection, bleeding, and diagnostic uncertainty, each complicated by the others. Because of the need for haste before an effective anesthesia was known, the danger of bleeding during surgery was high, and only cursory evaluation of the nature and extent of pathology could be made. The problem of infection was increased by foreign bodies, so that tying off bleeding arteries had its own dangers. For many centuries cautery with hot irons or boiling oil was preferred to tying of bleeding vessels. In the half century from 1850 to 1900 this entire constellation of problems was solved, enabling the development of surgery for many clinical conditions. Discovery of the effectiveness of ether as an anesthetic in 1846 almost immediately made painless surgery a practical reality. Control of the pain was not merely humanitarian. It allowed unhurried safe operating techniques, careful control of bleeding, appraisal of the situation for better diagnosis, and introduction of complicated procedures that would have been out of the question because of the necessary haste before the use of anesthesia.

With infections the solution was not so fortuitous. Surgeons had been aware of the importance of cleanliness since ancient times—though the lesson seems to have needed relearning many times throughout history. Yet, the extent and type of cleanliness necessary to prevent surgical infection could not be appreciated until bacteriology demonstrated the nature of the organisms involved and the means of eliminating them. Until Pasteur's work it was widely believed that suppuration of the wound was a natural consequence of almost any operation. Through most of history surgeons had been concerned not with preventing infection but with controlling it by in-suring proper drainage of the pus to reduce the chances of deeper sepsis. This was particularly the case with battle wounds, which were always dirty and accompanied by tissue damage, providing a perfect place for bacteria to grow.

In 1867, inspired by Pasteur's work, Joseph Lister attempted to "sterilize" wounds by washing the patient's skin and the surgeon's hands in carbolic acid and spraying the air over the wound. The rate of infections was re-duced, but the complications produced by carbolic acid and the misunder-standing of the infectious process, delayed the wider adoption of sterile techniques for another two decades. In 1886, after the discovery of the im-portance of bacterial spores and the insensitivity of many bacteria to dis-infectants, Ernst von Bergman introduced the steam sterilization of surgical equipment. By 1891 this aseptic procedure of modern surgery was generally accepted (Singer & Underwood, 1962).

Once pain and infection could be controlled, many areas of surgery never before dared were soon successfully developed. In Vienna Theodor Billroth, an early follower of Lister's method, began excising abdominal tumors (stomach and bowel) between 1872 and 1894, and opened up the entire field of gastrointestinal tract surgery, hitherto uniformly unsuccessful. In 1879 William Macewen of Glasgow began removal of subdural hematomas (blood clots due to head injuries), brain abscesses, and tumors, initiating neuro-surgery. Macewen also performed the first successful removal of a lung for tuberculosis in 1895. Corrective orthopedic (bone) surgery was also begun in the 1880s, as was more extensive kidney, bladder, and gynecological sur-gery.

The applicability of surgery was still limited to conditions that could be detected with the hands (e.g., large tumors), with the stethoscope, or by means of a few simple laboratory tests like blood cell counts or urinalysis until better diagnostic methods were developed. After Wilhelm Roentgen's discovery of x-rays in 1895, their use to diagnose ulcers and small tumors of the gastrointestinal tract as well as lung and brain lesions quickly made much greater preoperative knowledge possible and accelerated the expan-sion of surgical intervention into new areas.

The accomplishments of bacteriology and aseptic surgery, together with reform in nursing, began to have a major effect on hospitals and subse-quently on all medical care (Abel-Smith, 1964). In 1870 anyone entering a hospital still did so in desperation. There was an immense danger from exposure to the diseases and infections of other patients. In 1788 the death rate of patients at the Hotel Dieu in Paris was 25%, while that of surgeons and attendants was 6 to 12%, and things had not improved much by 1870. When Ignaz Semmelweiss investigated the causes of "childbed fever" in Vienna in 1848, he found that the maternal mortality rate in one hospital was 10% because infection was being carried from one patient to the other by careless physicians. The discovery of the bacterial nature of infection and the possible routes of contamination, along with the introduction of aseptic techniques in surgery, changed the hospital in a very brief time from a literal death house into a place where lives could be saved and diseases cured (Churchill, 1964).

This seemingly miraculous transformation was also based on organizational changes in the way hospitals were run, the most important being the reform of nursing (Bullough & Bullough, 1974). Florence Nightingale is best known for this development, but it was an idea whose time had come. The combination of enlightened humanitarianism, a puritan concern for cleanliness and well-ordered organization of public affairs, and the scientific use of vital statistics to demonstrate the relationship between disease and filth was leading to widespread pressure for hospital reform. Nightingale actually learned of the potential for improving nursing in 1836 by visiting the Kaiserswerth Deaconesses, a religious order devoted to nursing, in Germany. But it was her dramatic use of the ideas to organize nursing services during the Crimean War (1854–1856) and the subsequent success of her school of nursing in London that led to widespread recognition of the need for improved nursing. She awakened the medical world to the importance of sanitary techniques in hospitals, the institution of proper organization and administration of patient care, and the professional training of nurses. Without this organizational reform the knowledge about the bacterial nature of infection would have been almost useless because of the necessity that the aseptic routines and precautionary rules be scrupulously carried out.

THE FRUITION OF PHYSIOLOGICAL RESEARCH

Looking back it is easy to gain the impression that physiology in the seventeenth century was on the way toward establishing itself on a firm empirical foundation—as anatomy and physics did at that time. William Harvey demonstrated the circulation of the blood by a series of brilliant experiments between 1614 and 1626, the same time that Galileo was writing his great work on astronomy. Anton van Leeuwenhoek invented the microscope and began the study of microorganisms during the same period. Using it, Marcello Malphigi discovered capillary circulation in 1651, completing the work of Harvey. Yet physiology was not able to maintain the momentum of progress begun by Harvey and Malphigi, and it degenerated into a number of "systems" or schools of theory, each based on certain unifying principles but with little empirical basis (Shryock, 1969). "Iatrophysicists,"* fol-

* *Iatros* is the Greek word for physician.

lowing the direction of Rene Descartes and Guisseppi Borelli, believed that organisms could be considered as mechanical systems, and they spent their energies attempting to measure bodily forces, temperatures, and so forth. "Iatrochemists," following in the direction set by Paracelsus, J. B. van Helmont, and Franciscus Sylvius, believed that organisms could be viewed as chemical systems, which meant essentially an interplay of acids, bases, and salts. "Vitalism," a reaction against the first two schools, stressed the importance of so-called vital forces manifested by the sensitivity (excitability) of organisms to subtle stimuli and of the rapid decomposition of the body after death (Singer & Underwood, 1962). In fact there turned out to be some truth in each of the schools of physiological theory. But, unlike physics, physiology did not yet have a unifying paradigm to fit the different partial truths together into an overall working model of physiological processes. Such a theoretical model was necessary to direct physiological research and applications effectively. Experimental physiological research did continue during the eighteenth century, but it produced few results that had an impact on the medical world.

Two steps were necessary before physiology could begin to make rapid strides. First was the development of systematic knowledge and theory in chemistry, electricity, and thermodynamics, all of which provided techniques and understanding necessary for the advancement of scientific physiology (Nordenskiold, 1928). In the early nineteenth century these three disciplines graduated nearly simultaneously from haphazard collections of observations into systematic sciences built around unifying theories. The second step necessary for the emergence of scientific physiology was the development of a comprehensive theoretical working model (paradigm) for physiology itself (Holton, 1975). François Magendie of Paris grasping the significance of the breakthrough occurring in the basic sciences, turned away from the bedside, dissecting room, and pathological laboratory to establish the first modern physiological laboratory. More important than his own investigations of the nervous system was the precedent and his critique of "vitalism," which dominated French medical thinking and made physiological research impossible.

This prepared the way for his student, Claude Bernard, who established physiology as a mature experimental science by creating a model that could integrate the previously unsystematic chemical, electrical, mechanical, and thermodynamical observations about living organisms. This model provided the unified problem solving approach to physiological research and its application to clinical medicine. Bernard discovered that the liver acts to preserve a constant sugar concentration in the blood by converting absorbed glucose to glycogen after a meal and then by reconverting the glycogen to glucose later as needed. He speculated that the chemistry of the body might generally be understood in terms of mechanisms that maintain the constancy of body fluids, necessary for normal function. Each organ or mechanism was to be studied for its role in maintaining the normal equilibrium state of the body. This functional, so-called homeostatic, paradigm provided a way of ordering scientific thinking about physiology and applying many of the complex discoveries of the new basic sciences (Bernard, 1865).

The homeostatic functional model of physiology also provided a research framework for investigating the action of drugs. Investigators identified and made available chemical agents found in the body (and some that are not) that affect the physiological systems, blocking, stimulating, or modifying certain functions. Pharmacology developed rapidly, leading to many new drugs which for the first time were effective and could be used rationally to control or support bodily functions. Physiological research not only produced further understanding of the body's functions, but it also provided powerful tools for diagnosis and therapy in clinical medicine. For example, studies of metabolism produced techniques for measuring the levels of various metabolites and other chemicals in the blood that became valuable diagnostic tools for estimating a patient's physiological status. Investigations of the immunological response led to therapeutic antisera, but also to studies of white blood cells by means of microscopy with analine dye stains (Singer & Underwood, 1962). Today examination of stained smears of blood cells is one of the most frequent procedures for determining the presence of infections, certain malignancies, and other disorders. Karl Landsteiner's study of the immune reaction in regard to blood groups yielded the method of matching blood types that made safe routine blood transfusions possible. Walter B. Cannon's investigation of the digestive process by means of x-rays introduced diagnostic radiology of the gastrointestinal tract. As a result of such discoveries physiological research introduced many precise laboratory methods into clinical medicine and provided powerful means of therapy such as hormones, kidney machines, organ transplants, revolutionizing the potential of medical treatment.

The concepts of "normality" and "functionalism" in physiology were immediately important for clinical medicine. They provided a framework within which dysfunction and disease symptoms could be understood as interference with normal physiological processes. This approach made it possible to seek cures through repair of the defect (e.g., combatting the invading microorganisms). In addition knowledge of normal function also enabled devising means of supportive or substitutive therapy when a function usually accomplished by some part of the organism is damaged.

In the process of perfecting Sydenham's disease-entity model, the physiological interference theory of disease also subtly modified it. A specific underlying agent or defect in the body was still postulated as "causing" the disease. However, unlike Sydenham's assumption that the clinical pattern of a disease was a direct manifestation of the underlying entity, today we assume that symptoms and signs arise because the agent or defect interferes with the normal physiological mechanisms in a consistent and predictable way. This defect alters some functions and brings about changes in others through compensatory reactions (which are simple extensions of normal homeostatic functions under the altered circumstances). Such a defect may be the blocked function of a lung in pneumococcal (bacterial) pneumonia, the specific enzyme deficit or endocrine imbalance in metabolic diseases, or the anatomic defect and physiological consequences of the overgrowth of cells in a malignancy.

The need to consider more than the disease agent in developing effective clinical strategies, led to further expansion of the specific-defect model soon after its introduction. The incidence and course of a disease was also seen to be a product of the susceptibility or resistance of the human host, and of the environment influencing the likelihood of contagion. Physicians began to use a triple-causal model of disease taking into account the interaction between agent, host, and environment (Leavell & Clark, 1958). Discovery of nutritional diseases, hormonal disorders, and the role of genetic defects, dietary factors, toxic substances, carcinogens, and even psychological stress in causing specific diseases forced physicians to enlarge the disease "agent" concept to include many types of "specific defects" besides infectious organisms (Rosen, 1975). A disease is still viewed as a dysfunctional disturbance in a normal physiological system, but this system is no longer considered as just a passive substrate in which the agent simply produces the disturbance. The physiological system is itself a complex active entity whose parts interact with the agent in ways that modify the disease process—sometimes blocking it, sometimes intensifying it, sometimes changing it in other ways. These parts of the physiological system vary from one person to another and may themselves be modified as an additional means of controlling disease, for example, by immunization or suppression of overreaction. The environment is also a variable factor in the disease equation—on the one hand involved in the process of transmission, on the other hand a contributing factor that, like the host's physiology, may block, intensify, or modify the disease. The diet or the environment may also be the source of influences like carcinogens or stress that predate but eventually lead to the actual pathological "agents" such as malignant cell growths and arteriosclerosis.

Whatever the specific defect, the logic of diagnosis and treatment remains the same. The pattern of disturbance is recognized as a specific functional deviation against the normal baseline. By comparison with other similar cases, this pattern allows a conclusion about the nature of the defect causing the disturbance.* The logic of treatment is equally straightforward. Since a specific defect is assumed to be responsible for the dysfunctional pattern of altered physiology, the treatment must consist of removing, repairing, or in some way compensating for the causal defect. The logic of prevention is similar; where possible, it seeks to forestall the specific defect from occurring.

* If the primary defect can be verified by direct observation or laboratory methods, the certainty is greater, but this is not necessary to diagnose the disease because of the assumption that similar specific-disturbance patterns are due to similar specific defects, the "causes" of the disease.

Because the new paradigm serves as the fundamental conceptual framework for almost all medical thinking about causation, prevention, treatment, and research, it has a profound influence on physicians' behavior, attitudes toward patients, and orientation toward the mode of care to be rendered. It tends to focus attention on the disease rather than the patient or his adjustment to the illness. It emphasizes technical methods of dealing with the specific causal defect or physiological malfunction. As is shown in Chapters 5 and 6, these physician attitudes and orientations engendered by the specific-defect disease paradigm are increasingly less appropriate for dealing with the new pattern of chronic illnesses that has emerged since 1930 in this country. Despite this growing inappropriateness, the new paradigm and its associated attitudes are held tenaciously by the medical profession and show little sign of being significantly modified in the foreseeable future. Before leaving the history of its development, therefore, it is worthwhile examining features of that evolution that help explain this tenacity.

A first factor is the tremendous success that the profession has enjoyed from the scientific revolution in medicine based on that paradigm. Much of the prestige of the profession is now a product of its ability to intervene in the disease process using technology whose function is understood in terms of the new disease model. The scientific research necessary to develop the technology likewise depends on the new paradigm as a framework.

A second reason for the tenacious commitment to that paradigm is its close relationship to the prestige, ideology, incentive system, and vested interests of the university faculties and teaching hospitals. Certain features of academic medicine were major forces in shaping the development of the particular logical form of the specific-defect model and help explain its perpetuation. The objectivizing approach to disease and physiological mechanisms derives from the scientific ideology of academic medicine. This approach stressed research based on reproducible (objective) laboratory methods where technological manipulation of factors is possible. The learned profession has a vested interest in the use of such technology and in studying the kinds of diseases and patient problems that are amenable to these techniques—those that have a well-defined causal nature, like infectious diseases and hormonal disorders. The hospital base of medical faculties, where patients are isolated from their usual social situations, naturally focuses concern on the aspects of diseases that can be studied in such isolation rather than on the functional problems of patients in response to illness—which are much more influenced by their social conditions. Thus, the specific-defect model of diseases developed in a way that was logically consistent with the organization, social incentives, and professional ideological forces acting on the learned tradition.

This does *not* mean that the model was arbitrarily determined by medical scientists, so to speak, "to fit their own interests." The paradigm also *had to work* effectively in dealing with the common diseases. Its success in allowing physicians to understand, prevent, and treat the infectious diseases, which were most prevalent at the time, was crucial to its acceptance. This success was responsible for the tremendous growth in prestige and authority that medicine came to command in the ensuing decades. But such effectiveness does not mean that the specific-defect model was the only one that could be used in understanding and treating illness. Rather, the model had the effect of selecting out for special emphasis those illnesses or aspects of illness that could be most effectively dealt with in the framework of the paradigm. Quite a different model might be required for understanding and treating other medical conditions, for example, problems like mental illness and the chronic, behaviorially and socially caused conditions that are more characteristic of today's medical practice. The presently accepted model for understanding diseases is consonant with the present organization, attitudes, and behavior of the profession. To deal effectively with the new medical problems a new more comprehensive model of the disease process is required, which takes into account the entire field of social, behavioral, and environmental forces acting on the patient and his community (Miller, 1972). Such a model would necessarily entail adjustment of the attitudes, behavior, vested interests, and organization of the medical profession. Because such changes threaten significant dislocations for physicians, suggestions for revising the paradigm are apt to be met with serious resistance (Kuhn, 1962).

THE IMPACT OF SCIENTIFIC MEDICINE ON HEALTH STATUS

Since 1900 the health of Americans has improved remarkably by almost any measure (Erhardt & Berlin, 1974). The average life expectancy in this country reached 74 years in 1977 compared to 47 years at the turn of the century. The age-adjusted mortality rate from all causes declined from 1700 to 666 per 100,000 population during the same period. Infant mortality decreased by 90% from about 150 to 14 per 1000 live births. Maternal mortality declined by 99%. Gains in regard to certain infectious diseases were even more impressive. Mortality from infectious diseases as a group fell by 95%, but most of the remaining infectious disease deaths are from influenza and pneumonia, which strike down the debilitated aged with chronic heart or lung disease and infants, again usually as complications of other problems (Dauer et al., 1968). Diphtheria, typhoid fever, measles, dysentery, whooping cough (pertussis), and scarlet fever, which together accounted for almost one-third of the deaths in children between the ages of 1 and 15 in 1900, have been virtually eliminated as causes of death. Tuberculosis, which ranked second as a cause of death in 1900 has been reduced by 97% and now ranks only fifteenth among the causes of mortality. On the other hand, the mortality from cancer has increased steadily during the same period, and mortality from heart disease, strokes, and accidents has declined much less rapidly than from other causes. These four problems have now become the leading causes of death, together accounting for 80% of all fatalities (USPHS, 1979).

The most direct and obvious effect of the decreased mortality from infectious and other acute diseases has been an improved life expectancy and an increasingly higher percentage of older people in the population. In 1900 less than 4% of the population was 65 or older. In 1940 this reached 6.8%, and in 1976 11% (U.S. Bureau of Census, 1978). Increasing the percentage of persons who reach old age is highly desirable, not only for humanitarian reasons but also for socioeconomic ones in advanced industrial society. The difference in the pattern of mortality between the preindustrial and the premodern societies (prior to the changes resulting from scientific public health, preventive, and clinical medicine) was primarily the decline of deaths in the first few years of life that were due to poor nutrition, hygiene, and sanitation (Susser & Watson, 1971).

From a humane point of view this infant mortality in preindustrial societies is a terrible waste of life; but economically it is easily compensated for. Since it takes place before society has made a major investment in educating and training the individuals, merely increasing the birth rate, as such societies do, provides the same input to the work force at little extra social cost. On the other hand, the waste of young adult lives could not be compensated for by simply increasing the birth rate. This loss of productive life would be a heavy burden to a technologically advanced society because it takes place during the years of maximum productive input to the economy—after a major investment has been made by society in educating, training, and supporting these individuals during their youth. This loss would be even more severe in advanced industrial society than for early industrial society because productive life is extended longer since physical stamina is no longer the major qualification for working effectively. Knowledge and experience acquired over many years play an increasingly important role in contributing to society.

As shown in Chapter 2, until nearly 1900 the improvements in the health of society were almost entirely the result of changes in life style, standards of living, and social structure that took place in the course of historical development. From about 1890 on somewhat more of the improvement in health can be attributed to the intervention of health professionals. This improvement was based on scientific knowledge and medical techniques for action against particular diseases and for interrupting general modes of transmission responsible for numerous diseases. Yet, even after medical science made it possible to take some specific measures against particular diseases, the major part of the improvement in health during the twentieth century was still due to the continuing rise in the general standards of living and nonspecific measures like better nutrition and sanitation, carrying forward trends established in the nineteenth century (McKeown, 1965; McKinlay & McKinlay, 1977).

Even the impact of scientific medicine on diseases was not a homogeneous development. The control of most infectious diseases passed through a number of phases as the application of the new model of diseases produced successive levels of understanding and more sophisticated means for effective intervention—first in public health, then in preventive medicine, and finally in clinical medicine. This temporal sequence was a result of the different approaches to the disease problem used by these three subdivisions of health services.

Public health employs very general measures that affect large numbers of people and often many diseases at the same time, primarily by interrupting the means of transmission of contagion. These prophylactic measures generally are not dependent on sophisticated knowledge of the physiology involved in the diseases. Classic public health methods have been sanitation, water purification, and food inspection. As soon as the bacterial nature of certain important diseases was established, the epidemiological mode of transmission could be more precisely determined. Public health departments were immediately able to use the administrative machinery already available for monitoring diseases and sanitation to enforce more effective means of disease control. For example, their food and water inspection units simply added bacteriological laboratories to monitor contamination more accurately. Using their already established authority, they instituted filtration and chlorination of water supplies, pasteurization of milk, and so forth. As a consequence of these measures the incidence of typhoid fever and milk-borne tuberculosis dropped precipitously between 1910 and 1920 (Kilbourne & Smillie, 1969).

Another area where the public health approach was extremely successful was in the control of diseases transmitted by mosquitos and other insect vectors. Yellow fever and malaria were still major causes of mortality and morbidity in the Southern United States in 1900—as they had been even in New York and other northern cities during the nineteenth century. Mosquito control in agricultural areas was too large-scale an operation for local health departments and was primarily accomplished by the federal government. Although the U.S. Public Health Service was not established until 1912, the U.S. Army Medical Corps worked together with the Army Engineers as an effective instrument against many forms of epidemic and endemic diseases in the United States and its outposts. In 1900 Major Walter Reed and co-workers discovered the mode of transmission of yellow fever, which was plaguing operations in Puerto Rico and Cuba. Swamp drainage and mosquito control by military engineers rapidly decreased its incidence and mortality, as well as that of malaria (Rosen, 1958).

As distinguished from public health, *preventive medicine* is usually defined as the use of specific intervention techniques to prevent the occurrence of particular diseases through protection of individual persons. Immunization is the best known method of preventive medicine, but nutritional supplementation (especially in infants) and early presymptomatic detection of diseases through mass screening (secondary prevention) have become equally important. Preventive medicine depends on specific knowledge about individual disease processes and bodily responses in order to devise strategies for disease prevention. Once this knowledge was available, it could be applied almost immediately, in many cases by simply piggy-backing on public health organizations and programs already in effect (Rosen, 1975).

Prevention programs do have to reach individual persons, but this can be done on a mass basis (as with public health) since the approach to different patients does not have to be particularized by sophisticated diagnosis to meet individual circumstances and conditions—as with clinical medicine. Because of common organizational needs, public health and preventive medicine essentially merged in the period of their greatest success and most rapid growth between 1900 and 1930. The institution of mass immunization of school children against diphtheria was started by the New York City Health Department in 1920 and spread rapidly to other large cities of the world; it was followed soon by similar protection against whooping cough (pertussis) and tetanus. These programs brought a major reduction in early childhood mortality (Duffy, 1974). Much more recently the development of immunization techniques against poliomyelitis and measles has enabled similar reductions in the incidence of these viral illnesses.

Clinical medicine deals with diseases in progress in individuals and uses specialized therapy chosen to fit both the particular disease and the particular person. The treatment requires accurate diagnosis of the disease type, determination of the cause, removal or neutralization of the cause, and repair of the effect in the individual so that normal function can be restored. This necessitated the new physiological disturbance model of the disease process which allows the physician to think about the relation between these elements accurately. But, clinical medicine could only have a significant impact on the pattern of mortality in society when techniques had also been developed for intervention in individual cases to eliminate the cause without harming the patient. Between 1930 and 1960 effective means of clinical treatment were discovered for many acute diseases. For the first time in human history, medical intervention could make a significant difference in the outcome of an illness.

Probably the most important new therapeutic tools were the antibacterial agents: the sulfonamides (1936), then penicillin (civilian use, 1945), and later the so-called broad-spectrum antibiotics (McDermott, 1969). Almost immediately it became possible to cure most bacterial pneumonias, scarlet fever, streptococcal infections (and therefore diminish the sequellae including rheumatic fever and glomerulonephritis) as well as sepsis associated with childbirth and abortions. Together these had been the remaining principal causes of mortality among children and young adults (Shapiro et al., 1968). Other clinical advances contributed to reduction in mortality after 1930. Even before sulfonamides and penicillin were available, maternal mortality began to decline rapidly—probably as a result of the much better trained obstetricians coming out of the new medical education programs (Chapter 6), the availability of blood transfusions, wider use of hospital delivery, and improved prenatal care. The latter was made possible by the establishment of maternal and child health units with federal funding under the Sheppard-Towner Act and later programs (see Chapter 11).

The major component of the improvement in mortality between 1900 and 1970 was the reduction in deaths from infectious diseases (see also Table 5.1 in Chapter 5). The control of even this single group of diseases involved and continues to require interplay among all three types of health services, public health, preventive medicine, clinical medicine as well as changes of social factors. Each infectious disease has a different natural history, and a different series of factors was involved in the process of its control. Examining the history of a few of the typical major diseases illustrates the general principles and indicates the range of ways that the various factors came together in determining reduction of incidence and mortality (McKeown, 1976a, 1976b).

Typhoid fever was endemic in all larger American cities throughout the nineteenth century, and major epidemic outbreaks occurred somewhere almost every summer. It ranked seventh as a cause of death in the United States in 1900. As soon as the causative organism had been identified and the water contamination route of transmission determined, the strategy of intervention was clear. The construction of water filtration plants and the chlorination of the water supply in major cities between 1910 and 1920 brought about an immediate marked decline in incidence. By 1925 to 1930 mortality was reduced by 95% from the 1900 level (Kilbourne & Smillie, 1969). Sporadic but appreciable incidence and deaths continued, however, because of a second route of transmission in milk from infected cows and in food from asymptomatic carriers of the disease. Milk transmission was soon stopped by inspection of dairy herds and enforced pasteurization of milk. Food handlers who were typhoid carriers were gradually tracked down by epidemiological detective work and treated or at least prevented from further disseminating their disease. In the 1950s the antibiotic chloramphenicol was found to be active against typhoid, finally making it possible to treat quickly and effectively the occasional cases that still occurred (Clark & MacMahon, 1967).

Diphtheria was the fourth most common cause of infectious disease death in the United States in 1900, striking children especially hard. It was second only to the pneumonia-influenza group and tuberculosis as a cause of death in the 5 to 15 age group (Dauer et al., 1968). Von Behring's antitoxin was developed in 1891 and became widely available a decade later, when its use began to reduce case mortality considerably; but diphtheria remained a major cause of childhood death until active immunization techniques were more universally employed. In 1909 toxin-antitoxin immunization was discovered; the first major field trials were conducted in New York City in 1915. In 1920 a mass immunization campaign was started by the New York

City Health Department (switching to the improved toxoid technique in 1923), and by 1928 over half the school children in the city were immunized (Duffy, 1974). The strategy was soon applied in other cities (and other countries). By 1940 diphtheria cases were occurring only sporadically, and by 1960 the disease had been virtually eliminated. In recent years, however, the decreased threat from diphtheria has diminished emphasis on maintaining immunization levels in certain populations, and occasional outbreaks of the disease have begun to occur again. Public health officials are increasingly voicing their concern that unless more active immunization campaigns are again waged, serious epidemics could break out at any time (Hilleboe, 1968, 1972).

Scarlet fever (streptococcal respiratory infection) had been an even more frequent cause of death than diphtheria among children in the nineteenth century, but the death rate had already declined by 80% in 1900 and continued to fall gradually but steadily until 1945 when the availability of penicillin immediately reduced the case mortality almost to zero because of the marked sensitivity of the bacteria to the drug (McKeown & Lowe 1974). Penicillin therapy not only eliminated the remaining direct mortality from scarlet fever but also many of the complications of streptococcal infections, for example, middle ear infection and mastoiditis, which had been major sources of deafness and chronic morbidity in children. It also sharply dropped the incidence of rheumatic fever and glomerulonephritis, both of which are hyperimmune reactions to the streptococcal antigen—in the first case in the heart muscle and valves, in the second case in the kidneys. The prevalence of both these problems and their long-term consequences decreased tremendously after 1945.

The precise cause of the decline in mortality due to scarlet fever beginning in the midnineteenth century is debated. McKeown (1971) states that it was the result of changes in the virulence of the streptococcal bacteria. On the other hand, very similar long-term declines were occurring in the mortality rates from many other infectious diseases, including tuberculosis, whooping cough, and measles—all decades before the availability of any specific preventive or curative methods (Dubos & Dubos, 1952). In the cases of measles and tuberculosis it has been well established that the state of nutrition plays a major role in mortality. Among poorly nourished children in developing countries the case mortality rate for measles can be as high as 10 to 15%, while in the United States it had already dropped to much less than 1% long before the availability of penicillin to treat such complications as pneumonia (Kass, 1971).

Another problem area where preventive medicine techniques were effective was in the control of nutritional deficiencies. In 1900 *pellagra* (niacin deficiency) was rampant among the poor in the South of the United States. In certain states it was the second most common cause of death (Rosen, 1958). Although not an infectious disease, its cause and remedy were discovered by using essentially the same epidemiological techniques so successful for the infectious disorders. Pellagra was also due to a specific deficit, in this case nutritional, and therefore fit the specific-defect model for research and treatment. In 1914 Dr. Joseph Goldberger was assigned by the U.S. Public Health Service (USPHS) to study the problem. By 1920 he had determined from its pattern of incidence in relation to economic status and seasonal variation that it must be a consequence of the diets. The tenant farmer victims were at the mercy of marginal subsistence from seasonal crops. Goldberger guessed that it was probably due to lack of a specific dietary factor since they were not actually starving (Goldberger, 1914). Some years earlier in Java it had been discovered that beri-beri was a consequence of thiamine deficiency from a diet of polished rice. By 1929 Goldberger and Sydenstricker had shown that pellagra can be prevented by diet supplementation with meat and fresh vegetables (Terris, 1964). A program of mass health education was undertaken by the USPHS with the cooperation of the Agricultural Extension Service, and considerable progress was made in reducing the incidence of the disease. But because the economic conditions did not change appreciably, pellagra remained a serious problem in the South until World War II. Distribution of food surpluses (begun in the 1930s), mandated vitamin enrichment of bread, and the improved standard of living as a result of industrialization of the South after World War II finally brought the problem under control.

A similar nutritional problem with *rickets* (vitamin D deficiency) was encountered among children in northern industrial cities. Unlike pellagra, rickets was not a direct cause of death, but it did produce crippling disabilities due to bone deformities of the legs. In addition, deformities of the chest increased susceptibility to childhood pneumonias, and rickets of the pelvis increased maternal mortality when normal childbirth became impossible because of the narrowed pelvic outlet. Recognition of the problem by public health officers and discovery of the cause led to its eradication between 1920 and 1940 by use of codliver oil supplements and mandated addition of vitamin D to milk (Rosen, 1958).

One of the most important nutritional problems was moderate *protein deficiency* in infants. It only came to be recognized and understood long after it had ceased to be a problem in the United States—where it was largely eliminated indirectly through measures that were undertaken for other reasons and as a consequence of the general improvements in the standards of living. In 1900 infant mortality in the United States was between 140 and 150 per 1000 live births, 10 times the present rate. Approximately half of these deaths were due to the so-called weanling diarrheas and nonspecific pneumonias that still plague infants in underdeveloped nations. These have since been shown to be a product of poor protein nutrition combined with early exposure to bacteria and viruses that are not disease-producing in better nourished children.

Partly as an effort to control milk-borne tuberculosis, typhoid fever, and other diseases and partly as an outgrowth of the general philosophy of the child welfare movement, free milk dispensories were established early in the century by the New York City Health Department with the cooperation of voluntary groups. The system was copied in other cities and succeeded in improving infant nutrition among the poor. As massive immigration stopped after 1920 and most poor groups began to work their way up the economic ladder, infant nutrition continued to improve even though the milk stations were discontinued. By 1930 infant deaths from these two closely related causes had declined by 80% and by 1945 had almost disappeared—accounting for the largest part of the improvement in infant mortality from 1900 to the present (McDermott, 1969). Another large portion of the decline in infant mortality was due to the control of diphtheria and whooping cough through immunization and to decreased prematurity through better prenatal care. Nutrition, hygiene, and preventive care, in turn, depend very much on socioeconomic status and family structure (especially whether the pregnancy is in or out of wedlock). The major remaining differentials in infant mortality between groups seem to be a product primarily of these variables rather than medical care in the narrower sense (USPHS, 1979).

For *maternal mortality,* on the contrary, the improvement in prenatal care as a result of federal-state maternal and child health (MCH) programs and clinical care seem to have been the major factor in the marked reduction between 1930 and 1960 (Shapiro et al., 1968). The last major improvement in death rates due to childbirth had taken place between 1860 and 1880 because of the prevention of "childbed fever" (puerperal infection) by the introduction of sterile techniques in obstetrics. After that, little further improvement occurred, and the maternal mortality rates remained nearly constant—around one death in 200 births—from 1880 until 1930. Then maternal deaths began to decrease rapidly again, and by 1960 the rate had fallen by 95% from the 1930 level (Lerner & Anderson, 1963). Throughout most of this period, maternal mortality was probably a good indicator of the effectiveness of clinical care in general. Essentially the same factors were necessary for good maternity care as for clinical services of other kinds—competence in detecting, diagnosing, and treating medical problems, and the availability of adequate, appropriate techniques to correct them. This included availability of antibiotics, blood transfusions, improved surgical techniques, and major breakthroughs in the treatment of toxemias of pregnancy and of complicating medical problems during pregnancy, like diabetes and rheumatic heart disease. Today, however, as with most health problems, the residual differences in maternal mortality from one group to another are due more to social factors that determine life style, nutrition, and family structure, as well as the access, organization, and quality of the clinical care (Shapiro et al., 1968; Kitagawa & Hauser, 1973).

THE DOMINANCE OF CLINICAL MEDICINE

All three approaches to health care have made essential contributions to the conquest of infectious and nutritional diseases. The largest reductions in mortality came from public health and then from preventive medicine techniques. Each discipline quickly approached its maximum effectiveness against most infectious disorders soon after scientific techniques were developed for acting within its framework. Only the three disciplines working together could achieve the maximum reduction in mortality and morbidity. Within the triad of health disciplines, however, clinical medicine occupies a special position. Although it has contributed least to the reduction of mortality from infectious diseases and has achieved much less dramatic changes in the mortality rates from noninfectious diseases than preventive techniques did for infectious diseases, 95% of health care expenditures go to support clinical services. If there is any rational justification for this distribution of resources relative to outcomes, it must be sought in the impact on the quality of life for those who are sick rather than changes in the incidence or mortality from diseases.

The most fundamental and probably the strongest reason for the highly preferential allocation of health care resources to clinical medicine is the individualistic, humanitarian value perspective of our society. We place a greater emphasis on the individual good as opposed to or even at the expense of the collective good. We are strongly moved to action by humanitarian concern for the urgent need of a person already suffering or in danger. We are less moved by the high *probability* that many will suffer in the future when it is not certain who will actually be the ones to suffer—even if the total suffering in the collective is certain to be many times that of the individual who is presently in difficulty. We pay without question the high cost of care for persons struck by paralytic poliomyelitis but have great difficulty mustering the effort and budget to wage intensive immunization campaigns to prevent such needless cases from occurring. Public health and preventive medicine deal in future probabilities. Their success is measured in the abstract reduction of such probabilities or incidence of certain diseases—that is, in terms of what does *not* occur. These reductions represent a clear collective good but are difficult to appreciate as a distributive good for individuals. Not even at the height of their success in dealing with the major infectious diseases were preventive medicine and public health as glamorous, dramatic, or publicly visible as clinical medicine, neither did they seem to have as direct an impact on the lives of individuals.

The successes of clinical medicine, on the contrary, are very visible, personal, often dramatic, and humanitarianly appealing—real suffering, already in progress, is visibly alleviated. The immediacy of individual need for clinical care in times of illness and the moral belief that care cannot be denied anyone when it might be a matter of life and death have led to making such services accessible through insurance, charity, or public programs. As a consequence, the budgets for clinical care have grown steadily while budgets for prevention have barely kept up with inflation. As we discuss more extensively in Chapters 12 and 14, the differences in systems for financing medical services add to the disproportionate emphasis given to clinical medicine by providing much higher and more open-ended funding for clinical than for preventive care. Although both public health and clinical services are largely paid for indirectly, only public health services are (almost entirely) financed by fixed annual budgets that are prospectively set in competition with other public services like schools and fire departments. Since tax funds are always short, this process limits the financing available for public health and preventive services provided by health departments (Miller, 1975).

Clinical services, on the contrary, are largely financed by the insurance mechanism (even where tax funds are used), which provides open-ended funding by entitlement to a specified set of benefits as needed rather than a fixed budget. Since it is advantageous both to the health professionals who make the decisions about services and to the patients who seek them, there are strong incentives to increase utilization and costs. The insurance automatically reimburses, enabling the larger budget after the fact. (The only fiscal brake is any co-payment required from the patient, and this probably only has an effect on the decision for the first contact with a physician in any episode of illness. After this the decision-making passes to the provider of care.) Ironically, preventive services provided in a physician's office are poorly covered by insurance so that market constraints play a larger role in restricting financing for these services than for most clinical care. Thus the differences in financing, resource allocation, and utilization decision processes create a powerful bias in favor of clinical medicine over preventive medicine and public health.

There are also other factors that weight health service expenditures and resource allocation in the direction of clinical medicine. Despite the fact that public health and preventive medicine were first to apply techniques of scientific medicine effectively, the clinical approach is culturally much older and more deeply ingrained as a social institution. It still bears the priestly mantle of the medical profession as the socially mandated functional role that arose very early in response to the anxiety and suffering from illness (Chapter 3). Based on this cultural role, clinical medicine carries a much higher prestige than do preventive medicine and public health, which are viewed by society as functionary institutions without the priestly charisma associated with the magic of healing (Arnold, 1962; Ben-David, 1958). This prestige and power differential has been further augmented in recent times because the accomplishments of modern technology in clinical medicine are much more visible and dramatic than the successes of preventive medicine or public health. Heart transplants, life support systems, and even routine surgery or effective use of antibiotics seem to verge on the miraculous, while protection of a city's water supply and immunization of its children seem to be routine technical functions (Hall, 1959).

The tendency to play down the importance and prestige of preventive medicine is not limited to the lay public. Within the medical profession the highest prestige and the greatest professional rewards go to clinicians because of the belief that individual responsibility for patients is more difficult and important than the management of programs necessary to assure preventive care for a population (Freidson, 1970). This attitude is supported by the dominant ideology of the profession, which values independent decision-making and collegial regulation of standards while deprecating the bureaucratic hierarchical organization of practice necessary to implement preventive and public health programs. As a result physicians themselves tend to look somewhat condescendingly on the work of preventive medicine, public health, and administrative medicine, all necessary to make prevention work (Colombotos, 1969). Teaching of these subjects receives a low priority in most medical school curricula, and they are given little systematic attention by practicing clinicians (Coker et al., 1959, 1966). Physicians who eventually become involved in these specialties usually do so as a result of experiences gained after medical school and even after formal residency training (so-called secondary career choice; Coker et al., 1966). As a result entry into these fields is usually haphazard with little chance for the kind of extended, intensive training that most specialists receive. This tends to perpetuate the attitude among physicians that those who enter public health do so because they cannot make a go of it in clinical medicine (Back et al., 1958).

Still another factor contributing to the dominance of clinical medicine is the fact that public health and preventive medicine in their classic form quickly reached the limits of their accomplishments in regard to the types of diseases where they were successful. They have produced few dramatic breakthroughs since. Thus, although the *average* benefit per expenditure for public health and preventive medicine is much higher than for clinical medicine, the *marginal* benefit per expenditure from additional investment in the attempt to achieve further progress in prevention is not apt to be so striking (Weisbrod, 1961). Prevention of today's prevalent diseases would entail controversial social engineering and behavior modification, which are potentially very costly and difficult to achieve. With clinical medicine, on the contrary, the average benefit per expenditure has been much lower, but the limits of successful application of clinical techniques were not so immediately reached (Feldstein, 1979). Thus, marginal benefit increments have seemed to continue from additional increases in clinical medicine expenditures. Whether this is actually true of most clinical innovations today is beginning to be questioned and may require revision of our traditional approach to approving and financing new medical technology (see Chapter 10).

There are, moreover, many diseases where clinical medicine can make a significant difference in the quality of life—even if definitive cures are not possible. This includes maintenance techniques for chronic diseases and alleviating symptoms to improve the comfort of the patient in the face of both minor and serious illnesses. These two areas of activity in clinical medicine today account for the vast majority of expenditures and must be evaluated in reference to objectives and standards quite different from the major changes in morbidity and mortality that resulted from the efforts of health professionals between 1900 and 1960. Medicine today is confronted with a new constellation of problems in which the classical clinical approach can only provide one facet of the total strategy of care required. This new situation in regard to health and health care is a product of changes that have occurred in the pattern of diseases and in the organization of the health care system in the last 30 years.

REFERENCES

Abel-Smith, Brian, *The Hospitals, 1800–1948,* London: Heinemann, 1964.

Arnold, Mary F., "Perception of Professional Role Activities in the Local Health Department," *Public Health Reports,* 77(1):80–86, 1962.

Back, Kurt, Coker, Robert E., Jr., Donnelly, T. H., and Phillips, R. S., "Public Health as A Career of Medicine: Secondary Choice Within a Profession," *American Sociological Review,* 23:533–541, 1958.

Ben-David, J., "The Professional Role of the Physician in Bureaucratized Medicine, A Study in Role Conflict," *Human Relations,* 11:255–274, 1958.

Berlant, Jeffrey L., *Profession and Monopoly: A Study of Medicine in the United States and Great Britain,* Berkeley: University of California Press, 1975.

Bernard, Claude, *An Introduction to the Study of Experimental Medicine* (1865, translator, Henry C. Green), New York: Dover, 1957.

Bronowski, J., and Mazlish, Bruce, *The Western Intellectual Tradition,* New York: Harper, 1960.

Bullough, Bonnie, and Bullough, Vern L., *The Emergence of Modern Nursing,* New York: Macmillan, 1974.

Churchill, Edward D., "The Development of the Hospital," in Faxon, Nathaniel W., Ed., *The Hospital in Contemporary Life,* Cambridge: Harvard University Press, 1949.

Clark, Duncan, and MacMahon, Brian, *Preventive Medicine,* Boston: Little, Brown, 1967.

Coker, Robert E., Jr., et al., "Public Health as Viewed by the Medical Student," *American Journal of Public Health,* 49:601–609, 1959.

Coker, Robert E., Jr., Kosa, John, and Back, Kurt, "Medical Careers in Public Health," *Milbank Memorial Fund Quarterly,* 44(April, Part 1): entire issue, 1966.

Colombotos, John, "Physicians' Attitudes Toward a County Health Department," *American Journal of Public Health,* 59(1, January): 53–59, 1969.

Dauer, Carl C., Korns, Robert F., and Schuman, Leonard M., *Infectious Diseases,* Cambridge: Harvard University Press, 1968.

deKruif, Paul, *Microbe Hunters,* New York: Harcourt, Brace & World, 1926.

Dubos, Rene, and Dubos, Jean, *The White Plague: Tuberculosis, Man, and Society,* Boston: Little, Brown, 1952.

Duffy, John, *A History of Public Health in New York City, 1866–1966*, 2 vols., New York: Russell Sage Foundation, 1974.

Erhardt, Carl L., and Berlin, Joyce E., *Mortality and Morbidity in the United States*, Cambridge: Harvard University Press, 1974.

Feldstein, Paul, *Health Care Economics*, New York: Wiley, 1979.

Freidson, Eliot, *Profession of Medicine*, New York: Dodd, Mead, 1970.

Goldberger, J., "The Cause and Prevention of Pellagra," *Public Health Reports*, **29**:2354–57, 1914.

Hall, Oswald, "Half Medical Man, Half Administrator: An Occupational Dilemma," *Canadian Public Administration*, **2**:185–194, 1959.

Hilleboe, Herman E., "Public Health in the United States in the 1970s," *American Journal of Public Health*, **58**:1588–1610, 1968.

Hilleboe, Herman E., "Preventing Future Shock: Health Developments in the 1960s and Imperatives for the 1970s," *American Journal of Public Health*, **62**:136, 1972.

Holton, Gerald, "On the Role of Themata in Scientific Thought," *Science*, **188**:328–338, 1975.

John E. Fogarty International Center for Advanced Study in the Health Sciences, *Preventive Medicine, U.S.A.*, New York: Prodist, 1976.

Kass, Edward H., "Infectious Disease and Social Change," *Journal of Infectious Diseases*, **123**(1):110–114, 1971.

Kilbourne, Edwin D., and Smillie, Wilson G., *Human Ecology and Public Health*, London: Macmillan, 1969.

Kitagawa, Evelyn M., and Hauser, Philip M., *Differential Mortality in the United States: A Study in Socioeconomic Epidemiology*, Cambridge: Harvard University Press, 1973.

Kuhn, Thomas S., *The Structure of Scientific Revolutions*, Chicago: University of Chicago Press, 1962.

Leavell, Hugh K., and Clark, E. Gurney, *Preventive Medicine for the Doctor in His Community: An Epidemiologic Approach*, New York: McGraw-Hill, 1958.

Lerner, Monroe, and Anderson, Odin W., *Health Progress in the United States, 1900–1960*, Chicago: University of Chicago Press, 1963.

Lilienfeld, Abraham M., *Foundations of Epidemiology*, New York: Oxford University Press, 1976.

McDermott, Walsh, "Demography, Culture and Economics and the Evolutionary Stages of Medicine," in Kilbourne, E. & Smillie, W., Eds., *Human Ecology and Public Health*, London: Macmillan, 1969.

McKeown, Thomas, *Medicine in Modern Society*, New York: Hafner, 1965.

McKeown, Thomas, "A Historical Appraisal of the Medical Task," in McLachlan, G., and McKeown, T., Eds., *Medical History and Medical Care*, New York: Oxford University Press, 1971.

McKeown, Thomas, *The Modern Rise of Population*, London: Edward Arnold, 1976a.

McKeown, Thomas, *The Role of Medicine: Dream, Mirage or Nemesis*, London: Nuffield Provincial Hospitals Trust, 1976b.

McKeown, Thomas, and Lowe, C. R., *An Introduction to Social Medicine*, 2nd ed., Philadelphia: Lippincott, 1974.

McKinlay, John B., and McKinlay, Sonja M., "The Questionable Contribution of Medical Measures to the Decline of Mortality in the United States in the Twentieth Century," *Milbank Memorial Fund Quarterly/Health and Society*, **55**(3):405–428, 1977.

Miller, Alfred E., "The Expanding Definition of Health and Disease in Community Medicine," *Social Science and Medicine*, **6**(Fall):1972.

Miller, C. Arden, "Issues of Health Policy: Local Government and the Public's Health," *American Journal of Public Health*, **65**:1330, 1975.

Nordenskiold, Erik, *The History of Biology* (translator, Leonard Eyre), New York: Tudor, 1928.

Newman, Sir George, *Thomas Sydenham, Reformer of English Medicine*, London: 1924.

Payne, J. F., *Thomas Sydenham*, London: 1900.

Rosen, George, *A History of Public Health*, New York: MD Publications, 1958.

Rosen, George, *Preventive Medicine in the United States 1900–1975: Trends and Interpretations*, New York: Science History Publications, 1975.

Rosenstock, Irwin M., "What Research in Motivation Suggests for Public Health," *American Journal of Public Health*, **50**:295–302, 1960.

Shapiro, Sam, Schlesinger, Edward R., and Nesbitt, Robert E. L., Jr., *Infant, Perinatal, Maternal, and Childhood Mortality in the United States*, Cambridge: Harvard University Press, 1968.

Shryock, Richard H., *The Development of Modern Medicine: An Interpretation of the Social and Scientific Factors Involved*, New York: Hafner, 1969.

Singer, Charles, and Underwood, E. Ashworth, *A Short History of Medicine*, Oxford: Clarendon Press, 1962.

Sigerist, Henry E., *The Great Doctors*, Garden City, N.Y.: Doubleday Anchor, 1958.

Sigerist, Henry E., *On the History of Medicine*, New York: MD Publications, 1960.

Susser, Merwyn W., and Watson, W., *Sociology in Medicine*, New York: Oxford University Press, 1971.

Terris, Milton, Ed., *Goldberger on Pellagra*, Baton Rouge: Louisiana State University Press, 1964.

U.S. Bureau of the Census, *Statistical Abstract of the United States*, Washington, D.C.: Department of Commerce, 1978.

U.S. Public Health Service, *Healthy People: The Surgeon General's Report on Health Promotion and Disease Prevention*, Washington, D.C.: DHEW(PHS) Publ. No. 79-55071, 1979.

Weisbrod, Burton, *Economics of Public Health*, Philadelphia: University of Pennsylvania Press, 1961.

CHAPTER FIVE

Problems of Post-Clinical Medicine

The decline of infectious diseases between 1900 and 1960 was unfortunately paralleled by increasing incidence of other diseases that were previously much less common (Lerner & Anderson, 1963; Table 5.1; Figure 5.1). Morbidity and mortality from chronic debilitating disorders like heart disease and cancers have risen. So has the incidence of traffic accidents and other violence which often produces prolonged disabilities. As recently as 1940 the typical patient seen by a physician was suffering from some acute disease. He could usually be returned to full health and activity if the causal agent or specific defect could be remedied—either by medical intervention or by allowing it to run its course with some support from the physician. If the defect could not be repaired or overcome by the body's defenses, the course of the disease was often rapidly downhill. Today the situation is almost reversed. The major and increasing portion of sickness is due to chronic diseases for which no definitive cure exists or seems possible. These diseases require continuing care and support as long as the patient lives (McKeown & Lowe, 1974; USDHEW, 1979).

In 1978 heart disease accounted for 38% of all deaths compared to only 8% in 1900. Cancer is responsible for 20% of deaths now compared to less than 4% then; and strokes account for 10% now compared to 6% then (Erhardt & Berlin, 1974). Accidents and violence cause 7% of deaths (compared to 4% in 1900), but they account for 15% of the productivity lost due to health disability because they tend to occur among the young, and because the disabilities, such as paraplegia, are often long lasting. Diabetes, cirrhosis of the liver, and chronic lung disease together account for another 5% of total mortality. Thus, chronic diseases and disabilities today make up the overwhelming portion of social loss due to health impairment and health care costs (Fuchs, 1974). Except for routine checkups, they also make up the major portion of adult medical practice (USDHEW, 1979). The resulting pattern of diseases and health care problems today is just as characteristic of post-industrial society, and just as far-reaching in its social consequences as were the patterns of disease in tribal, agrarian, and early

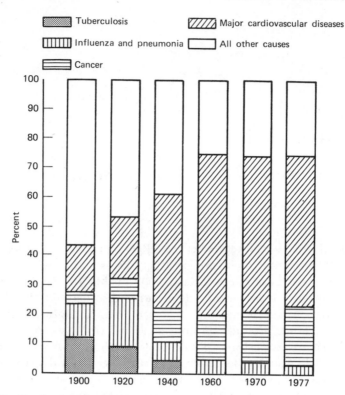

Figure 5.1. Deaths for selected causes as a percent of all deaths: United States, selected years, 1900–1977. Note: 1977 data are provisional; data for all other years are final. Source: USDHEW, 1979a.

industrial societies (White, 1973; Kass, 1971). This new pattern requires very different methods of prevention and a very different organization of health care, which can be referred to as "post-clinical medicine."

The term "post-clinical medicine" is meant to be understood in the sense of "post-industrial society" (Bell, 1973). The latter does not imply that industry has ceased to play an essential role in the economic or social structure. Post-industrial society is necessarily built on a continuing and growing industrial economic base. Yet the role of industry is modified by the massive expansion of the service sector required by changes in the structure of society and the needs generated by products and effects of industries themselves. Similarly post-clinical medicine does *not* imply the decline of clinical medicine or its importance. It does imply an *expansion* of need for supportive maintenance, patient management, and new kinds of preventive care. As with post-industrial society, these new needs are a product of changes in the nature of society as well as those generated by the effects of health care itself. Industry must be more efficient in order to support the new economic demands of post-industrial society. It must be more responsive to shifting

Table 5.1   Age-Adjusted Death Rates for Specified Causes (Per 100,000 Population)

	1977	1940–1944	1900–1904
Heart disease	210.4	288.9	180.8
Cancer	133.0	118.4	83.9
Stroke	48.2	87.6	134.2
Accidents	43.8	71.6	83.1
Diseases in Early Infancy and Birth Defects	16.8[a]	51.8[a]	81.6[a]
Influenza/Pneumonia	14.2	60.3	190.9
Liver Cirrhosis	13.1	8.7	15.9
Suicide	12.9	11.7	12.1
Diabetes	10.4	25.1	14.6
Homicide	9.6	5.7	1.2
Chronic Lung Disease	7.2	4.1	23.7
Kidney Disease	2.7	69.2	101.6
Tuberculosis	1.0	43.0	188.5
All other Infectious Diseases	0.7	46.4	206.4[b]

SOURCE: Erhardt & Berlin, 1974; National Center for Health Statistics, *Vital Statistics Rates in the U.S. 1940–1960,* USDHEW, 1968; *Monthly Vital Statistics Report,* 28 (1, Suppl.), May 1979.

[a] Not age-adjusted because almost all occur in first year of life.
[b] Age-adjustment approximated because of changes in disease classification.

social needs and social contexts if it is to provide solutions to problems of society rather than adding to them. Similarly, clinical medicine must become more efficient and better organized to fulfill its new and growing role in post-clinical medicine without creating intolerable costs. Otherwise, sufficient resources will not be available for meeting the expanding health care needs. Clinical medicine must become more responsive to the changing health needs and social context if it is to provide solutions to the health problems of society rather than adding to the burden.

CHARACTERISTICS OF TODAY'S PREVALENT DISEASES AND NEEDS OF POST-CLINICAL MEDICINE

The most prevalent diseases of today have a number of typical characteristics in common that shape the problems of post-clinical medicine. Unlike infectious diseases, today's degenerative and malignant diseases usually have a prolonged course requiring ambulatory and in-hospital care over many years. For every victim of a sudden unanticipated fatal heart attack, there are many patients who have repeated episodes of angina pectoris (chest pain due to inadequate blood flow to the heart, often leading eventually to a fatal coronary), nonfatal heart attacks, or congestive heart failure, all requiring prolonged care (DeBakey, 1964). For every stroke that leads to rapid death there are several victims of nonfatal strokes who require long periods of hospitalization, nursing home, or rehabilitation care for their paralysis or other disability. An increasing number of the aged suffer from diffuse brain degeneration from the same arteriosclerotic process; they gradually lose their ability to function in society and must finish out their unhappy days in nursing homes or the back wards of mental hospitals. Fatal cases of cancer require months or years of treatment before the end finally comes. In cases where cure is possible, treatment usually requires major surgery or intensive radiation or chemotherapy, with prolonged aftercare and rehabilitation (Powles, 1973).

The new pattern of diseases has arisen from two factors that must be distinguished in attempting to develop appropriate policy strategies for dealing with the problems of post-clinical medicine: the change in age distribution of the population because of greater longevity, and the change in incidence of diseases in each age group as a result of new life styles, new environmental factors, and a new social structure. As positive as greater longevity is for humane and economic reasons, the increased percentage of individuals reaching advanced age does present new problems that affect society as a whole and the health care system in particular (Shanas et al., 1968). Increased life expectancy does not mean immortality, and after the age of 65 the death rate rises rapidly—and the morbidity rate even more so—no matter how good the system of preventive or clinical medicine (Comfort, 1964). In part, then, the increasing prevalence of chronic diseases is simply a function of the greater number of older persons in the population, since the incidence of heart disease, cancer, and stroke rises dramatically with increasing age (Berg et al., 1970). Those over 65 make twice as many physician visits as those under 65, use 3.5 times as many days of hospital care per capita, and use virtually all of the nursing home care. As a result their rate of health care expenditures is four times as high as that for the rest of the population (USDHEW, 1979).

The major increases in life expectancy achieved for younger age groups have not been matched by such gains for the older groups. The mortality rate in the first 15 years of life is 95% lower today than in 1900. The (age-adjusted) mortality rate for those over 65 is only 30% lower than in 1900 (USPHS, 1979; Figure 5.2). In this group any improvement in longevity from a breakthrough in regard to one disease is quickly limited by the high mortality rate from others. Rice (1966) has estimated that if all cancers could suddenly be cured the gain in overall life expectancy would scarcely be two years, and even eliminating heart disease would only improve life expectancy by six years.

Yet, the problem is not simply that the inevitable fatal disease is postponed from youth or middle-age to old age. The increasing prevalence of

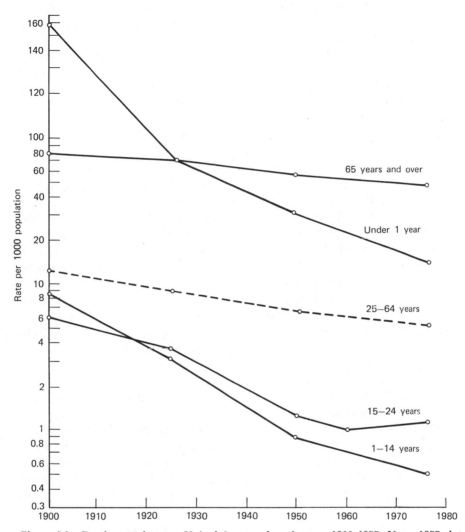

Figure 5.2. Death rates by age: United States, selected years, 1900–1977. Note: 1977 data are provisional; data for all other years are final. Selected years are 1900, 1925, 1950, 1960 (for age group 15–24 years only), and 1977. Source: USDHEW, 1979a.

chronic disease is more than just a residual phenomenon. Epidemiological studies point to the conclusion that changing life style, exposure to stress, and environmental pollutants in today's urban, industrial society are also major causal factors (Belloc & Breslow, 1972; Belloc, 1973). This new constellation of causal elements presents a set of problems for the prevention and treatment of diseases quite different from heretofore. The *behavior* patterns of individuals and socioeconomic communities have become much more important ultimate causes of today's major diseases than the biological and physiological factors that were primary in the past. To be effective, both prevention and treatment must deal with influences bound up in the socio-economic and cultural life style of the society—including the physical and social environment produced by this life style and its technology. Dealing with such diverse influences requires new degrees of sophistication in health education and "social engineering," involving problems that have not pre-viously been considered part of the province of medicine.

The major diseases today have *multiple causes*—and not just in the sense used in reference to infectious diseases where the host immunity system, the vector of the disease agent, and other environmental factors in transmission are often considered as "causal factors" in addition to the agent (Leavell & Clark, 1958). Multiple causation in the new sense involves a whole field of factors arising from diverse sources *no one* of which is a *sine qua non* or can be called the primary causal agent (Miller, 1972). Coronary heart dis-ease, cancer, and strokes are prime examples of diseases with such multiple causation. Genetic predisposition, diet, stress, personality type, environmen-tal pollution, and personal habits, such as smoking, are all important influ-ences on the incidence of these diseases, and many factors are probably in-volved within each of these categories. The situation is less well understood with accidents and violence, but a similar pattern seems to be unfolding from epidemiological studies of these conditions. As a result of this multiple causation there is often no clear target against which preventive or clinical medicine can intervene.

The *causation* of today's diseases, as well as their treatment, is also *ex-tended* over long periods of time. The average duration from beginning exposure to carcinogens until the development of clinically recognizable tumors is 30 to 40 years for many kinds of malignancies. Arteriosclerotic changes apparently take place over much of a lifetime. In the diseases that were important in the past, a causal agent acutely, but usually reversibly, distorted the normal physiological processes of the body in a recognizable way. Today's dominant diseases come about as a result of slow but cumula-tive and irreversible changes in the structure and physiology of the body. Since there is no clear time of onset, both preventive efforts and early de-tection must be organized to work reliably over long periods of time. By the time the damage is discovered, little can be done to remedy the under-lying condition. Thus long-term management, supportive care, and con-tinuing surveillance over the disease process are necessary.

These characteristics of today's prevalent diseases present major new problems of disease prevention, treatment, health planning, and health policy. The multiplicity of causation, together with the environmental and behavioral factors underlying these diseases, makes prevention a very differ-ent affair than in the days of infectious disease. In order to have a signifi-cant impact beyond its classical role, prevention must enter a new phase. The Secretary of the U.S. Department of Health, Education and Welfare (HEW) has referred to this as the need for the "second public health revolution in the history of the United States" (USPHS, 1979). To make a major difference in mortality, prevention will have to be targeted against coronary heart disease, strokes, cancer, accidents, and personal violence—besides continuing its traditional efforts with infectious diseases. There are also major needs for new preventive strategies to reduce morbidity, disability, and social loss from certain nonfatal problems such as veneral disease and unwanted pregnancies (particularly among teenagers), alcoholism, drug abuse, child abuse, and other behavioral problems. In regard to prevention these disorders present many of the same problems as the major causes of death.

The principal contributing factors and causes of both groups of disorders are direct or indirect consequences of personal, social, and economic life style and thus beyond the traditional realm of public health and preventive medicine. Modification of personal and social behavior to change nutritional, exercise, and smoking habits contributing to heart disease and cancer require much more effective health education than we have been capable of in the past. To achieve the degree of impact needed it may be necessary to resort to economic incentives and penalties, or legal sanctions. This raises a host of political and ethical problems unfamiliar to traditional health educators. It also runs head-on into vested economic interests and resentment of government regulation or intrusion into private lives.

The factors influencing the incidence of the major diseases in post-clinical medicine and the changes necessary to reduce them are intertwined with other social factors essential for the socioeconomic well-being of today's society. Therefore improvement or even maintenance of health levels may require difficult *economic tradeoffs* and *political compromises* with other social goals and priorities. For example, reducing carcinogen exposure from industrial pollution is often costly to the economy and may lead to loss of employment opportunities in some places. A great deal of progress has been made in identifying environmental and food carcinogens in recent years, and major legislative efforts have made some important beginnings in their control. However, as countervailing pressures mount, such as unemployment, economic recession, and energy shortages, maintaining the resolve to increase our efforts in this direction becomes difficult. The payoffs seem so distant compared to the immediately pressing economic and social problems. These are the kinds of alternatives that will confront future preventive health policy decisions. Tradeoffs among social values and goals will become primary issues of policy making.

The difficulties in making adequate evaluations for such decisions are immense because we still know so little about the social factors determining the health status of a population. Developing better methods for producing "health impact statements" should be a major priority for health policy strategists who take the initiative in the "second public health revolution." Such assessments, as with environmental impact statements, would attempt to predict the outcome for the health of various groups from one project or pattern of spending as opposed to another. We need to compare the health effects of decreased employment with the impact of pollution from plants needed to maintain employment. We must be able to assess the influence on health of the inflation generated by subsidies to pay for pollution control compared to the effect of the pollution. We must try to predict the potential health improvement from a given investment in mass transit or job training as opposed to an equivalent investment in new health centers or medical technology.

The *social* environment also contributes heavily to some major health problems of today, such as personal violence, alcoholism, drug abuse, venereal disease, unwanted pregnancies, child abuse, and automobile accidents (by way of alcoholism and transportation patterns based on demography and economic life style). Decreasing their incidence might call for restructuring our metropolitan areas or greater restriction of personal freedom to take risks than has been acceptable in this country until now (Ford, 1976). We do not know as much as we need to about the "social engineering" necessary to modify social environments to alleviate these health problems. There are also many moral and political issues to evaluate before we are ready to use such techniques. At this point health policy becomes inextricably interwoven with social planning and social policy in general. Health professionals can play an advocacy role, but the primary arena for debate passes outside their realm in these cases. Social policy has traditionally been left to the political process in this country, not to professional groups—and that is clearly the way it has to be in our political system. To have a significant impact on today's health problems, preventive strategies will have to work more effectively through and within the political arena.

Many epidemiologists and policy analysts have become concerned about the implications of the new pattern of causal relationships of today's prominent diseases. Some have suggested the need for a new more relevant conceptual model for describing the causation of chronic illnesses and identifying policy strategies to control them. The classic clinical and preventive epidemiological model of disease evolved as the key to the scientific revolution in medicine in the late nineteenth century. It assumed a single specific agent or physiological defect with a one-to-one causal relationship to particular diseases. This model was effective in devising strategies to block the transmission of agents or repair physiological defects. Today, even where specific agents or defects such as carcinogens or hypertension can be identified as *immediate* causes of a disease, the *deeper* causes lie in the more diffuse behavioral, social, and environmental factors. The latter must be the targets of effective prevention and more encompassing treatment strategies to make an appreciable difference in the health of the population.

To help decide where to concentrate efforts at prevention and health promotion in this new situation, a so-called health field concept of disease causation has been proposed. This model divides the causal factors into fields (related groups) characterized as: biological, environmental, life style, and health care factors (Laframboise, 1973). It was adopted by the Ministry of

Health of Canada as a useful typology for classifying the factors to be dealt with in considering possible health policy strategies (Lalonde, 1974). The model is not meant to replace the classical one, which is still essential for research and intervention in regard to specific factors where they can be identified and influenced directly. Rather, it is an adjunct to the standard model intended to provide insight and evaluation of strategies for intervention when the causal basis is identifiable only in terms of risk factors whose reduction lowers the *probability* of a disease.

The causal fields defined in this model correspond to areas where particular *strategies of intervention* may be possible and effective rather than to the kind of final physiological deficit. For instance, factors in the life-style field may be influenced by health education and incentives to encourage or discourage particular habits or behavior patterns. Environmental factors might be impacted by legislation and regulation to control or encourage certain features of industry or other social behavior. Biological factors call for more classical preventive or therapeutic approaches but also for such social and behavioral approaches as genetic counseling. Medical care inadequacies call for planning, organizational, and financing reform to assure adequate access and appropriate services.

Causes of diseases in the traditional sense are often influenced by factors in all four fields. For example, the cause of coronary heart disease, occlusion of an artery of the heart due to atherosclerosis, is the result of a biological process entailing some degree of genetic predisposition (Russek, 1959). Life-style characteristics such as diet, exercise, and smoking are major risk factors influencing mortality rates. Environmental features, particularly social stress but also carbon monoxide and other air pollutant levels, have been shown to play a role. Finally, there is some evidence that emergency resuscitation and medical care services make a difference in the immediate outcome of coronary attacks. The model makes it possible to determine the extent to which factors in each of these categories influence the incidence and outcomes. For example, men in the 45 to 65 age group who are heavy smokers have a cardiac mortality rate four times as high as nonsmokers. If 50% of the men in this age group were smokers and all other factors were equal between smokers and nonsmokers, the excess mortality due to smoking in this group would account for 60% of cardiac mortality. Actually many other factors tend to parallel smoking behavior so that it is necessary to standardize for these factors using the same basic statistical techniques. Thus, smoking alone may not account for the entire 60%. On the other hand, if all known life-style factors are taken into account, about 75% of the mortality may be explained (Dever, 1976).

For most diseases the data are insufficient to make as sound estimates as for coronary heart disease. However, for some of the major cancers we have reasonably good evidence to estimate the extent of influence from certain habits, such as smoking, or certain environmental factors. Using similar techniques where data are available and educated estimates for those dis-

Table 5.2   Relative Importance of Disease Causal Factors Compared
to Distribution of Expenditures

Field of Factors	Percent of Mortality Attributable to Field	Percent of Expenditures Targeted for Field
Human biological factors	20	6.9
Environmental hazards	20	1.5
Behavioral factors and life style	50	1.0
Health care inadequacies	10	90.6

SOURCE: USPHS, 1979; Dever, 1976.

eases where it is not, the Surgeon General has estimated how the causation
for the 10 leading causes of death can be apportioned among these "fields"
(Table 5.2). When the distribution of importance of causal factors is compared with the distribution of health related expenditures, the contrast is
startling.

To be sure, such an aggregate estimate has little concrete meaning and
must be interpreted with great caution. Nevertheless, it does suggest that
far too much is expended on medical care compared to the extent of the
problem that lies there and far too little on promotion of healthy life
styles.*

To evaluate the appropriateness of health policy strategies we need to
know the extent of social loss attributable to each disease group—and
therefore the potential benefit to be gained in controlling them (Coase,
1960). Rice (1966) has developed a method for evaluating the loss due to
various disease groups from the cost of treatment and the cost of lost pro-

---

* A more precise analysis of proper resource allocation would require more than simply
balancing expenditures against the portion of the problem represented by each area. According to economic theory, optimum allocation of limited resources is achieved when
the marginal benefit of each additional dollar spent in one way is just equal to the benefit
of the same dollar spent in an alternative way. A proper attempt to optimize expenditures
of resources for health would require cost-benefit analysis of each specific strategy to improve health. The greatest increase of spending, then, should be for those strategies that
produce the greatest benefit per additional dollar. This allocation strategy should continue
until diminishing returns reduce the marginal benefits of the new investment to equal
those of other areas. In implying that the allocation of budget should be proportional to
the extent of the problem, the implicit assumption is being made that resources spread
out in proportion to the problem will tend to have the same marginal benefit everywhere.
Another equivalent assumption is that more resources can be effectively spent where the
greater part of the problem lies. This assumes a uniformity of diminishing returns for resources expended in relation to the extent of the problem to be overcome. There are no
quantitative data to support or refute either of these assumptions. Yet, intuition and general experience suggest there is some justification for such a rule of thumb. At least it
seems reasonable to conclude that spending 90% of our health resources for clinical services, whose deficiencies account for only 10% of the problem, is unlikely to be cost-
efficient.

ductivity (Cooper & Rice, 1976). The latter cost is a product of the morbidity and mortality of each disease in each age group and the loss of immediate and probable future productivity suffered as a result of death or disability at the given age. Relative social cost provides a rough indicator to set priorities for resource allocation in regard to health problems. To select strategies for best using the resources we also need to know the major factors contributing to the most important diseases in order to evaluate potential methods for reducing incidence or decreasing disability. Unfortunately, precise methods for such evaluation are not available in regard to most health problems. The diseases responsible for most morbidity and mortality vary greatly from one age group to another, as do the strategies necessary to prevent or treat them. Considerable insight can therefore be gained into the relative nature of the various problems by examining the major health problems in each age group and the factors influencing their incidence (Table 5.3).

INFANT MORTALITY—PREVENTING LOW BIRTH WEIGHT

After leveling off in the late 1960s and early 1970s, infant mortality rates (age 0 to 1) have improved rapidly again in the past few years. The mortality from diarrhea and infant pneumonias had already been nearly eliminated prior to 1960 largely as a result of improved nutrition and living conditions (Chapter 4; Shapiro et al., 1968; Anderson, 1958). The major remaining risk factor to infants is low birth weight (with or without a shortened period of gestation). Two-thirds of all infant deaths occur in those weighing less than 5.5 pounds (2500 gms) at birth, and infants in this group are 20 times more likely to die within the first year. A large part of the reduction in infant mortality during the past 10 years can be attributed to the decreased portion of low weight births (USPHS, 1979). Subnormal birth weight, in turn, is highly correlated with poor maternal nutrition or immaturity, out-of-wedlock pregnancy, low socioeconomic status, smoking, alcohol and drug abuse, and lack of prenatal care—all of which tend to be highly intercorrelated. Twenty-five percent of mothers under age 15 have low-weight infants (three times the rate of older mothers), and 70% receive no care during the first months of pregnancy. The incidence of low birth weight is inversely proportional to socioeconomic status of the mother. Low socioeconomic status probably influences birth weight through poorer maternal nutrition, bad housing, more stressful living, and less likelihood of receiving early prenatal care.

Preventive programs to improve infant mortality will have to operate on a number of social, behavioral, educational, and health care organizational fronts (Morris & Heady, 1955). Continued efforts to improve economic status and nutrition of certain segments of our population, such as food stamp programs and reducing unemployment, may well be the major factor in de-

Table 5.3 Causes of Death by Life Stages, 1977

Problem	Infants (Under 1) Rank	Rate[a]	Children (1–14) Rank	Rate[b]	Adolescents/ Young Adults (15–24) Rank	Rate[b]	Adults (25–44) Rank	Rate[b]	Adults (45–64) Rank	Rate[b]	Older Adults (Over 65) Rank	Rate[b]	Total Population (All Ages) Rank	Rate[b]
Chronic diseases														
Heart disease			7	1.1	6	2.5	2	25.5	1	351.0	1	2334.1	1	332.3
Stroke			8	.6	9	1.2	8	6.1	3	52.4	3	658.2	3	84.1
Arteriosclerosis											5	116.5	9	13.3
Bronchitis, emphysema, and asthma									10	12.2	8	69.3		
Cancer			3	4.9	5	6.5	1	29.7	2	302.7	2	988.5	2	178.7
Diabetes mellitus					10	.4	10	2.4	8	17.8	6	100.5	7	15.2
Cirrhosis of the liver							7	8.6	4	39.2	9	36.7	8	14.3
Infectious diseases														
Influenza and pneumonia	5	50.6	6	1.5	8	1.3	9	3.0	9	15.3	4	169.7	5	23.7
Meningitis			8	.6										
Septicemia	6	32.7												
Trauma														
Accidents														
Motor vehicle accidents			2	9.0	1	44.1	3	23.1	7	18.3	10	24.5	6	22.9
All other accidents	7	27.7	1	10.8	2	18.4	4	18.5	5	25.5	7	78.1	4	24.8
Suicide			10	.4	3	13.6	5	17.3	6	19.1			9	13.3
Homicide			5	1.6	4	12.7	6	15.6						
Developmental problems														
Immaturity associated	1	407.7												
Birth-associated	2	294.4												
Congenital birth defects	3	253.1	4	3.6	7	1.6								
Sudden infant deaths	4	142.8												
All causes		1412.1		48.1		117.1		182.5		1,000.0		5288.1		878.1

SOURCE: USDHEW, 1979a.
[a] Rate per 100,000 live births.
[b] Rate per 100,000 population in specified group.

creasing the differentials in infant mortality between various social and ethnic groups. Decreasing smoking, alcohol, and drug abuse during pregnancy could make a major contribution toward reducing low birth weights and infant mortality. Recent studies suggest that smoking may be a significant factor in 20 to 40% of low-birth-weight infants (USPHS, 1979a).

Reducing teenage pregnancy through improved family planning and outreach programs to get pregnant women into prenatal care at an earlier stage could significantly cut the rate of low-birth-weight infants and therefore mortality. Seventy percent of teenage pregnancies are undesired, 85% occur out of wedlock, and 40% end in abortion. Yet a third of all teenage girls who are sexually active use no contraception (Zelnick & Kantner, 1978). The easier availability of safe legal abortions (though increasingly restricted for certain groups as a result of the cutoff of medicaid funding for abortions) has appreciably lowered the birth rate among teenagers and may be the major factor in the recent new improvement of infant mortality rates—as it certainly has been in the reduction of maternal mortality rates (USPHS, 1979b). The rapid decline of infant mortality among low-income groups in recent years suggests that the outlook for improvement is not as bleak as once thought (Richmond & Filner, 1979). Yet, the structure of preventive services and the organization of health care is far from adequate to overcome the persistent problems responsible for most infant mortality today. For example, an adequate program to prevent the pregnancies would have to involve girls in an ongoing physician-care or counseling relationship closely tied to the health care and prenatal care systems. In this way contraception, abortion services, or early prenatal care and nutritional counseling could be made available as soon as the need arises. All these approaches require significant modification of behavior among groups that have previously been very hard to reach using traditional health education programs (Kessner, 1973, 1974).

CHILDHOOD HEALTH PROBLEMS— CREATING SAFER LIVING ENVIRONMENTS

Children (aged 1 to 14) are another group where tremendous improvement in mortality and morbidity has been and continues to be made. Their death rate has decreased by 95% since 1900 and by 50% since 1950. This is primarily due to control of infectious diseases as a result of better sanitation, nutrition, housing, immunization, and antibiotics. Today measles complications account for the greatest remaining mortality from infectious diseases in this age group. Yet, measles, as well as polio, could be completely eradicated by proper immunization. Clearly continued efforts are still necessary to maintain immunization levels and other traditional public health measures against preventable diseases.

Today, however, accidents are the largest single cause of death among children, accounting for 45% of childhood mortality—20% from motor vehicle accidents alone, 8% from drowning, 6% from fires. Little can be done about these problems by either traditional clinical pediatrics or classical prevention programs. Major improvement would have to come from better safety behavior of other age groups and safer living environments generally. (Early swimming instruction and water safety training might make a difference in the large drowning mortality rate.)

The major preventive emphasis aimed at this age group itself must center on nutrition, growth and development problems, learning and behavioral problems—more to prevent future morbidity and disability rather than immediate. Again, most of these problems lie outside the areas of traditional clinical pediatrics or classical prevention. Effective help in regard to learning, behavior, or child abuse problems requires coordination between schools, counseling services, social welfare services, and clinical care of a kind seldom achieved even for short-lived experiments where major resources have been focused on small groups. More limited but well institutionalized programs, like Headstart, have been shown to make a difference, particularly for the poor. However, major improvement in the health status of American children will require reorganization and commitment of a full spectrum of human services dealing with their welfare and education.

ADOLESCENT AND YOUNG ADULT HEALTH PROBLEMS— MODIFYING ACCIDENT-PRONE BEHAVIOR

An even higher portion of adolescents and young adults (age 15 to 24) die of accidents than do younger children. Seventy-five percent of deaths are a result of violence in some form: 40% from motor vehicle accidents alone among whites and almost as high a rate from homicide among blacks. This is the only age group where mortality rates have actually been increasing since 1960. American adolescent death rates are almost twice those of England, Sweden, and Japan. Death rates for males are three times as high as for females in this group. Violent death and disability from injury represent an epidemic of major proportions among America's youth (Iskrant & Joliet, 1968). The situation for adolescents and young adults differs from that of young children primarily in that the preventive efforts must be more directed toward the young persons themselves rather than just the parents.

Excessive speed was a factor in half of all teenage motor vehicle fatalities compared to 35% for older drivers. Eighty percent of teenage drivers fail to use safety belts, which can reduce fatalities and serious injuries by half in accidents (Robertson, 1975, 1976). Risk-taking behavior is a major contributor to death and injury among young males in this country. The challenge to prevention is to find safer ways to channel such behavior or to decrease it. Half of all fatal auto accidents involve drivers who had high levels of alcohol in their blood (Kilbourne & Smillie, 1971). Most of them were already known to the police because of previous incidents of drunken or reckless driving. Although alcoholism is frequently considered a medical problem today, traffic accidents resulting from it are not. A more encompassing and appropriate view of preventive medicine in today's world will have to consider traffic accidents as a very central concern (Selzer et al., 1967).

A great deal could be done to reduce motor vehicle fatalities: safer highways, better enforcement of speed limits, safer vehicles with some kind of automatic crash restraints, programs to curb drunken driving. The highly disproportionate incidence of highway deaths among young males indicates a serious need for professional concern with ways of influencing behavior in order to prevent such a major cause of death and disability. As with the other problems of post-clinical medicine, accident prevention calls for new understanding and techniques other than those that have been classically used in preventive or clinical practice. Adequate health care for the coming era would have to include measures for moderating major behavioral causes of death during the most productive years of adult life (Baker & Hadden, 1974).

Many complex and difficult-to-change factors likewise contribute to the high homicide rate in this country: economic deprivation, family instability, drug and alcohol abuse, glamorizing violence in the media and in our cultural tradition. Yet one simple measure, gun control, could have an appreciable impact on the homicide rate. Sixty-five percent of homicides involve the use of handguns. Most of these occur as a result of personal disagreements among family or acquaintances, not in the course of robbery, assault, or the like. Since these incidents tend not to be premeditated, handgun control could reduce the availability of a suitable weapon and thus lower the homicide rate—and probably also the suicide rate. There is evidence that when the preferred means of suicide is not available, potential victims do not readily turn to alternative means (Baker & Dietz, 1979).

Although they are not causes of death in this age group, a number of serious health problems among teenagers and young adults are equally in need of major preventive efforts. Because of the epidemic proportions they have reached their toll in morbidity, ruined lives, and later mortality makes them afflictions of first magnitude. Alcoholism and drug abuse, uncommon among teenagers in 1950, now occur at shocking rates. Besides contributing to the incidence of motor vehicle accidents and other violent deaths, they have serious long-range health consequences and create social problems, such as crime and family disruption. The indirect health damage resulting from the social impact may far surpass the direct results like cirrhosis. Most smoking, which contributes to 30% of deaths in this country, starts in this age group (USPHS, 1979). Unlike adult males, teenagers are smoking at a higher rate than ever before, and girls are taking up the habit as rapidly as do boys (USPHS, 1979a). The long-range health implications of these trends are ominous.

The major venereal diseases were seemingly on the road to eradication after World War II as a result of the introduction of effective treatment with penicillin. Today gonorrhea has again reached epidemic proportions, and 75% of the cases occur in this age group. Each year an estimated 75,000 women become sterile as a result of gonorrheal pelvic infections (USPHS, 1979). In addition, certain newly recognized sexually transmitted diseases (such as genital herpes and nongonococcal urethritis), have become rampant. Teenage pregnancy is a problem likewise arising from the new life style of younger Americans. Each year 10% of all teenage girls become pregnant, and 25% have at least one pregnancy by age 19. Seventy percent of the pregnancies are out of wedlock and 40% end in abortion. For those carried to term, the consequences for mother and child are often tragic because of the discontinuation of education that usually occurs and the socioeconomic disruption into which it plunges them.

All these problems are primarily results of life style, social behavior, and economic instability rather than the traditional kinds of disease agents dealt with by preventive or clinical medicine. The present health care system has little to offer toward alleviating them. Yet, they constitute the major health problems facing this age group. Fundamental changes in health priorities and in our preventive and treatment strategies are necessary if the health system is to be responsive to the real needs of this population.

MORTALITY IN EARLY MATURITY—
CANCER AS A SOCIAL DISEASE

In the midadult group (age 25 to 44) accidents and violence begin to decline in frequency and are surpassed by cancer and heart disease (in that order) as the primary causes of death. Cancer (malignant tumors, or neoplasms) is not a single disease, but rather a category of diseases (like infectious diseases). Each type has a different set of symptoms, a different clinical course, occurs predominantly at a different age, and probably has different causes. Nevertheless, there are a number of features common to many of the malignancies so that they can be discussed as a group for certain purposes. The basic pathological process in all cancers is an uncontrolled overgrowth of cells of some particular type. These spread and encroach on normal cells in the body's organs, interfering with necessary physiological functions. Just what causes the uncontrolled growth is poorly understood and may be different for each kind of tumor. The incidence of most types of cancers increase with advancing age although there is a group (e.g., certain leukemias) that peaks in childhood, and another group with highest incidence in early maturity. Much accumulated epidemiological evidence indicates that malignancies are not just degenerative processes (where the normal mechanisms of control simply break down as a result of increasing chances of failure with advancing age), as was once believed. The difference in rates of occurrence of various kinds of cancer in different population groups is too marked to make this a tenable explanation (Schneiderman, 1975).

It has been known for many years that certain malignancies are due to exposure to particular agents in the environment. In 1775 Percival Potts (an English physician) described the high incidence of cancer of the scrotum among chimney sweeps, and suspected that it was due to irritation from the coal tars they were exposed to. This correlation could be demonstrated more precisely only many years later (Singer & Underwood, 1962). Nevertheless, Potts was able to decrease the incidence considerably by instituting a careful system of cleansing after work. A similar discovery was made in regard to cancer of the urinary bladder among analine dye workers toward the end of the nineteenth century, cancer of the bone among radium paint workers, and leukemia among X-ray technicians still later. In these cases it was possible to protect workers by limiting the levels of exposure, but in most instances the malignancies develop many years after exposure to the carcinogen. Consequently, as the number of agents to which workers are exposed increases, it becomes more difficult for occupational medicine to keep up with new potential dangers and devise methods of protecting workers and other exposed populations. Every year nearly 1000 new chemicals are introduced into industry. Only a handful of these can be thoroughly studied for their possible toxic and carcinogenic effects (Lehmann & Kelmar, 1979). Two industrial carcinogens now known to be serious occupational hazards are asbestos fibers causing certain types of lung cancer, and vinyl chloride causing cancer of the liver. Although steps have been taken to reduce further exposure of workers, it is anticipated that because of the long time lag thousands of deaths will occur in coming years from the exposure to these agents that took place over the past 40 years (Selikoff & Hammond, 1978).

In recent years it has also been discovered that agents reaching a much more general population (than industrial carcinogens do) may account for many malignancies. The best known case is cigarette smoking. In 1958 Hammond demonstrated that the incidence of lung cancer is much higher among heavy cigarette smokers than among nonsmokers or light smokers (Hammond, 1966). In retrospect it is possible to correlate the rise in incidence of lung cancer almost exactly with the increasing amount of cigarette smoking during the twentieth century—with a lag of about 30 to 40 years. Smoking is now known to account for the vast majority of deaths from cancer of the lung (bronchus), which has now become the most common malignancy among American men, accounting for almost 25% of all male cancer deaths (overtaking cancer of the stomach, which has decreased dramatically). A similar trend is now being seen among women who took up cigarette smoking considerably later than men. It is difficult enough to stop exposure to industrial carcinogens, but those that are widespread in the population as a result of cultural habits present an even greater problem for public health and preventive medicine. In spite of warnings printed on all packs of cigarettes and educational programs attempting to stop people from smoking, prevalence of smoking among young people has continued to rise. The group of persons who seem to have taken the danger most seriously is physicians themselves, among whom the percentage of cigarette smokers dropped from 75 to 25% in the last 15 years (USPHS, 1979a). There is also an encouraging decline among adult male smokers generally. However, the difficulty experienced in achieving overall reduction in smoking bodes ill for the prevention of other cancers that result from sociocultural habit patterns where the source of the offending agent is much less obvious and dispensable than smoking.

The great differences in incidence rates of certain malignancies and their time trends among sociocultural groups suggests that personal habits or cultural mores and general environmental exposures must play a major role in causing cancers, even when the precise carcinogenic agent cannot be identified (Cairns, 1979). For example, the incidence of cancer of the colon is much higher among some national, ethnic, and socioeconomic populations than others. Incidence is closely correlated with variations in the richness of the diets. Cancers of the colon and rectum have been increasing in most industrialized countries in recent years. Immigrants from less affluent nations (where the colon cancer rates are lower) begin to approach the United States incidence rates. It is suspected that diets high in animal fat and low in plant fibers, or other socioeconomic or culture-related factors, may be the cause, but no specific factors have been demonstrated. Thus social behavior seems to be the major factor determining variations in incidence. Modification of dietary customs would be necessary if primary prevention is to be achieved.

In many other types of tumors major variations and trends in incidences occur with even less indication of the underlying causes. For example, cancer of the stomach, which used to be the most common cause of cancer death among males (and third most common among females), has declined precipitously during the past 40 years—by 60% in white males, by 72% in white females, and to a lesser degree among blacks (Lilienfeld et al., 1972). Mortality rates for cancer of the stomach are higher in most other countries where such statistics are available, but immigrants to the United States from those countries have a rate closer to that of native born Americans. This strongly suggests that there are factors in the diet or environment causing stomach cancer and that it has been changing for the better in the United States in recent years. What these factors are remains completely unknown.

Similar class, ethnic, geographic, or historical trend differences in incidence and mortality rates occur for nearly all types of malignancies. Many epidemiologists assume that differences in cancer mortality rates between various sociocultural groups, or groups with certain habit patterns or particular occupational situations are the result of exposure to specific carcinogenic agents. Postulating that the excess mortalities (differences) between such groups are potentially preventable by discovering and eliminating the exposure, they calculate that between 75 and 90% of all cancers could conceivably be avoided (Schneiderman, 1975). In general it is not yet known what carcinogens or precisely what sociocultural behavior patterns underlie these epidemiological facts. When they are discovered, the problem of removing the "agents" where there is widespread exposure, or of changing the behavior pattern, entails projects in health education and/or social engineering that are formidable.

The second way that cancer deaths can be reduced is through early detection and treatment. The most widely used cancer screening test is for cancer of the cervix, which can be cured in most cases if it is discovered by Papanicalaou smear in the preinvasive stage. If every woman over the age of 30 had an annual Pap smear with good follow up, deaths from this disease could probably be dramatically reduced. Yet thousands of women still die from cervical cancer each year. This is an indication of the inadequacy of our present system of health care for dealing with the diseases of postclinical medicine. Self-examination for breast nodules and annual physical examination for rectal and prostate cancer and for certain changes in routine laboratory tests like blood counts, urinalyses, and tests for hidden blood in the feces are also valuable screening methods for early detection of cancer. Immediate investigation of any unusual symptoms is also essential for early detection of tumors.

Progress is being made in the more traditional clinical approach to treatment of malignant diseases. Some malignancies such as certain leukemias and Hodgkins disease can now be cured in a fair number of cases. There is hope that chemotherapeutic agents for specific malignancies will be found for other kinds of cancer, with effectiveness similar to those for infectious diseases. If this happens, a much better system will still be needed for detection and for the organization of the chronic care and rehabilitation that would be necessitated by such advances in medical technology.

MIDDLE-AGE MORTALITY—LIFE STYLE AND CORONARY HEART DISEASE

Heart disease is the largest single cause of death in the United States and in most other advanced industrial countries, accounting for 38% of all deaths in this country in 1977. Among mature adults (age 45 to 64), especially males, heart disease increases rapidly with age as a cause of mortality and disability, surpassing cancer as the number one cause. Its incidence continues to rise with increasing age. A large part of this mortality is sudden, and most of it occurs at a rather advanced age. Consequently, only 10% of direct health care expenditures went for treatment of heart disease in 1972 (Cooper & Rice, 1976) and only 14% of productivity lost due to disability can be attributed to it. Sudden death due to "heart attacks" (cardiac infarcts, severe damage of a section of heart muscle due to plugging of a coronary artery supplying it with blood) is the most dramatic and best known form of heart disease. Nevertheless, much coronary heart disease (CHD) does not result in sudden death. Instead, it leads to chronic illness and disability with frequent, prolonged, and expensive hospitalization and physician care over many years.

CHD, by far the most common type of heart disease today,* is due to narrowing of the coronary arteries from deposits of cholesterol. It is a poorly understood, slowly cumulative process whose onset cannot be readily detected—nor can its progress be medically controlled. CHD is primarily a disease of men, who die of it five times more frequently than do women in the United States. Its incidence begins to rise steeply after the age of 45. Almost one-third of all deaths in the United States occur from this cause alone. About one and a quarter million Americans suffer heart attacks each year and over one-half million deaths result, 60% of these occur suddenly, another 10 to 15% without going to a hospital (Moriyama et al., 1971). For those admitted to hospitals the case mortality rate is about 35%. There is heated debate among health professionals whether intensive coronary care units in hospitals reduce in-hospital mortality (Office of Technology Assessment, 1978; Mather et al., 1971; Martin et al., 1974). The overall reduction of mortality is minimal, however, because the chances of another attack are five times higher after the first coronary. Such recurrences result in a 30% death rate in the five years following the first attack (age 45 to 60) (Wright & Fredrickson, 1973).

The general (age adjusted) mortality from CHD in the population rose steadily until almost 1970. However, since 1970 there has been a slight but significant and encouraging decline (Moriyama et al., 1971; U.S. Bureau of the Census, 1978). This decrease is probably largely attributable to decreased smoking among adult males, some decrease in cholesterol intake, and decreasing prevalence of high blood pressure (USPHS, 1979). Besides the tremendous loss of life, coronary artery disease is the cause of a great deal of disability. Today six to eight million Americans suffer from angina (pain in the chest that limits physical activity, as a result of partial occlusion of a coronary artery but short of a real heart attack), weakness, or shortness of breath after recovery from a heart attack. Ten percent of all persons over age 65 have such disabilities from coronary disease (Moriyama et al., 1971). Recently, bypass of obstructions in coronary arteries by surgical

---

* Besides coronary or arteriosclerotic heart disease, there are three other major categories of heart disease classified according to cause: hypertensive heart disease, congenital heart disease, and rheumatic heart disease. Each of these has quite different trends and presents different problems for health care delivery, policy, and planning. Other types of heart disease are either rapidly disappearing, such as syphilitic disease of the heart valves and aorta or tuberculous constrictive pericarditis, or else they are rare and poorly understood disorders, such as subendocardial fibrosis and nonrheumatic myocarditis.

grafts has gained great popularity. Although the procedure has had some success in reducing symptoms, it has not improved the overall mortality rate appreciably if the high surgical mortality rate is taken into account (Preston, 1977; Murphy et al., 1977).

With such high mortality rates and little evidence that clinical therapy can make such difference, the key problem is to prevent development of the underlying arteriosclerosis before coronary occlusion occurs (Ross, 1975). The fact that such tremendous variations in incidence are found among different groups encourages professionals to believe that effective measures can be taken to reduce its incidence and mortality (Marmot, 1975; Moriyama et al., 1971). For example, the death rate from CHD among males in Japan (age 45 to 64) is only one-sixth of that in the United States. There are differences of the same order of magnitude in CHD mortality between smokers and nonsmokers. Although genetic predisposition undoubtedly plays a role in CHD, four conditions have been identified as major risk factors contributing to increased incidence of CHD: cigarette smoking, rich diets high in cholesterol and other fats (meat, eggs and dairy products), high blood pressure, and diabetes (or prediabetic elevated blood sugar) (Kannel & Gordon, 1974). All these problems can potentially be controlled and their reduction has been shown to lower mortality rates by as much as 50%—even after evidence of arteriosclerotic disease has appeared. If the first three factors occur together, the risk of CHD is five to six times as high as in groups where they are absent (USPHS, 1979).

High blood pressure occurs in 15 to 20% of the United States adult population (USPHS, 1978). It is a major contributing risk factor in both CHD and strokes. Thus the indirect mortality from hypertension makes it a health problem of first magnitude. High blood pressure can arise from certain specific conditions: kidney disorders, congenital narrowing of the artery to a kidney, and certain hormone-secreting tumors of the adrenal gland and elsewhere (Beeson & McDermott, 1969). Where these specific defects occur, they can and should be detected and, if possible, corrected to prevent the eventual consequences of the high blood pressure on the heart, kidneys, and arteries of the brain.

However, far and away the largest percentage of cases today are so-called "essential" hypertension, that is, high blood pressure arising from no other identifiable biological cause (Eyer, 1975). It is widely believed that this kind of hypertension results from the stress of the modern competitive life style and from frustration due to blocked striving for achievement. Many of the same social factors that contribute to arteriosclerotic heart disease also influence the development of hypertension (Fejfar, 1967). High blood pressure is much more prevalent among blacks than whites, among the lower socioeconomic groups than middle or upper, and is sightly more common among females than males. Social and environmental rather than biological factors seem to be the crucial ultimate causes. There is indirect evidence that the incidence of high blood pressure has declined markedly during the past 20 years. For example, the mortality rate from hypertensive heart disease (as opposed to CHD) has declined by 50% during that period, long before effective hypertension treatment was widely employed (Moriyama et al., 1971). The reasons for this decline are not well understood but seem to be related to improved living standards.

Early detection and treatment of high blood pressure by antihypertensive drugs can appreciably decrease this risk element for CHD as well as for strokes (Veterans Administration, 1967, 1970). To have a major impact, systematic mass screening is required, plus careful follow-up, long-term supervision, and maintenance therapy (Weinstein & Stason, 1976). Demonstration programs where such services are provided have succeeded in reducing morbidity and mortality. Without such special efforts, however, routine screening alone in the context of ordinary clinical or preventive care programs has been much less effective. Thus, optimal prevention and treatment of both CHD and strokes would call for reorganization of the health care system to overcome the unsystematic and episodic orientation to screening and follow-up that now exists.

Several other factors also may influence the mortality and morbidity rates from CHD: sedentary life style, obesity, and stress. Population groups with a very active life style seem to have lower mortality rates from CHD, but very stringent and continued exercise programs are necessary to reduce the incidence appreciably in other groups (Breslow & Buell, 1960). Nevertheless, regular jogging may lower the incidence of recurrent heart attacks (Bruce, 1974). It is popularly believed that CHD is primarily an affliction of hard-driving, affluent executives, and in fact in the past there was some degree of positive correlation between social class and the incidence of CHD (Friedman & Rosenman, 1974). More recently, however, this relationship has disappeared or even reversed so that the incidence is slightly higher today among the working class than the upper classes (Cassel, 1969). Theories about the relationship between particular personality types or stress and CHD persist although most have not stood up to more careful analysis (Friedman & Rosenman, 1974; Paffenberger & Hale, 1975).

With the exception of high blood pressure, which requires long-term medical treatment and surveillance, decreasing the risk factors that contribute to CHD demands changes in life style and personal habits, especially diet and smoking (Ross, 1975). The most important role of health care in regard to this disease would be health education for prevention, and early detection together with programs of countermeasures. Yet clinical medicine's primary concern has been traditionally with treatment of already established diseases rather than with prevention. The actual role of most physicians today is either in short-term intensive care of persons hospitalized with acute myocardial infarctions (heart attacks) or in the care of the chronic, advanced stage of the disease by means of expensive maintenance, hospitalization, rehabilitation, or long-term nursing care (USDHEW, 1979).

HEALTH CARE OF THE ELDERLY— STROKES AND LONG-TERM CARE

Heart disease and cancer continue to be the major causes of death among senior citizens (age 65 and over), but in this age group the incidence of strokes also begins to climb rapidly. Strokes (cerebral vascular accidents) are the result of damage to some part of the brain due to occlusion of a blood vessel or rupture of one with bleeding into brain tissue. They produce partial paralysis and other neurological damage such as loss of speech or blindness. Multiple tiny "strokes" without a single incident massive enough to be noticed are probably the cause of much of the loss of memory, "dementia," or "senility" (degeneration of thinking ability) common in older persons. Occasionally strokes occur in younger persons as a result of the rupture of blood vessels (aneurysms) in the brain due to congenital defects, but the overwhelming portion results from the same kind of arteriosclerotic changes in the arteries of the brain that lead to coronary heart disease.

Strokes account for 10% of deaths in the United States, but there is an additional nonfatal stroke for each fatal one. Hospitalization is lengthy, and the rate of serious residual disability after such incidents is very high. Consequently strokes take up a larger proportion of health care expenses in relation to incidence than do heart attacks—6.3% of all direct costs in 1972 compared to 10% for heart disease, while the latter accounted for almost four times as many deaths. It is estimated that there are always one to two million Americans chronically disabled as a result of strokes (DeBakey, 1965). In 1977, 36% of nursing home beds were occupied by patients with diagnoses of stroke, arteriosclerosis, or chronic brain syndrome—most such cases probably result from the same basic pathological condition (USDHEW, 1979). On the other hand, since strokes tend to occur at an older age, the indirect cost from lost productivity is much lower from strokes than from heart disease (Cooper & Rice, 1976). Unlike CHD, the incidence of strokes is approximately the same for males and females. The age-adjusted incidence of strokes has been declining gradually but steadily for the past 50 years. High blood pressure is the major factor contributing to increased stroke risk and raises the probability of occurrence in all age groups about five times. The effect of smoking and diet are less clear than with CHD. The only known effective preventive measure in regard to strokes is the detection and long-term drug control of high blood pressure.

The major task of the health care system in dealing with stroke problems is the rehabilitation and maintenance care of patients who have residual paralysis. This requires intensive physiotherapy, occupational therapy, and the continued custodial or supportive care of those who are unable to return to an independent life, often involving nursing homes or supportive home care. The fact that our present system of clinical care is poorly organized to provide these functions promises to intensify these problems as the population continues to age.

NEW NEEDS FOR HEALTH CARE—
THE PARADOX OF PROGRESS

The new pattern of diseases that has emerged during the past 50 years has created a corresponding new set of health care needs typical of post-clinical medicine: growth in the *amount* of health care required, need for *different kinds* of health services than before, and need for *new organizational* structure of health care.

The decrease in infectious diseases and the new preponderance of chronic diseases and disabilities presents a "paradox of medical progress"—while mortality rates have decreased during this century, the amount of sickness in society has actually increased. For example, the number of bed disability days per capita per year increased from 6.3 in 1965 to 7.1 in 1978. The number of persons with limitation of activity due to chronic conditions grew from 9.8% in 1958 to 14.2% in 1978. Similarly the days of restricted activity per capita for health reasons increased from 15.6 in 1965 to 18.8 in 1978 (U.S. National Center for Health Statistics, 1977, 1978, 1979). This increased morbidity is reflected in the steady rise in the per capita utilization of clinical services. In 1900 there were 55 general hospital admissions annually per 1000 population. By 1950 the rate had doubled to 110 per 1000, and in 1977 it reached 163 per 1000 population. Similar changes have occurred in utilization of physicians' services. In 1930 it was estimated (Committee on the Costs of Medical Care, 1933) that the average American made 2.6 physician visits per year. In 1977 this had risen to 4.8 visits per year (USDHEW, 1979).

Undoubtedly part of this growth in health care utilization is due to causes other than sickness such as greater availability, easier financial access to care, unnecessary utilization as a result of maladapted organization of care, and use-inducing professional incentives. Such factors are considered in detail in Chapters 6, 8, 12, and 13. A significant amount of the increase, however, does reflect the real need for more services due to the growth in the actual amount of sickness in society at any time. This is largely a product of the greater prevalence of chronic diseases that extend over longer periods of time and create more person-days of illness. As noted, a major factor in the rising prevalence of chronic disease is the inceased number of aged persons in the population. The elderly suffer from more "degenerative diseases" like heart disease, strokes, disabling arthritis, as well as rising incidence of cancer. The large portion of the increased utilization due to senior citizens is seen from the fact that 27% of all health expenditures today are incurred by the 11% of our population over age 65 (Gibson, 1979).

Yet hospital admission and physician visit rates have risen in every age group except for those under 15 (USDHEW, 1980). This reflects the increased prevalence of chronic diseases in nearly all age groups. The increased frequencies of heart disease, cancer, strokes, and accidents are major contributors to need for prolonged care (McKeown, 1971). Ironically, improvements in clinical medicine are partly responsible for the growing prevalence of chronic illness by converting many previously fatal acute diseases into nonfatal chronic ones that require lifelong medical care or maintenance therapy. This adds to the number of persons who are sick at any given time. In many cases such maintenance therapy yields further useful and happy life in spite of the chronic illness with dependency on continuing treatment, and the result is a net gain for both the individual and society. Diabetics, for example, comprise one large group of such patients. As long as diabetics take their insulin conscientiously and carefully control their diets, they are able to lead essentially normal lives, although they are still more susceptible to early onset of certain degencrative disorders such as arteriosclerosis than are non-diabetics.

The expenditures that may be involved in maintenance of patients with otherwise fatal diseases can be enormous. It is only hinted at by estimates of subsidies that may be necessary under the Medicare program for patients requiring hemodialysis and/or kidney transplants to substitute for lost kidney function. The cost of this one program will be over one billion dollars in 1980, and this is only the tip of the iceberg (Rettig, 1979). For example, a major breakthrough in the feasibility of organ transplants or satisfactory mechanical heart substitutes could create a catastrophic budgetary crisis in health care. As more such expensive life-saving techniques become possible, there will be tremendous pressure on Congress to provide financial support for everyone who can be maintained by such technology. In still other cases, such as traumatic "brain death" or terminal cancer, life may be extended by highly sophisticated technology, prolonging an illness at great financial and personal cost to patient, family, and society without any hope of returning the patient to a useful life. Some very difficult ethical and social priority decisions may be necessary concerning the development and use of such expensive services in coming years (Katz & Capron, 1975).

Another reason for increased utilization of health services is the higher expectation about the benefits to be obtained from medical care. This creates an escalation of demand for care out of proportion to the actual increase in the amount of illness in the population. This "revolution of rising expectations" (Somers & Somers, 1961) is just as inherently a part of post-clinical medicine as is the increased prevalence of chronic illnesses. In the process of overcoming most infectious diseases and many other acute medical and surgical problems, medicine and public health made use of many sophisticated scientific discoveries and techniques. These technological successes captured the public's interest much more than the improvements in living standards, nutrition, and sanitation which undoubtedly were responsible for more of the improvement in health. Highly publicized, dramatic medical interventions such as heart transplants, artificial life support systems for critically ill patients, and massive surgical or chemotherapeutic attacks on cancer cases have inflated the public image of potential effectiveness of medical treatment—whether such advanced technologies have any significant impact on the overall outcome of these diseases or not. Popularized by the mass media, medical science came to be viewed as a panacea, intensifying a widespread inclination to hope for technological solutions to problems and raising unrealistic hope in regard to medicine's capacity to improve longevity and the quality of life (Kisch, 1974).

Certain features of American society have augmented this development of growing public demand for medical services. The rising affluence of the economy after World War II and the transition to a post-industrial society placed growing emphasis on the service sector (Bell, 1973). As the basic provision of food, clothing, shelter, and industrial commodities came to demand less of the total national production, it was possible to concentrate more effort on the residual problems like health care and other personal services that were once viewed as luxuries primarily for the well-to-do. The development of many voluntary "health lobbies" also enhanced the political popularity of these issues (Strickland, 1972a; Spingarn, 1976) and helped channel billions of public and private dollars into medical research. In waging campaigns to raise the funds for research and new services, such lobbies often evoked the illusion of virtual immortality just around the corner. This was exaggerated by an uncritical faith in science and unrealistic hope for the potential of technological progress held by many people during this period.

These overly high expectations intensified the growth of demand for guaranteed access to medical services. This was expressed in collective bargaining for health insurance to assure financial access (Chapter 11) and political pressure to make the most advanced technological services available to all through construction of new facilities and training of more manpower. Federal funding through programs like Medicaid, Medicare, and neighborhood health centers removed additional barriers to medical care. The new expectations encouraged the laity to espouse the medical profession's perspective in regard to diseases and to accept uncritically the judgments of health professions about all matters relating to health care. This provided a virtual blank-check endorsement to recommendations for expansion of facilities or acquisition of new equipment. Public opinion promoted the general assumption that the most specialized and technologically sophisticated care possible was the best. It encouraged the continuing growth of specialism and residency training programs without critical assessment of true need (Chapter 6).

Some health professionals have sought to encompass certain behavioral or social problems such as alcoholism, drug addiction, and some learning disabilities in children within the realm of medicine. Hoping that such problems would be treated more humanely as diseases than as social deviance, they encouraged "medicalization" of many behavioral problems. Any physiological component in the problem served as a justification for classifying them as "diseases" and therefore in the realm of medical care. In many instances laymen go even further than physicians in urging the application of medical approaches to social or behavioral problems because they are less aware of the limitations of the medical techniques. The tendency of the public to favor medical solutions to such problems often thrusts health professionals into a position of dealing with situations for which there are no well established medical treatments and where the primary factors are actually behavioral, social, or even political. The adoption of the medical perspective by the laity can serve as an excuse to abdicate personal or public responsibility by defining certain conditions as "diseases" and placing the task of handling them in the lap of the medical profession (Szasz, 1961, 1970).

Urbanization and sociogeographic mobility have led to the breakup of extended families and close-knit supportive communities, making it difficult to care for aging parents at home. The resulting demand for nursing homes as a means of caring for them has been justified by defining "senility" as a disease. The medicalization of care for the aging precludes the planning and organization of social and personal support services, which might be possible if the moral dilemma were more openly faced (Kasl, 1972). These same changes in social structure also intensify the demand for physicians to be personal counselors and sources of general social support, which are not easily obtained elsewhere in our depersonalized society. The unrealistic expectation that such problems of post-industrial society can simply be turned over to medicine neglects the underlying causes, which have to be dealt with at the socioeconomic and political levels. The hope that they can be overcome by pure technological means defers the personal and public responsibility of facing the more difficult dilemmas of socioeconomic tradeoffs necessary to cope with these problems or of making the behavioral and life-style changes needed to improve health.*

In order to meet this rising demand for care, the health care system must be able to supply an increasing amount of services. To keep the cost of the increase affordable, we must find ways to do so more efficiently. With so much *necessary* increase in utilization, it is all the more important to reduce waste and *unnecessary* utilization. We return to these questions in Chapters 12, 13, and 14.

Besides demand for *more* care, today's new pattern of diseases creates a

---

* There is also danger that the public's exaggerated expectations regarding the medical profession's abilities may change into disillusion, dissatisfaction, and alienation when these expectations cannot be met. This discrepancy between expectation and reality is probably a major factor in the growing impatience, suspicion, and open hostility toward the health care system in recent years and may well be an important cause of the increasing incidence of malpractice litigation and escalating cost of malpractice insurance.

set of needs for new *kinds* of care quite different from the services provided by the traditional system of health care. In earlier times when most diseases had a clear acute onset, the task of clinical medicine was set in motion by the patient's arriving in search of relief from symptoms. The job of the physician was to make a diagnosis, determine the cause and intervene, if possible, to correct the cause and restore the patient to health. Today this model is applicable for only a small fraction of health care. Because of the slow onset, symptoms are often present only at a stage of the disease when it is too late to reverse its course. The cumulative or irreversible nature of the underlying pathological process means that *care* (compensatory support and maintenance) rather than *cure* by removing the cause or repairing the defect is usually the only clinical strategy possible (Cochrane, 1971). In order to have an impact on diseases with a long asymptomatic onset, clinical medicine needs to adopt much more of the preventive medicine approach. Regular periodic screening for early detection of developing disorders and counseling to encourage healthier life style require as much emphasis as traditional diagnosis and therapy (Baric, 1969; Schenthal, 1960). Where there is evidence of early abnormalities such as high blood pressure or elevated serum cholesterol, specific preventive countermeasures need to be instituted. Although such preventive services could be and often are provided in separate programs organized exclusively for this purpose, there are good reasons to integrate them more completely into clinical care.

Pediatrics is the sector of medicine where this model is already best developed. The importance to children of preventive care, such as immunization and early detection and correction of abnormalities in growth and development, always gave the preventive medicine approach an important role in pediatrics. Because the incidence of traditional diseases declined most dramatically in the pediatric age group, pediatricians were left with more time to increase their emphasis on preventive services. The general success of preventive care in pediatric practice demonstrates how effectively it can be given within the framework of an ongoing primary care relationship. Many children who would never be brought to special programs receive preventive services in this way. Patient motivation to seek preventive care is in general much lower than for clinical care. Pediatricians use the occasion of unimportant clinical visits to update preventive care for their patients. Mothers honor notices for an inconvenient preventive checkup for the sake of the ongoing relationship with their pediatrician for future clinical care.

Preventive care for adults would also be more reliably attended to within the framework of an ongoing primary care relationship. If it depends on the resolve of the patient to visit a preventive program for those services alone, postponement is much more likely. Unlike childhood immunization, however, for many forms of adult preventive care a single procedure does not take care of the problem. Screening is only the first step. Any positive finding must be referred for further diagnostic testing and appropriate action. These necessarily take place in a clinical setting. When screening is separate from follow-up services, there is a much greater chance that the urgency of the next steps may not be communicated and that necessary follow-up may not take place.

Hypertension screening and treatment is a good example. Of patients found to have significant blood pressure elevation by routine screening programs, three-fourths were still hypertensive at a later screening examination—one-fourth because they had stopped taking prescribed medication without the advice of a physician and half because their drugs were insufficient to keep them under adequate control (U.S. National Center for Health Statistics, 1976). By contrast, a special program with intensive follow-up and educational efforts was able to achieve adequate control in 80% of the cases (USDHEW, 1977). If similar intensive follow-up were built into an ongoing primary care relation with a personal physician, it seems likely that even better success rates could be achieved.

The problem of long-term maintenance therapy for patients with chronic progressive or irreversible diseases requires much the same integration of preventive care into clinical services. Patients with chronic diseases are particularly prone to develop complications that may exacerbate their disabilities. Diabetics are a good example. Besides insulin regulation and dietary control, it is equally vital to prevent foot infections due to arteriosclerosis of the legs, urinary infections in the face of poor blood sugar control, and hypertension secondary to kidney damage. Regular preventive surveillance programs and patient education can significantly reduce these complications.

The chronic disability associated with much of today's disease means that supportive care and improvement in the quality of life are as important as intervention of the traditional clinical kind (Sun Valley Forum; 1972). To meet these challenges medicine also has to modify its approach to care. Treatment today is often largely a holding action or a patch-up operation where the principle objectives are to slow the progress of the disease, to alleviate symptoms, and to help patients live as well as possible within the limitations of their disabilities. This calls for very different strategies of care than in the heyday of curative clinical medicine. Effective treatment for these disorders requires dependable patient management, maintenance, and social support that provides for many diverse aspects of a patient's life needs. For example, after acute care a stroke patient may require physiotherapy, speech therapy, and occupational therapy as an inpatient. After hospital discharge he may need homemaking assistance, nutritional support, social counseling, and aid in finding living arrangements that allow a maximum degree of independence. Services or assistance are needed for whatever activities of daily living the patient or family alone cannot accomplish. Adequate surveillance and follow-up must be assured so that the patient does not develop unnoticed, irreversible muscle contractures, bed sores, or social withdrawal and deterioration out of proportion to the actual physical impairment. The support that physicians give patients to increase their functional capacity and comfort or to help them cope with their illness and disability is as crucial as the purely technical therapy.

Even if major progress in disease prevention is achieved, increased longevity is not immortality, and all body systems are not apt to reach their mortal limit at the same time. Thus, short of a morally unacceptable decision not to treat failure of body systems after specified ages, we will inevitably have increasing numbers of chronically ill patients requiring long-term maintenance and support. It is necessary to restructure health care to provide more effective and efficient maintenance for these chronically ill patients (Chapter 9).

Few physicians in private practice today have the resources at hand to provide the supportive services or assure the surveillance of preventive and maintenance care needed for post-clinical medicine. Consequently, a *new organization* of health care is also needed. As the importance of preventive care grows, the need for its integration into clinical medicine increases. Easy availability of primary care is essential for its preventive and health promotional potential through the ongoing personal physician relationship—as well as to meet consumer demand for access to physician services (Chapter 8). To assure necessary screening, health surveillance, and health education functions, however, more than simple availability of primary care is needed. Continuity of the patient's relationship to the system of care would require permanent enrollment for the kind of records and information system needed for notification and repeated attempts at follow-up. These are essential when preventive services are missed or when positive findings are not followed up. Similarly, to provide supportive services for patients with disabilities, something more than a solo or fragmented group practice arrangement is needed.

Many health care analysts have pointed out the problem of inappropriate utilization of services, its cost and even danger to patients. A major element of the problem is the use of inappropriate levels of care. Hospitalization is used where the care could be given just as well on an ambulatory basis. Institutional long-term care is used where supportive services at home would be adequate and more beneficial to the patient's morale and social well-being. Physician time is used for services that could be provided by skilled paraprofessionals. Only a system that includes a complete spectrum of such services and includes incentives to optimize their use is apt to improve the present waste and inappropriateness of services.

A well-organized comprehensive *team* system of care would be appropriate using nurses, physician-associates, home-care workers, technicians, physical and occupational therapists, and social workers to provide much of the routine treatment and health surveillance. The special diagnostic and treatment expertise of highly trained physicians would be used only where these skills are really needed (Glazier, 1973). For effective coordination these team members would have to be linked by a comprehensive administrative system. Clinical health care would become as much a planning, surveillance, and integration (information processing) problem as a diagnostic and treatment problem in the narrower sense. As with any complex planning and management problem, it could no longer be run by a single individual, like the solo physician, attempting to make all the decisions. A system of divided responsibility and decision-making would have to be employed merging the different kinds of expertise and coordinating them by means of effective patient management information systems (e.g., computerized record and scheduling systems; Barnett, 1972).*

Health maintenance organizations (HMOs) are one such organizational model (Chapter 10). A number of health-care experts (Glazier, 1973; Rutstein, 1974; Maxman, 1976) have proposed even more sweeping reorganizations of clinical care into comprehensive, integrated systems with team practice and computerized guidance systems for patient and community health care management. Such reorganization would be necessary to bring about appreciable improvement in health in the face of the problems of post-clinical medicine—as the factors influencing disease continue to increase along present trends. Reorganization of health services along these lines, however, faces obstacles and problems that are formidable.

MISMATCH OF THE PRESENT SYSTEM OF HEALTH CARE WITH TODAY'S HEALTH PROBLEMS

The health care system has undergone tremendous changes in the past 50 years as a result of the revolution in medical science. But in many ways the product of these changes is poorly matched to the needs of post-clinical medicine. Until the end of the last century, medicine had little to offer technically that could make much difference in the outcome of diseases. The major function of practitioners was using their priestly mandate to allay the anxiety of illness by reassuring patients and making it possible to carry on a workable social order in the face of the disruption created by illness (Chapter 3). Today, medicine has a technology that can make a real difference in the outcome of some diseases. The application of this powerful technology has become the primary concern of medical practice (Chapter 6). The personal and social supportive functions that dominated the former physician role have fallen victim to the technological revolution in medicine.

Yet, managing today's chronic illness optimally would require more rather than less attention to the nontechnical needs of patients in order to improve the quality of their lives in the face of continuing disability. Chronic illness often leads to alienation from family, friends, and social groups (Chapter

* The advantages of the information and surveillance systems necessary to implement the chronic care management would have to be weighed against the dangers of potential invasion of privacy and possible unwanted organizational intervention in the lives of individuals, communities, and society.

9). The personal counseling and social expediting role of the health professionals is important in helping patients to maintain normal social interaction up to the limits of their physical abilities. Chronic illness calls for aid in arranging living situations in which patients can function as well and as independently as possible. Lacking a comprehensive system of care to make these arrangements, physicians need to serve as ombudsmen to expedite the necessary supporting services.

Because of the increased emphasis of physicians and institutions on technology, utilization of high-technology care is far out of proportion to its effectiveness in improving health outcomes. This is very costly and sometimes even dangerous to the patient. Whatever technology is available for diagnosis or treatment of a condition tends to be used whether its efficacy and need have been demonstrated or not. The cost-benefit relationship of a procedure is virtually disregarded in making decisions about use of such care. Professional standards and practice attitudes demand that whatever *can* be done *must* be done—the so-called technological imperative (Fuchs, 1972). This leads to an inappropriate allocation of the available resources and health care budget, particularly for the care of patients with chronic illnesses. Massive technological intervention in the treatment of such diseases seldom makes a major difference in their long-term course and does little to improve the quality of patients' lives (Chapter 10). Yet, the major part of health expenditure goes for such services while resources are often lacking for the maintenance services that could significantly add to patients' well-being.

Parallel to the developing emphasis on the technological approach to medical care, a number of shifts have occurred in the structure of the health system that are poorly suited to today's health problems. Emphasis on high-technology care inevitably leads to growth in specialization. The large percentage of physicians trained as specialists is a direct result of the need to limit the range of complex medical technology one has to master in order to apply it to very particular problems. Eighty percent of physicians today list themselves as specialists compared to only 20% in 1930 (Chapter 6). Yet today's diseases call for increased emphasis on primary care into which preventive care, surveillance, and long-term maintenance for chronic illness can be built. The continuing trend toward specialization means fewer primary care physicians to provide such integrated care. In particular there is a shortage of primary physicians with specialized training for geriatric care. The abundance of specialists also increases the utilization of the technology that they are trained to employ—in many cases clearly beyond the real need for its use. The oversupply of surgeons, for example, perhaps the most technology oriented group of all, very probably contributes to the incidence of unnecessary surgery (Chapters 8 and 12).

Technology oriented care concentrates attention on the *acute episodes* of a disease rather than the longer course of illness or the maintenance of the patient. The scientific model of disease, within which today's technology has developed, assumes a definable, clearly caused episode or specific physio-logical defect to be diagnosed and remedied. Medical technology is most effective in dealing with such episodes of illness, especially where the cause is reversible through specific intervention. Technology oriented care, there-fore, tends to keep physicians focused on the episodes of illness. Yet, a cen-tral requirement of post-clinical medicine is the long-range comprehensive view of illness to enhance the preventive approach and to assure continuity for maintenance—precisely to minimize such acute episodes in the course of chronic diseases. Acute episodes do arise within chronic illnesses for which high-technology care is appropriate. Certain stages of some cancers can be aided by complicated surgery, chemotherapy, or radiation. Acute episodes in heart disease may need intensive specialized treatment. Diagnosis of cer-tain disorders can be assisted by complex procedures to determine the na-ture of the illness and enable more appropriate therapy. Yet, for most care of chronic illness today, this sophisticated technological approach is in-creasingly less appropriate. The major elements of care that can contribute appreciably to a patient's overall well-being are continuity, surveillance to prevent complications, and supportive care to improve the quality of life. All these require focusing on the long-term course of the patient and his illness rather than on the individual acute episode using specialized inter-vention. The technological orientation of most modern medicine com-pletely reverses this emphasis by focusing on the disease process and its acute episodes, which it is best equipped to treat. In so doing it leads to neglect of the overall course of the patient, representing a serious mismatch with today's needs for care.

The complexity of medical technology has encouraged *fragmentation* of the health care system into many specialized units for different elements of medical care (Chapter 8). Hospital clinics and medical specialties are the most obvious examples, but the same problem permeates other parts of the health system as well, for example, the financing methods and planning mechanisms (Chapters 10 and 11). There is no overall means of coordinating these components into a unified whole for ensuring a complete spectrum of services needed by any patient. Patients are left to negotiate their way through the maze with little guidance and often fail to get the needed ser-vices, adequate follow-up, or supportive care to improve their ability to cope in the face of chronic illnesses. Preventive services are provided in special-ized programs that often have little relation to the clinical services essential for follow-up. Supportive services like social work and homemaking op-erate out of separate organizations which must be specially solicited when needed—if someone thinks about it. Long-term care is poorly integrated into the system so that nursing homes become dead-end custodial institu-tions rather than part of a continuum for integrating the disabled patient into society to as great an extent as possible (Schulman & Galanter, 1976; Chapter 9).

The cost and complexity of high-technology care has required its *central-*

ization into hospitals. The emphasis on the use of technology has therefore meant increased concentration of medical practice into hospitals and over-use of hospital care. Yet, precisely the opposite—greater availability and use of ambulatory care—is needed for the maintenance and supportive care of chronic illnesses. Forty percent of health care expenditures today go for hospital care (Chapter 12). Thirty-five percent of physicians now practice in hospital based settings (Chapter 8). As a result fewer office based physicians are available to provide the kind of primary preventive and supportive care needed. The technology oriented approach drives far more medical care into hospital settings than is necessary. Comparable patient groups enrolled in HMOs, for example, can be cared for with only half as much hospitalization as those in the standard organization of care (Luft, 1978).

The overabundance of specialists and the centralization of technology into hospitals, both of which tend to be located in urban areas, produces serious *maldistribution* of medical resources (Chapter 8). Because availability of services largely determines their utilization, there is overuse of services in some areas and underservice in others. This misallocation of health manpower and resources contributes to the soaring cost of care while leaving tremendous gaps in availability of services. As a result resources are also overcommitted for medical care in relation to other sectors of the economy where their use might be more effective in improving the health of the population. A prime example is the unbridled growth of hospital budgets where an increasing portion of health care dollars are expended (Chapter 12). The organizational mismatch also exacerbates the tendency to use inappropriate levels of care: too much hospital care, too little ambulatory; too much nursing home care, too little home care; too much intensive care, too little supportive service. Thus the mismatch between the structure of the health care system and the patern of diseases profoundly effects virtually every aspect of health care. It lies at the root of many of the more obvious problems facing health policy makers today: overspecialization, maldistribution of manpower and resources, fragmentation of care, overuse of hospital care, unnecessary utilization of services, and runaway costs.

Why did such a mismatch arise and why does it continue to intensify when it is apparently dysfunctional for the needs of the majority of patients and for society? There is no *single* reason for this perverse state of affairs. A number of interrelated causes that reinforce each other are responsible. Collectively this mutual reinforcement creates a momentum that carries the system in a direction little influenced by the needs of society.

First, scientific medicine and its associated technology contributed to the conquest of infectious diseases and have enabled dramatic successful clinical intervention in some other circumstances. These successes endowed the technological approach with a prestige far out of proportion to its actual continuing contribution to the improvement of health. The resulting prestige, the associated public expectation, and the financial rewards that accompany it are the driving incentives governing the behavior of the medical profession. That prestige continues despite the fact that the pattern of diseases for which it was most successful has long since disappeared. Attempting to apply the same technological approach to today's dominant diseases usually leads instead to the development of what Lewis Thomas (1972) has called "half-way technologies." These are techniques that palliate symptoms or partially substitute for impaired physiological functions without really changing the course of the disease. Based on a specific-cause model inappropriate for today's diseases, they use a quasi-curative orientation to treatment without being able to effect a cure. Confronting such situations, the technological approach is costly and inefficient. By focusing ever more intensive treatment on the effects and symptoms without eliminating or fundamentally repairing the underlying causes, it is possible to expend almost limitless resources (Chapters 10 and 12).

Second, almost every aspect of the present health care system reinforces the specialized, high-technology approach to practice: medical education, the professional prestige system, financial incentives, the organization of the health system increasingly centered around hospital practice, the reimbursement system. The medical profession has developed a professional socialization process during medical education, a professional reward and sanction system, and vested interests in the specialized technology, all of which perpetuate and intensify the technological orientation (Chapters 6 and 8). Hospitals as organizations built around the use of complex medical technology likewise have an institutional momentum that continues to drive medical practice in the direction of increasing utilization of technology (Chapter 7). The interaction between physicians and hospitals reinforces both these tendencies (Chapter 8).

Finally, because of the unpredictable, high cost of hospitalization and sophisticated high-technology medical care, a system of health insurance was developed to protect patients from these potentially catastrophic financial burdens. The evolution of the insurance system as the principal means of paying for care and the unique reimbursement system created a financing system that further reinforced the use of hospitals and high-technology specialized care (Chapter 12). The system of reimbursing hospitals on the basis of their costs incurred in the treatment of beneficiaries provides them open-ended revenues with little restriction on their level of expenditures. This removes any financial brakes on hospital investment in increasingly sophisticated technology—whether it is shown to be cost-effective in treatment or not. As a result, hospitals compete for patients and staff physicians by trying to offer the most sophisticated facilities and equipment rather than competing through lower prices (Chapter 12). Similarly, physicians are reimbursed on the basis of their customary fees, which tends to reward hospital visits and high-technology procedures at a higher rate per unit time than office visits or simple hands-on procedures. The resulting financial incentives encourage greater use of high-technology care (Blumberg, 1979).

Because of this array of mutually reinforcing forces it is unlikely that the present inappropriate orientation and health care organizations will change unless major changes are made in the professional incentive structure, organization of the delivery system, and reimbursement methods. Left to their own course the present trends, both in the pattern of chronic diseases and in the nature of medical care, are likely to continue. This will intensify the functional mismatch unless vigorous measures are taken to intervene in the present dynamics. Policy makers must deal with these deep-seated roots of the more apparent problems if they are to succeed in improving the function of the health system. Simply pouring additional resources into the present system will accomplish little except to increase costs (Auster et al., 1969; Benham & Benham, 1975). They will be absorbed without significant improvement in services or health outcomes unless something is done to bring the health system into a better fit with needs and to solve its structural problems (McKeown, 1976, 1976a).

Achieving the kind of reorganization called for by the problems of post-clinical medicine would entail overcoming serious professional and political obstacles. Some obvious problems stem from the vested interests of physicians, hospitals, and insurance companies, but other barriers to change are more invisibly embedded in the dynamics of the established system, for example, the cultural role of physicians, their commitment to a disease model less than ideal for today's problems, and a financing system riddled with internal inconsistencies. Even if it were clear what the ideal health care system should be, we do not have the option of starting over *de novo* to construct it according to some preconceived plan. The internal dynamics of the medical profession and of the organization and financing of health care, as they now exist, create powerful forces reinforcing the present trends. Any realistic plans to reform the system must take these forces into account. Much of the rest of this book is therefore devoted to analyzing the basis of these trends so that in the final chapters we can attempt to assess the chances of success for various reforms that are being considered.

REFERENCES

Abelson, Philip H., "Changing Climate for Medicine," *Science*, 188:1888, 1975.

Anderson, Odin W., "Infant Mortality and Social and Cultural Factors: Historical Trends and Current Patterns," in Jaco, E. Gartly, Ed., *Patients, Physicians and Illness*, New York: Free Press, 1958.

Auster, Richard, Levenson, Irving, and Sarachek, Deborah, "The Production of Health: An Exploratory Study," *Journal of Human Resources*, 4:411–436, 1969.

Baker, Susan P., and Haddon, William, "Reducing Injuries and Their Results: The Scientific Approach," *Health and Society*, 52:377, 1974.

Baker, Susan P., and Dietz, Park E., "Injury Prevention," in *Healthy People: The Surgeon General's Report on Health Promotion and Disease Prevention, Background Papers*, Vol. 2, Washington, D.C.: USPHS No. 79–55071A, 1979.

Baric, L., "Recognition of the 'At-Risk' Role: A Means to Influence Health Behavior," *International Journal of Health Education*, 12:24–34, 1969.

Barnett, G. Octo, *Computer Stored Ambulatory Record*, Boston: Massachusetts General Hospital, Laboratory of Computer Science, 1972.

Becker, Marshall H., Ed., *The Health Belief Model and Personal Behavior*, Thorofare, N.J.: Slack, 1974.

Beeson, Paul B., and McDermott, Walsh, *Textbook of Medicine*, Philadelphia: Saunders, 1969.

Bell, Daniel, *The Coming of Post-Industrial Society: A Venture in Social Forecasting*, New York: Basic Books, 1973.

Belloc, Nedra B., "Relationship of Health Practices and Mortality," *Preventive Medicine*, 2:67, 1973.

Belloc, Nedra B., and Breslow, Lester, "Relationship of Physical Health Status and Health Practices," *Preventive Medicine*, 1:409, 1972.

Ben-David, J., "The Professional Role of the Physician in Bureaucratized Medicine, A Study in Role Conflict," *Human Relations*, 11:255–274, 1958.

Benham, Lee, and Benham, Alexandra, "The Impact of Incremental Medical Services on Health Status, 1963–1970," in Andersen, R., Kravitz, J., and Andersen, O., Eds., *Equity in Health Services*, Cambridge: Ballinger, 1975.

Berg, Robert L., Browning, Francis E., Hill, John G., and Wenkert, Walter, "Assessing the Health Care Needs of the Aged," *Health Services Research*, 4:36–59, 1970.

Blumberg, Mark S., "Rational Provider Prices: An Incentive for Improved Health Delivery," in G. K. Chacko, Ed., *Health Handbook*, Amsterdam: North Holland, 1978.

Breslow, Lester, "A Quantitative Approach to the World Health Organization Definition of Health: Physical, Mental and Social Well-Being," *International Journal of Epidemiology*, 1:347, 1972.

Breslow, Lester, and Buell, Phillip, "Mortality from Coronary Heart Disease and Physical Activity of Work in California," *Journal of Chronic Disease*, 11:421–444, 1960.

Bruce, Robert A., "The Benefits of Physical Training for Patients with Coronary Heart Disease," in Franz J. Ingelfinger, Richard V. Ebert, Maxwell Finland, and Arnold S. Relman, Eds., *Controversy in Internal Medicine, II*, Philadelphia: Saunders, 1974.

Buell, Philip, and Breslow, Lester, "Mortality from Coronary Heart Disease in California: Men Who Work Long Hours," *Journal of Chronic Diseases*, 11:615–626, 1960.

Cairns, John, "Cancer: The Case for Preventive Strategies," in *Healthy People: The Surgeon General's Report on Health Promotion and Disease Prevention, Background Papers*, Vol. 2, Washington, D.C.: USPHS No. 79–55071A, 1979.

Cassel, Eric J., "New and Emergent Diseases," in Kilbourne, E., and Smillie, W., *Human Ecology and Public Health*, London: Macmillan, 1969.

Coase, R., "The Problem of Social Cost," *Journal of Law and Economics*, No. 3, 1960.

Cochrane, A., *Effectiveness and Efficiency*, London: The Nuffield Provincial Hospitals Trust, 1971.

Comfort, Alex J., *The Process of Ageing*, New York: Signet, 1964.

Committee on the Costs of Medical Care, *Medical Care for the American People*, Chicago, Ill.: University of Chicago Press (Reprinted, USDHEW, 1970), 1932.

Cooper, Barbara S., and Rice, Dorothy P., "The Economic Cost of Illness Revisited," *Social Security Bulletin*, (February): 21–36, 1976.

Dauer, Carl C., Korns, Robert F., and Schuman, Leonard M., *Infectious Diseases*, Cambridge: Harvard University Press, 1968.

DeBakey, Michael, *President's Commission on Heart Disease, Cancer and Stroke, A Na-*

tional Program to Conquer Heart Disease, Cancer and Stroke, Washington, D.C.: Government Printing Office, 1964.

Defensive Medicine Project, "The Medical Malpractice Threat: A Study of Defensive Medicine," *Duke Law Journal,* December: 939–993, 1971.

Dever, G. E. Alan, "An Epidemiological Model for Health Policy Analysis," *Social Indicator Research,* 2:453–466, 1976.

Donabedian, Avedis, "An Examination of Some Directions in Health Care Policy," *American Journal of Public Health,* 63:243, 1973.

Elinson, Jack, Ed., "Sociomedical Health Indicator," *International Journal of Health Services,* 6: entire issue, 1976.

Engel, George L., "The Need for a New Medical Model: A Challenge for Biomedicine," *Science,* 196:129–136, 1977.

Erhardt, Carl L., and Berlin, Joyce E., *Mortality and Morbidity in the United States,* Cambridge: Harvard University Press, 1974.

Eyer, Joseph, "Hypertension as a Disease of Modern Society," *International Journal of Health Services,* 5:539–558, 1975.

Fein, Rashi, "Some Healthy Policy Issues: One Economist's View," *Public Health Reports,* 90:387, 1975.

Feinstein, A., "Symptoms as an Index of Biological Behaviour and Prognosis in Human Cancer," *Nature,* 109:241, 1966.

Fejfar, Zdenek, "Some Aspects of the Epidemiology of Arterial Hypertension," in Stamler, J., Stamler, R., and Pullman, T., Eds., *The Epidemiology of Hypertension,* New York: Grune & Stratton, 1967.

Ford, Amasa B., *Urban Health in America,* London: Oxford University Press, 1976.

Frank, J., "Mind-Body Interactions in Illness and Healing," presented at the May Lectures, *Alternative Futures for Medicine,* April 4, 1975, Airlie House, Airlie, Virginia, 1975.

Freymann, John G., *The American Health Care System: Its Genesis and Trajectory,* New York: Medcom Press, 1974.

Friedman, Meyer, and Rosenman, Ray H., *Type-A Behavior and Your Heart,* New York: Knopf, 1974.

Fuchs, Victor R., Ed., *Essays in the Economics of Health and Medical Care,* New York: Columbia University Press, 1972.

Fuchs, Victor R., *Who Shall Live?: Health, Economics, and Social Choice,* New York: Basic Books, 1974.

Gibson, R. M., "National Health Expenditures, 1978," *Health Care Finance Administration Review,* 1(1):1–36, 1979.

Glazier, William H., "The Task of Medicine," *Scientific American,* 228: 1973.

Hammond, E. C., "Smoking in Relation to Death Rates of One Million Men and Women," in *National Cancer Institute Monograph,* 19:127–204, Bethesda: National Cancer Institute, 1966.

Harman, W., "New Images of Man: What to Do until the New Paradigm Arrives," presented at the May Lectures, *Alternative Futures for Medicine,* April 4, 1975, Airlie House, Airlie, Virginia, 1975.

Hiatt, Howard H., "Protecting the Medical Commons: Who is Responsible?" *New England Journal of Medicine,* 293:235, 1975.

Higginson, J., "A Hazardous Society? The Role of Epidemiology in Determining the Individual versus Group Risk in Modern Societies," *American Journal of Public Health,* 66:359, 1976.

Hilleboe, Herman E., "Preventing Future Shock: Health Developments in the 1960s and Imperatives for the 1970s," *American Journal of Public Health*, **62**:136, 1972.

Holton, Gerald, "On the Role of Themata in Scientific Thought," *Science*, **188**:328–338, 1975.

Iskrant, Albert P., and Joliet, Paul V., *Accidents and Homicide*, Cambridge, Mass.: Harvard University Press, 1968.

Jenkins, C. David, Rosenman, Ray H., and Zuzanski, Stephen J., "Prediction of Clinical Coronary Heart Disease by a Test for Coronary-Prone Behavior Pattern," *New England Journal of Medicine*, **290**:1271–1275, 1974.

John E. Fogarty, International Center for Advance Study in the Health Sciences, *Preventive Medicine, U.S.A.*, New York: Prodist, 1976.

Kannel, W. B., and Gordon, T., Eds., *The Framingham Study, An Epidemiological Investigation of Cardiovascular Disease*, Section 30, Washington, D.C.: USDHEW (NIH) 74–599, 1974.

Kasl, Stanislav V., "Physical and Mental Health Effects of Involuntary Relocation and Institutionalization on the Elderly—a Review," *American Journal of Public Health*, **62**: 377–384, 1972.

Kass, Edward H., "Infectious Disease and Social Change," *Journal of Infectious Diseases*, **123**(1):110–114, 1971.

Katz, Jay, and Capron, Alexander M., *Catastrophic Diseases: Who Decides What?* New York: Russell Sage Foundation, 1975.

Kelman, Sander, "Toward the Political Economy of Medical Care," *Inquiry*, **8**(3):30–38, 1971.

Kessner, David M., *Infant Death: An Analysis by Maternal Risk and Health Care*, Washington, D.C.: Institute of Medicine, National Academy of Sciences, 1973.

Kessner, David M., et al., "Assessing Health Quality—The Case for Tracers," *New England Journal of Medicine*, **288**:189, 1973.

Kessner, David M., et al., *Contrasts in Health Status, 3: Assessment of Medical Care for Children*, Washington, D.C.: Institute of Medicine, 1974.

Kilbourne, Edwin D., and Smilie, Wilson G., *Human Ecology and Public Health*, London: Macmillan, 1971.

Kisch, A., "The Health Care System and Health: Some Thoughts on a Famous Misalliance," *Inquiry*, **11**:269, 1974.

Kitagawa, Evelyn M., and Hauser, Philip M., *Differential Mortality in the United States: A Study in Socioeconomic Epidemiology*, Cambridge: Harvard University Press, 1973.

Laframboise, Hubert L., "Health Policy; Breaking it Down into More Manageable Segments," *Journal of the Canadian Medical Association*, (February 3): 1973.

Lalonde, Marc, *A New Perspective on the Health of Canadians: A Working Document*, Ottawa: Government of Canada, 1974.

Last, John M., and White, Kerr L., "The Content of Medical Care in Primary Practice," *Medical Care*, **7**:41–48, 1969.

Leavell, Hugh K., and Clark, E. Gurney, *Preventive Medicine for the Doctor in His Community: An Epidemiologic Approach*, New York: McGraw-Hill, 1958.

Lehmann, Phyllis, and Kalmar, Vicki, "Improving the Quality of the Work Environment," in *Healthy People: The Surgeon General's Report on Health Promotion and Disease Prevention: Background Papers*, Vol. 2 Washington, D.C.: USPHS No. 79–55071A, 1979.

Lerner, Monroe, and Anderson, Odin W., *Health Progress in the United States, 1900–1960*, Chicago: University of Chicago Press, 1963.

Leventhal, Howard, "Fear Communications in the Acceptance of Preventive Health Practices," *Bulletin of the New York Academy of Medicine*, **41**:1144–1167, 1965.

Lilienfeld, Abraham M., Levin, Morton L., and Kessler, Irving I., *Cancer in the United States,* Cambridge: Harvard University Press, 1972.

Lilienfeld, Abraham M., *Foundations of Epidemiology,* New York: Oxford University Press, 1976.

Luft, Harold S., "How do Health Maintenance Organizations Achieve Their 'Savings'?" *New England Journal of Medicine,* **298**:1336–1343, 1978.

Marmot, Michael G., *Migrants, Aculturation and Coronary Heart Disease,* Bethesda, Md.: National Heart and Lung Institute, 1975.

Martin, Samuel P., Donaldson, Magruder C., London, C. David, Peterson, Osler L., and Colton, Theodore, "Inputs into Coronary Care during Thirty Years: A Cost Effectiveness Study," *Annals of Internal Medicine,* **81**:289–293, 1974.

Mather, H. G., et al., "Acute Myocardial Infarction: Home and Hospital Treatment," *British Medical Journal,* **3**(August 7):334–338, 1971.

Maxman, Jerrold S., *The Post-Physician Era,* New York: Wiley-Interscience, 1976.

McKeown, Thomas, *Medicine in Modern Society,* New York: Hafner, 1965.

McKeown, Thomas, "A Historical Appraisal of the Medical Task," in McLachlan, G., and McKeown, T., Eds., *Medical History and Medical Care,* New York: Oxford University Press, 1971.

McKeown, Thomas, and Lowe, C. R., *An Introduction to Social Medicine,* 2nd ed., Philadelphia, Pa.: Lippincott, 1974.

Mechanic, David, "The Right to Treatment: Judicial Action and Social Change," in D. Mechanic, *Politics, Medicine, and Social Science,* New York: Wiley-Interscience, 1974.

Miller, Alfred E., "The Expanding Definition of Health and Disease in Community Medicine," *Social Science and Medicine,* **6**:573–582, 1972.

Miller, C. Arden, "Issues of Health Policy: Local Government and the Public's Health," *American Journal of Public Health,* **65**:1330, 1975.

Moreland Act Commission, *Regulating Nursing Home Care: The Paper Tigers,* Albany, N.Y., October, 1975.

Moriyama, Iwao M., Krueger, Dean E., and Stamler, Jeremiah, *Cardiovascular Diseases in the United States,* Cambridge: Harvard University Press, 1971.

Morris, J. N., and Heady, J. A., Social and Biological Factors in Infant Mortality," *Lancet,* **1**:343–349, (February 12), 1955.

Murphy, Marvin L., et al., "Treatment of Chronic Stable Angina," *New England Journal of Medicine,* **297**:621, 1977.

Newhouse, Joseph P., "Determinants of Days Lost from Work Due to Sickness," in Herbert E. Klarman, Ed., *Empirical Studies in Health Economics, Proceedings of the Second Conference on the Economics of Health,* Baltimore: Johns Hopkins University Press, 1970, pp. 59–70.

Office of Technology Assessment, *Assessing the Efficacy and Safety of Medical Technologies,* Washington, D.C.: Congress of the United States, 1978.

Paffenbarger, Ralph S., and Hale, Wayne E., "Work Activity and Coronary Heart Mortality," *New England Journal of Medicine,* **292**:545–550, 1975.

Parsons, Talcott, and Fox, Renee, "Illness Therapy and The Modern Urban American Family," *Journal of Social Issues,* **8**(4):2–3, 31–44, 1952.

Parsons, Talcott, "Definitions of Health and Illness in the Light of American Values and Social Structure," in Jaco, E., Ed., *Patients, Physicians, and Illness,* New York: Free Press, 1958.

Parsons, Talcott, "Social Change and Medical Organization in the United States: A Sociological Perspective," *The Annals of the American Academy of Political and Social Science,* 346:21–33, 1963.

Patrick, D. L., Bush, J. W., and Chen, Milton M., "Toward an Operational Definition of Health," *Journal of Health and Social Behavior,* 14:6–23, 1973.

Phillips, Donald F., "Long Term Hospital Care," *Hospitals, Journal of the American Hospital Association,* 47(13):46–49, 1973.

Pollard, William E., Bobbitt, Ruth A., Bergner, Marilyn, Martin, Diane P., and Gilson, Betty S., "The Sickness Impact Profile: Reliability of a Health Status Measure," *Medical Care,* 14:146–155, 1976.

Powles, John, "On the Limitations of Modern Medicine," *Science, Medicine and Man* 1(April):1–30, 1973.

Preston, T. A., *Coronary Artery Surgery: A Critical Review,* New York: Raven Press, 1977.

Rettig, Richard A., "End-Stage Renal Disease and the 'Cost' of Medical Technology," in Sun Valley Forum on National Health, *Medical Technology: The Culprit Behind Health Care Costs?,* Washington, D.C.: USDHEW (PHS) No. 79–3216, 1979.

Rice, Dorothy P., *Estimating the Cost of Illness,* Washington, D.C.: USDHEW, Division of Medical Care Administration, 1966.

Richmond, Julius, and Filner, Barbara, "Infant and Child Health: Needs and Strategies," in *Healthy People: The Surgeon General's Report on Health Promotion and Disease Prevention, Background Papers,* Vol. 2, Washington, D.C.: USPHS No. 79–55071A, 1979.

Rivlin, Alice M., *Social Policy: Alternate Strategies for the Federal Government,* Washington, D.C.: The Brookings Institution, 1974.

Robertson, Leon S., "Factors Associated with Safety Belt Use in 1974 Starter-Interlock Equipped Cars," *Journal of Health and Social Behavior,* 16:173–177, 1975.

Robertson, Leon S., "Estimates of Motor Vehicle Seat Belt Effectiveness and Use: Implications for Occupant Crash Protection," *American Journal of Public Health,* 66:859–864, 1976.

Rosen, George, *Preventive Medicine in the United States 1900–1975: Trends and Interpretations,* New York: Science History Publications, 1975.

Rosenstock, Irwin M., "What Research in Motivation Suggests for Public Health," *American Journal of Public Health,* 50:295–302, 1960.

Ross, R. S., "The Case for Prevention of Coronary Heart Disease," *Circulation,* 51:May, 1975.

Russek, H. I., "Role of Heredity, Diet, and Emotional Stress in Coronary Heart Disease," *Journal of the American Medical Association,* 171:503–508, 1959.

Rutstein, David D., *Blueprint for Medical Care,* Cambridge: MIT Press, 1974.

Schenthal, J. E., "Multiphasic Screening of the Well Patient," *Journal of the American Medical Association,* 172:1–4, 1960.

Schneiderman, M., "Cancer—A Social Disease?" Interagency Collaborative Group on Environmental Carcinogenesis, Bethesda, Md.: National Institutes of Health, 1975.

Scitovsky, Anne A., and McCall, Nelda, "Changes in the Costs of Treatment of Selected Illnesses, 1951–1971," Health Policy Discussion Paper, San Francisco: University of California School of Medicine, 1975.

Selikoff, Irving J., and Hammond, E. C., "Asbestos-Associated Disease in United States Shipyards," *CA-A Cancer Journal for Clinicians,* 28(2):87–99, 1978.

Selzer, Melvin L., Gikas, Paul W., and Huelke, Donald F., Eds., *The Prevention of Highway Injury,* Ann Arbor: Highway Safety Research Institute, University of Michigan, 1967.

Shanas, Ethel, Townsend, Peter, Wedderburn, Dorothy, Friis, Henning, Milhoj, Poul, and Stehouwer, Jan, *Old People in Three Industrial Societies,* New York: Atherton, 1968.

Shapiro, Sam, Schlesinger, Edward R., and Nesbitt, Robert E. L., Jr., *Infant, Perinatal, Maternal, and Childhood Mortality in the United States,* Cambridge: Harvard University Press, 1968.

Shulman, D., and Galanter, R., "Reorganizing the Nursing Home Industry: A Proposal," *Health and Society,* 54:129, 1976.

Sigerist, Henry E., *Medicine and Human Welfare,* College Park, Md.: McGrath Publishing Co., 1970.

Simmons, Roberta G., Klein, Susan D., and Simmons, Richard L., *Gift of Life: The Social and Psychological Impact of Organ Transplantation,* New York: Wiley-Interscience, 1977.

Singer, Charles, and Underwood, E. Ashworth, *A Short History of Medicine,* Oxford: Clarendon Press, 1962.

Silver, Morris, "An Economic Analysis of Variations in Medical Expenses and Work Loss Rates," in H. Klarman, Ed., *Empirical Studies in Health Economics,* Baltimore: Johns Hopkins University Press, 1970.

Smith, Kenneth R., Miller, Marriene, and Golladay, Frederick L., "An Analysis of the Optimal Use of Inputs in Production of Medical Services," *Journal of Human Resources,* 7 (Spring):208–224, 1972.

Somers, Herman M., and Somers, Anne R., *Doctors, Patients and Health Insurance,* Washington, D.C.: Brookings Institution, 1961.

Spingarn, Natalie D., *Heart Beat: The Politics of Health Research,* Washington, D.C.: Robert B. Luce, Inc., 1976.

Star, P., "The New Medicine," *The New Republic* (April 19):15, 1975.

Stewart, Charles T., Jr., "The Allocation of Resources to Health," *The Journal of Human Resources,* 6 (Winter):103–122, 1971.

Strickland, Stephen P., *U.S. Health Care: What's Wrong and What's Right,* New York: Universe, 1972.

Strickland, Stephen P., *Politics, Science, and Dread Disease: A Short History of United States Medical Research Policy,* Cambridge: Harvard University Press, 1972a.

Stunkard, Albert J., *The Pain of Obesity,* Palo Alto, Calif.: Bulletin, 1976.

Sun Valley Forum on National Health, "Medical Cure and Medical Care," *Milbank Memorial Fund Quarterly,* 50(4, Part 2): entire issue, 1972).

Susser, Merwyn, "Ethical Components in the Definition of Health," *International Journal of Health Services,* 4:539, 1974.

Susser, Merwyn W., and Watson, W., *Sociology in Medicine,* New York: Oxford University Press, 1971.

Szasz, Thomas S., *The Myth of Mental Illness,* New York: Hoeker-Harper, 1961.

Szasz, Thomas, *The Manufacturer of Madness,* New York: Harper & Row, 1970.

Terris, Milton, "Breaking the Barriers to Prevention: Legislative Approaches," *Bulletin of the New York Academy of Medicine,* 2nd Series, 51:242, 1975.

Thomas, Lewis, "Guessing and Knowing: Reflections on the Science and Technology of Medicine," *Saturday Review of Science,* 55(December 23):52–57, 1972.

Titmus, Richard M., *Social Policy: An Introduction,* New York: Pantheon Books, 1974.

U.S. Bureau of the Census, *Statistical Abstract of the United States,* Washington, D.C.: U.S. Department of Commerce, 1978.

USDHEW, *Health; United States, 1976–1977,* Washington, D.C.: USDHEW (HRA), 77–1232, 1977.

USDHEW, *Health; United States, 1978,* Washington, D.C.: USDHEW, (PHS) 78–1232, 1978.

USDHEW, *Health; United States, 1979,* Washington, D.C.: USDHEW, 79–1232, 1979.

USDHEW, *Health; United States, 1980,* Washington, D.C.: USDHEW, 80–1232, 1980.

U.S. National Center for Health Statistics, *Origin, Program and Operation of the U.S. National Health Survey,* Series 3–1, Washington, D.C.: USDHEW, 1963.

U.S. National Center for Health Statistics, *Vital and Health Statistics,* Series 10, No. 111, Washington, D.C.: USDHEW (PHS), 1977.

U.S. National Center for Health Statistics, "Limitation of Activity and Mobility Due to Chronic Conditions," *Vital and Health Statistics,* Series 10, No. 118, Washington, D.C.: USDHEW (PHS), 1978.

U.S. National Center for Health Statistics, "Current Estimates from the Health Interview Survey," *Vital and Health Statistics Series 10,* No. 130, Washington, D.C.: USDHEW (PHS), 1978.

U.S. National Center for Health Statistics," Hypertension: United States, 1974," *Advance Data,* No. 2, Washington, D.C.: USDHEW (HRA), 77–1250, 1976.

USPHS, *Healthy People: The Surgeon General's Report on Health Promotion and Disease Prevention,* Washington, D.C.: USDHEW (PHS), No. 79–55071, 1979.

USPHS, *Surgeon General's Report on Smoking,* Washington, D.C.: USDHEW, 1979a.

U.S. Senate Special Committee on Aging, Subcommittee on Long-Term Care, *Nursing Home Care in the United States: Failure in Public Policy,* Washington, D.C.: November, 1974.

Veterans Administration Cooperative Study Group on Antihypertensive Agents: Effects of treatment on morbidity in hypertension—results in patients with diastolic blood pressure averaging 115 through 129 mm. Hg. *JAMA,* **202**:1028–1034, 1967.

Veterans Administration Cooperative Study Group on Antihypertensive Agents: Effects of treatment on morbidity in hypertension. II. Results in patients with diastolic blood pressure averaging 90 through 114 mm. Hg. *JAMA,* **213**:1143–1152, 1970.

Weinstein, M. C., and Stason, W. B., *Hypertension, A Policy Perspective,* Cambridge: Harvard University Press, 1976.

Weisbrod, Burton, *Economics of Public Health,* Philadelphia: University of Pennsylvania Press, 1961.

White, Kerr L., "Organization and Delivery of Personal Health Services: Public Policy Issues," *Milbank Memorial Fund Quarterly,* **46**:225, 1968.

White, Kerr L., "Life and Death and Medicine," *Scientific American,* **23**: September 1973.

White, Kerr L., "Health and Health Care: Personal and Public Issues," Michael M. Davis Lecture, May 29, 1974, Chicago: University of Chicago, Center for Health Administration, 1974.

White, L. S., "How to Improve the Public's Health," *New England Journal of Medicine,* **293**:773, 1975.

Wilson, F. A., and Neuhauser, D., *Health Services in the United States,* Cambridge, Mass.: Ballinger, 1974.

World Health Organization, "The Constitution of the World Health Organization," *WHO Chronical,* **1**:29, 1944.

Wright, Irving S., Frederickson, Donald T., *Cardiovascular Diseases: Guidelines for Prevention and Care,* Washington, D.C.: USDHEW (NIH), 1973.

Zelnick, M., and Kanter, J. F., "Contraceptive Patterns and Premarital Pregnancy Among Women Age 15–19 in 1976," *Family Planning Perspective,* **10**:135, 1978.

PART TWO

ORGANIZATION AND BEHAVIOR OF THE HEALTH CARE SYSTEM

What Drives It In Its Present Direction?

Part 1 describes the origin of the mismatch between health problems and the system of care. Part 2 attempts to answer the question of why health care has failed to adapt to the new needs of society. It examines the various components of the health system to explain the mechanisms that drive it in a direction increasingly less appropriate for the chronic disease problems of post-clinical medicine.

Chapter 6 describes the system of medical education that grew out of the revolution in medical science. Physicians' training inculcates certain attitudes and patterns of behavior that are consonant with the technological approach to medicine—derived from the success of the modern conception of disease. Many of these attitudes and behaviors are counterproductive for the problems of post-clinical medicine. Yet medical education is more a mirror of the organizational forces and incentives acting on physicians in practice structured around the dominating technology rather than the ultimate cause of such behavior. The incentives and structure of practice would have to be the primary point of effective corrective change.

Chapter 7 examines the evolution of hospitals under the pressures of the medical technological revolution from custodial institutions of last resort into technical workshops for physicians and finally into complex organizational giants propelled by their own momentum. As the main institutions for bringing new medical technology to communities, hospitals have come to play a very central role in medical practice, but the social organization that evolved to operate the technology has become an end in itself. It drives hospitals in a direction often poorly fitted to the needs of post-clinical medicine and responsible for a large portion of the uncontrolled costs of medical care.

Chapter 8 analyzes the changing organization of the medical profession and the fragmentation of practice. This has transpired largely as a result of increasing specialization, which, in turn, is a consequence of the new technological approach to medicine. The increasing role of hospital care and the changing structure of urban areas have also contributed to the new pattern of practice poorly fitted for the needs of post-clinical medicine.

Patients' behavior is in part determined by the health care system, which defines their role and influences their actions. It is also molded in part by the social system in which patients function during their normal lives, as well as by the special needs they have individually as patients. This multiple determination of patient behavior leads almost inevitably to ambivalence and conflict examined in Chapter 9. Such conflicts, inherent in the patient role, are intensified by the situation of chronic illnesses, the changes of the health system described in the preceding chapters and the changing structure of society. As close-knit communities and extended families have given way to the urbanization and mobility of modern society, the problem of caring for the sick, once tended to by families, has increasingly been transferred onto the health care system.

Although little effort has been made to deal explicitly with the mismatch between the health system and the new problems of illness, several attempts at reform of health care delivery strive to remedy some of the obvious symptoms of this maladjustment. Chapter 10 examines three major strategies of health system reform: health planning, health maintenance organizations, and health care technology assessment. Health planning has the objective of rationalizing the allocation of resources, primarily by correcting the misallocation resulting from overemphasis on (high-technology) hospital care. Health maintenance organizations (HMOs) attempt to overcome fragmentation of care and overreliance on hospital care by changing the financial and organizational incentives influencing physicians' practice. Technology assessment scrutinizes the effectiveness and appropriateness of new modes of diagnosis and treatment before their uncontrolled dissemination, subjecting them to cost-benefit analysis as well as the usual standards of efficacy and safety. All these strategies tacitly acknowledge that health care has become too important and too expensive to be left entirely to the discretion of the individual physician. Certain tradeoffs with other social goals and needs have become necessary in order to maximize social welfare using the limited resources available.

CHAPTER SIX

Medical Education and
Professional Socialization

The reform of medical schools in the United States from 1880 to 1930* together with the continued advancement of medical technology produced
profound changes in the profession. The effects on the organization of medical practice and the structure of the profession (the subject of Chapter 8)
were gradual. They only became evident with the replacement of the older
generation of physicians. The effects on the type and quality of medical
training and the philosophy of medical care were felt immediately and are
the subject of this chapter.

Largely isolated from the mainstream of scientific and medical advancement in Europe during the nineteenth century, the medical profession and
medical care in the United States took a rather different course of development. Revolutionary changes occurred late in the century in the process of
catching up with Europe. Although much the same forces and influences
eventually came to dominate professional behavior and organization here
as in Europe, the process was modified in this country. American medicine
made the transition faster by building on the European example, and the
unique socioeconomic, ideological, and political forces in the United States
produced a different approach to the same problems of development.

In the early colonial period most medical care was provided by ships'
surgeons, apothecaries, and a few adventuresome English-trained physicians
(only about 10% of the practitioners in the colonies). These diverse types
of practitioners competed on an equal basis just as during the unregulated period of medical practice in medieval Europe before the ascendancy of the universities during the Renaissance (Chapter 3). By the late
colonial period more physicians trained in Edinburgh and London began
to practice in eastern seaboard cities. Consequently, American medicine was
closely associated with and influenced by the English medical tradition dur-

* Where not otherwise attributed, standard historical data used in this chapter are taken
from Stevens, 1971.

ing the resurgence of the guild element under the Royal College and during the institutionalization of bedside teaching. Since there were not enough physicians to supply the needs of the rapidly growing American population, however, the system of bedside teaching was often abbreviated into an informal apprenticeship, perpetuating much of the diversity and unregulated nature of the profession.

In 1765 the College of Philadelphia Medical School (later the University of Pennsylvania) was founded. It was followed by the College of Physicians and Surgeons in New York City in 1768 (later Columbia University's Medical School), and Harvard Medical College in 1783. But these early medical schools in the United States were essentially formalized extensions of the apprenticeship system. No university or even high school degree was required for enrollment. The curriculum consisted of only a few evening lectures on the basic medical sciences by part-time professors who were primarily private practitioners. In part this divergence from the British system occurred because there were still very few voluntary hospitals in America that could be used for bedside teaching. The Massachusetts General Hospital was not founded until 1821, 40 years after the Harvard Medical School, and Bellevue was essentially a poorhouse when the College of Physicians and Surgeons began training students (Stevens, 1971).

As the number of practitioners grew, colonial and state medical societies were established to protect guild interests, and pressure for medical licensure arose. New York established a medical licensing law in 1760, as did New Jersey in 1766, at the request of the colony's medical society. After the Revolution the power of licensure was commonly given to the state medical societies themselves or to the medical schools, or to both, following the pattern of dual licensure established in England. Before this system of licensure could develop very far, however, the combined influence of the extreme commitment to laissez faire principles and the Jacksonian Democratic anti-elitist philosophy produced a countertrend toward unregulated medical education and practice. In this unrestrained situation many third-rate proprietary and sectarian medical schools were established after 1800 (Stevens, 1971). There were only four functioning medical colleges in the United States at the turn of the nineteenth century, but more than 400 medical schools were founded during the nineteenth century. The better university medical schools were soon outnumbered by the new proprietary schools, and even the best schools found it difficult to maintain educational standards in the face of this new competition. The typical American physician in the nineteenth century was trained either by apprenticeship alone or attended a school with no formal bedside teaching, no laboratory instruction, and often no organized curriculum at all.

Parallel to the unbridled growth of new schools there was a trend to repeal the system of licensure and decrease regulation of medical practice by the state medical societies. By 1845 eight states had repealed all legislation in regard to medical licensure or regulation of medical practice, and many other states simply removed any penalty for practicing without a license (Shryock, 1967). This disenfranchisement of the medical societies resulted in part from public resentment against medical society fee schedules and in part from the growing public disillusion with the efficacy of medicine in general. Just as in Europe during the same period, patient dissatisfaction was reflected in the growth of sectarian systems of medicine like osteopathy, homeopathy, faith healing (e.g., Christian Science), and outright quackery. Morale within the medical profession reached a low ebb, leading among other things to the founding in 1847 of the American Medical Association (AMA) as a nonlicensing guild organization to work toward better standards of medical education and practice (Burrow, 1963). But little change was achieved until the scientific developments in Europe led to the potential for real pragmatic benefits for the public and the profession.

As reports of the new developments in pathology and statistically controlled clinical trials began arriving here in the second quarter of the century, a new generation of elite students traveled to Paris for medical education as their forefathers had journeyed to London and Edinburgh. Oliver Wendell Holmes studied under Pierre Louis in Paris, bringing back the healthy cynicism in regard to traditional methods of treatment for which he became famous. After the American Civil War, the forefront of scientific and medical progress moved to Germany, and student physicians flocked to Vienna and Berlin. This generation of European-trained physicians brought back the new microscopic pathology, bacteriology, and other laboratory methods. It became apparent that a medical revolution was taking place. Medical education and research in the United States needed to change radically if the fruits of this breakthrough were to be made available here.

Charles Eliot, the vigorous president of Harvard University, was quick to sense important new intellectual directions and place his school in the vanguard. In 1871 he summoned the faculty of the Harvard Medical School and outlined his program for restructuring medical education. This included a graded curriculum of study over three years, with regular written examinations, and entrance requirements of a previous college degree or qualifying examinations in a foreign language. Prodded by Eliot's threat to discontinue university recognition, the faculty complied and started the movement toward reform of medical education throughout the country. Harvard's lead was soon followed by other first-rank universities. In 1876 twenty-two of the better medical schools organized the Association of American Medical Colleges with the objective of upgrading the standards of medical education generally. At first they were unable to pressure even their own members to stiffen admission requirements because of the competition for students from the proprietary schools. Some years later, however, the leverage of endowment financing succeeded where exhortation alone had failed.

In the late nineteenth century large-scale philanthropy arose in the United States as a result of the fortunes made by the barons of industry following the Civil War. In 1893 Johns Hopkins University Medical School and Hospital were founded on the basis of a huge endowment. The school, built around the research and teaching hospital and modeled after the German university structure, provided not only intensive laboratory and bedside teaching for medical students but also postgraduate (specialty) residency training. Residencies made it possible for young physicians to acquire practical experience in their chosen specialty while still in a position to learn from their professors and to carry on clinical and laboratory research. With abundant financing, the new school recruited the best faculty available and established full-time endowed chairs so that professors could devote themselves entirely to teaching and research. The core faculty members became the giants of American medicine in their generation—William S. Halstead in surgery, Sir William Osler in medicine, William Henry Welch in bacteriology and pathology. Halstead's first surgical resident was Harvey Cushing, a giant in his own right, who then developed the residency system at Harvard (Shryock, 1953; Hughes, 1974). Almost overnight Johns Hopkins became the leading medical center in the United States setting the standard for the rest of the country.

There was no longer any question about the direction in which American medical education had to go. The better university medical schools rapidly adopted the pattern of combined laboratory and bedside teaching for undergraduates and the residency system of postgraduate specialty training as quickly as money could be raised for the facilities and faculty. Yet the problem remained of creating uniform standards throughout the country. Most physicians were still being trained by diploma mills, and the public had little means of distinguishing the well-trained from the poorly-trained physicians in practice. Even in the better schools the curriculum seldom contained much laboratory or clinical training, and the students were left essentially on their own to seek out what they hoped was important from textbooks. There was almost no full-time faculty and no hospital affiliation. The examination, if it existed, was strictly of book knowledge. State licensure was either nonexistent or accomplished simply by paying a registration fee. The actual learning of medical skills took place in the guild tradition through apprenticeship to an older physician whose ability often counted less than the size of his practice. Even this training opportunity was bypassed by many who moved into new areas and learned what they could from their own experience at the expense of their patients.

At the turn of the century, however, the growing faith in science and technology as forces to improve the quality of life, and the increasing concern brought on by muckraking journalism led to the liberal politics of the so-called Progressive Era (Hofstadter, 1955). These movements in public opinion began to cast doubt on the desirability of completely unbridled, unregulated businesses and services. Evidence of the growing ability of medicine to make a difference converged with the political climate to make the first decades of the twentieth century an opportune moment for reform.

With the urging of the AMA and under the auspices of the Carnegie Foundation, Abraham Flexner, a respected educator, visited 155 of the existing medical schools in 1909 to 1910 to survey their facilities and teaching methods (Hyde & Wolff, 1954; Burrow, 1963). The "Report" (Flexner, 1910) issued in 1910 put the official seal on the revolution in medical education that was already well underway in the better schools as a result of the pressure created by the Harvard and Johns Hopkins examples. Flexner gave detailed public exposure of the inadequate medical schools by name, describing the appalling conditions of most. He recommended that the number of schools be reduced from 155 to 31 by closure or merger. By 1915, under pressure from the public and the AMA Council on Medical Education, 40 schools closed and 52 others merged with stronger schools (Banta, 1971). The hope of foundation money was a strong incentive in this compliance. Implicit in Flexner's recommendations was the promise that foundation subsidies would enable the better schools to make the suggested improvements, leaving the noncomplying schools to fend for themselves in the increasingly expensive business of medical education (Stevens, 1971).

From this point on the AMA Council on Medical Education set the standards for medical training and rated the schools annually. The Johns Hopkins model was made the standard, with its combination of full-time staff, a low student-to-faculty ratio, laboratory and hospital facilities for teaching, and a close affiliation with a major university. Standards of premedical education for admission were also raised, and the requirement of at least a year of internship before licensure was added. The structure and quality of medical education had been revolutionized, but the output of physicians had also been cut in half. This was to have profound effects on the practice of medicine and the provision of health services in the years to come.

The so-called Flexner reforms also led to changes in the professional socialization process, in the power relationships of and within the profession, and eventually in the structure of the profession. Nevertheless, with the limited system for dissemination of medical information to the practicing profession, it was necessary to educate a whole new generation of physicians before the new scientific discoveries and technical developments could have a widespread impact on the practice of medicine in this country. Hospitals had to be constructed where surgery could be performed. The public needed reorientation to accept hospital care, which until then had been understood as nothing short of a death sentence or as custodial warehousing for the destitute. Only after 1930 did the improved medical education and new clinical techniques begin to make themselves felt.

The principle objective guiding the new system of medical education was to make each graduate into a competent scientist-clinician trained in the basic laboratory and clinical methods of diagnosis and patient care. Advances in medicine were making many illnesses susceptible either to direct clinical treatment or to systematic prevention, or both. Effective use of this new scientific medicine required the ability to identify the underlying pathological process (the disease) and also the disturbance in the normal physio-logical mechanisms in order to combat the disease agent and correct the physiological imbalance. The four years of medical school were intended to give students an understanding of the new knowledge and techniques and sufficient experience at the bedside to apply them effectively in practice. A very systematic curriculum provided intensive, highly structured, and ex-tremely demanding training during medical school, the year of internship, and two to five years of further specialty residency training—which came to be almost a standard part of the medical education sequence after World War II. Thus physician training became a logical progression from clini-cally oriented knowledge to graded responsibility in patient care.

Accompanying this planned acquisition of knowledge, skills, and experi-ence is a second learning process, referred to as "professional socialization." This is a less planned and less obvious process in which medical students gradually take on the attitudes, values, role behaviors, and identities that are typical of physicians: (1) an approach to illnesses strongly oriented to disease and less so to patients' personal problems; (2) an overwhelming ten-dency toward specialization; (3) professional authority behavior. The ac-quisition of these traits is just as much part of becoming a physician as is learning the requisite knowledge and skills. Both aspects of medical educa-tion are closely linked, and their present forms have been decisively influ-enced by the new technology. Both aspects of medical education in turn have influenced the nature of medical practice and the structure of the health care system.

THE MEDICAL SCHOOL CURRICULUM

Following the Flexner reforms until the 1960s, nearly all medical schools had very standardized curricula divided roughly into two preclinical years spent mostly in lectures and laboratories, and two clinical years spent pri-marily on the hospital wards. During the first two years students were ex-pected to acquire the basic knowledge of the biomedical sciences. In the second two years they learned to apply this knowledge to the care of pa-tients. Students entering medical school already had general knowledge of the basic physical and biological sciences, so that this could be immediately applied to learning the more specific elements of the biomedical sciences. The first year was devoted to acquiring a knowledge of the normal struc-ture and function of the human body including gross and microscopic anatomy, neuroanatomy and neurophysiology, biochemistry, cellular and organ physiology. These courses were taught in academic settings almost completely isolated from any clinical application or patient contact, and often with little attempt to integrate the functional (physiological) and struc-tural aspects—in many schools the structural elements were taught one se-mester and the functional the next. Thus the first year consisted of mastering a mass of factual material to be stored away for use in later course work and potential clinical application. This was done on a rigorous and highly regimented schedule. The volume of work led many students to question whether their time was well spent on so much basic science when there was so much practical material to be mastered.

In physiology students began work that came closer to clinical application. The laboratory consisted largely of experiments on the organ systems in living mammals. Since the mechanisms are essentially the same as in man, students could see the relevance of understanding the effect of the various drugs used in the lab for treating patients. Some of the experiments, such as those on digestion and breathing, were even done on fellow students, giving the first opportunity to begin learning techniques used on patients, such as drawing blood from veins, passing tubes into the stomach, or measuring the rate of oxygen uptake in the lungs. Nevertheless, most material was difficult to associate with patient care and tended to encourage a pure scientific attitude, dampening students' early enthusiasm for the service aspects of medicine.

The second year continued the acquisition of basic scientific knowledge for later clinical application, but the emphasis shifted to pathological changes in the body and their effects on the normal structure and function. Much of the pathology course was still spent in the laboratory examining microscopic slides of diseased tissues, but students also began learning about clinical diseases and their effects in a more functional way. In microbiology they acquired the techniques and theory for growing, identifying, and studying the various organisms that cause infectious diseases and the immunological responses of the body to these agents. They memorized the exotic names of dozens of strange parasites and marveled at their intricate life cycles, which tropical disease epidemiologists had traced out—but made no connection to the suffering of half the world's population doomed to short miserable lives because of such organisms. In laboratory diagnosis they learned tests to help discern the nature of the diseases in patients, such as blood cell counts, urinalyses, and blood chemistries. Pharmacology consisted largely of experiments on animals measuring the effects of various drugs on normal or impaired physiological systems.

By the fourth semester medical students were well into the application of scientific methods to clinical problems, if not yet in the clinical setting. This was capped by the course in physical diagnosis, when the students finally came into direct contact with patients after having learned the basic techniques such as percussion of chests, auscultation (using the stethoscope to listen to the heart and lungs), use of ophthalmoscope and otoscope to examine the eyes and ears, and so on, all by practicing on each other. Having memorized a long series of questions to be asked of patients for picking up possible indications of disease, having learned the routine for a complete physical examination, and having learned the rudiments of symptomatology for a few common diseases, students were sent forth on the hospital

wards to do their first complete "workup" (clinical history and physical examination).* This workup was both written out in standard form for the
patient's chart and presented orally to the clinical instructor for discussion
and critique.

During the remaining two years of medical school, the so-called clinical
years, the students spent the major part of their time on teaching hospital
wards or outpatient departments. There they did workups on patients, par-
ticipated in conferences where cases were presented and discussed, accompanied interns, residents, and attending staff physicians on ward rounds or
patient visits, and carried out minor diagnostic and therapeutic procedures
on patients.

They now become, in essence, apprentices who learn not by studying material
from books and lectures, but by doing under the supervision of those who are already doctors the things they will later do as doctors. (Becker et al., 1961)

Students continued to attend almost daily lectures throughout the third
year and less regularly in the fourth year, but their place of work was the
hospital ward and their identification was now clearly with the clinical
world of the teaching hospital. This transition was symbolized by the
white uniforms provided by the hospital. Throughout their third and
fourth years they were assigned to a series of so-called clinical clerkships,
tours of duty on clinical services where they functioned as part of the clinical team caring for the patients. These rotations included medicine, surgery,
pediatrics, obstetrics, psychiatry, and briefer exposure to the various specialty services such as ophthalmology, urology, dermatology, and so on. Students now lived on the hospital's schedule rather than on an academic one.
They might be expected to arrive on the wards at 6:30 A.M. to draw blood
from patients for laboratory analysis, start IVs (intravenous fluid infu-
sions), and carry out other necessary procedures before ward rounds at 7:30.
They spent nights in the emergency room to treat minor injuries and work
up emergency cases. On obstetrics they followed women through labor and
performed the deliveries whenever they occurred. On surgery they assisted
at the operations of the patients they had worked up.

This was the introduction to medicine experienced by most physicians
trained between 1930 and 1960—who still make up the majority of those in
practice—two years of intensive, highly structured exposure to the scientific
basis of medicine, storing away information; two years of intensive apprenticeship learning the skills of medicine and the application of the knowledge to clinical problems. This provided little opportunity in either period

---

* The patients for this are usually carefully selected, that is, known to be good-natured
about such things, since the first such undertaking might require one or two hours to
complete—something that the students accomplish in 15 to 20 minutes or less later in their
careers.

to raise questions on their own or to understand the wider context and social implications of what they were learning.

Since 1945 graduation from medical school has marked only the halfway point in medical education and professional socialization for most physicians. Three to six years of internship and residency lie ahead to qualify for their specialty and subspecialty board examinations. The structure and effect of such specialty training on new physicians and their practices are very much a product of changes in the organization of the medical profession from 1930 to 1950. We therefore defer discussion of residency training until Chapter 8.

RECENT CURRICULUM REFORMS

Today the course of study in most medical schools has been markedly changed and varies greatly from one school to another or from one year's class of students to the next as various experimental curricula are tried. There are a number of reasons for these modifications.

First, the most pervading problem has been the explosion of knowledge in the biomedical sciences. Previously it was believed that medical students could be given a basic body of knowledge that would serve as a foundation to understand medical problems for the rest of their careers, with minor modifications and updating. Each preclinical discipline was expected to distill out the essential information and present it to the students in the allocated teaching time. As new developments came at a more rapid rate, the faculty first simply tried to compress more material into the same amount of time without reevaluating the relative importance or cutting back on less relevant information. Then, whole new bodies of knowledge like molecular biology and modern genetics appeared. The result was a system overload that eventually made it apparent that some basically new approach to medical education was called for. Even if it had been possible to master the mass of facts known at the time of medical training, the rapid development meant that a large part of this information would be outmoded within a short time. The real problem was learning to keep up with the new information rather than mastering the old. It was as necessary to prepare the physicians to cope with ongoing learning after graduation as it was to become more efficient in teaching the mass of material. Medical education also had to discover a better balance between the various areas of knowledge and the needs of practitioners.

Second, numerous investigations of the medical education process during the 1950s, together with the impressions of those involved, suggested that there was too heavy an emphasis on the scientific approach to disease. This seemed to be creating insensitivity to patients' personal problems and a strong tendency toward overspecialization. There was also growing discontent and resistance on the part of students because of the long delay before contact with patients and the lack of relevance of the material during the early years of training.

Third, forces outside the profession and the medical schools also had an influence on curriculum policy. Public outcry about the disappearance of primary care physicians and the growing unresponsiveness of physicians to patients' personal concerns created pressure on medical schools by way of legislation to train more family practitioners and increase the overall output of physicians. The pattern of funding medical education also changed. After World War II research grants became a major source of faculty support and pushed the faculty composition in the direction of the basic sciences. Later direct government subsidization of medical education, which was tied to requirements for increased class sizes and more stress on family practice, restructured the faculty in the clinical direction again (Fein & Weber, 1971).

As a consequence of these pressures a number of innovative programs have been tried in the past 15 to 20 years. One of the first was the early exposure of students to clinical experience in the hope of increasing the relevance of the preclinical sciences. This was also intended as a counterforce against the student's tendency to lose sight of the patient as a person in the zeal to understand diseases from a scientific point of view. Some schools established special family-care clinics where students could follow families or a patient with a chronic disease problem over a period of three to four years during their medical school training. Other schools simply moved up physical diagnosis into the first year or started various hospital duties parallel to the study of preclinical sciences. Evaluation of the different types of programs has not yet given any clear indication of the relative advantages and disadvantages of the various methods of early clinical exposure. All have been enthusiastically welcomed by the students and seem to have mitigated their impatience with the delay in learning practical material during the first and second years of training (Lippard, 1971).

A second curriculum reform has been to bring the basic and applied science into better balance and into more meaningful relationship with each other. Nearly all schools have reduced the amount of time spent on gross anatomy and classical biochemistry while increasing emphasis on cellular biology and genetics (Lippard, 1971). Many schools teach the preclinical sciences by organ systems or functions such as circulation, respiration, digestion, and so on, rather than by the traditional disciplinary divisions, like anatomy and physiology. Each unit of this kind includes both normal and pathological anatomy, physiology, diseases occurring in that system, their clinical manifestations, and treatment. This approach captures students' interest by making the basic scientific knowledge about a body system immediately relevant in regard to disease states. Structure and function, disease processes and normal systems are seen in meaningful juxtaposition. On the other hand, the necessary integration of teaching disciplines has often been quite difficult and time-consuming and has met considerable faculty resistance. Many schools have planned for such curricula and then decided not to implement them. On the other hand, most of the new medical schools established in the last decade with younger faculties have adopted such a curriculum (Purcell, 1976).

Another widely used approach to improving medical education has been to give students the option of learning much of the material by independent study, assisted by audiovisual programs available at the discretion of the student, and monitored by self-administered examinations (plus parts I and II of the National Board of Medical Examiners examination). Many schools have also left more time open for the student to pursue elective work on or off campus. Besides accommodating to student discontent in regard to the previous overly structured curricula, electives and independent study are intended to allow students to learn how to learn by themselves. This acknowledges the lifelong need for continuing self-education to keep up with the advances in their field and to fill inevitable gaps in training as new problems are encountered. These programs have been quite successful with well-prepared students but have presented problems for those poorly prepared (Purcell, 1976).

In the late 1960s there was growing medical student concern in regard to social responsibility and community service as one part of the social movements and campus unrest of the time. As one response to meet these concerns behavioral science teaching was added to many medical school programs. Community medicine departments were also established; many sponsored community based family health clinics and other projects that involved students in direct social service in their neighborhoods (Lanthem & Newbery, 1970; Wise et al., 1974). In many instances medical students themselves were instrumental in setting up such programs and medical student organizations. The Medical Committee on Human Rights, the Student Health Organization, and the Student American Medical Association became active in civil rights and antiwar affairs bringing a new phase of social involvement to medical education. These movements have waned as the social issues changed and as the loss of funding for health centers and similar programs forced retrenchment of this kind of activism in medical schools. A new student preoccupation with personal success has emerged coincident with the greater economic hardships of the 1970s. Nevertheless, these social movements have left an imprint on medical education that continues to influence teaching. What the lasting effect will be on the attitudes and behavior of these younger physicians in practice, only the future can tell.

ADULT SOCIALIZATION

During the past 25 years much research has been done on the process of medical education and its effect on students as they pass from college to full membership in the fraternity of physicians. Much of this has been concerned with the way that students acquire the values, attitudes, and role behavior typical of physicians and how these affect relationships to patients. No attempt is made here to review this literature in detail, except where it applies to specific problems being considered (Bloom, 1965; Becker et al., 1972). The central question about any adult socialization process (of which professional socialization is a special kind) is how persons with diverse backgrounds and attitudes come to think and act in accord with the special norms of a particular social group—how homogeneous values, attitudes, and role behavior are achieved that are considered appropriate by the group, consonant with its objectives, and capable of dealing with the special problems it faces. Most studies of the mechanisms involved in reshaping behavior during adult socialization have been done in deviant subcultures, for example, delinquents or drug users. The contrasts existing in these situations make the forces at work more obvious than the subtle shifts in behavior and attitude during assimilation into socially approved adult subcultures. Yet, the stages and mechanisms are similar in both cases. To illustrate these mechanisms it is worth a brief examination of the process of deviant socialization shown in a classic study of becoming a drug user (Becker, 1963).

The sequence of events that Becker describes as a "career of deviance" provides an understandable route for the gradual reshaping of behavior and attitudes from a normal and accepted pattern into a totally deviant one without a sharp break:

1. Certain traits of the individual or his social background set the stage for entry into the deviant career—although these traits are within the normal range of variation and not deviant in themselves. For example, the person who is to become a drug user is apt to be more adventuresome or to live in a neighborhood with friends who are involved in risk taking activities and in conflict with some norms of adult society.
2. These factors lead to the initial opportunity to experiment with drugs.
3. Those who try drugs have a common experience of a new adventure that leads them to associate more with each other than with their peers who have not. This differential association strengthens the traits and attitudes supporting continued experimentation with drugs by mutual reinforcement.
4. To become more than an occasional experimenter requires learning how to go about it successfully, mastering a special "technology," and taking considerable risk in procuring the drugs. Accomplishing this represents an investment in the process, and according to the sociology of knowledge any such vested interest will lead to a redefinition of life situations in terms of how they affect the individual's new interests.
5. This redefinition of the situation is reinforced by emulation of a new reference group with whom the neophyte becomes associated, those who are already confirmed users. From them he learns a jargon that will help

admit him to the subculture. The jargon also embodies new norms of behavior and new perspectives on the world.

6. At some point a crucial event almost inevitably takes place if the individual remains on this course—he is arrested or his new behavior is in some way brought to public attention so that he becomes labeled as a user, an "addict." This label creates stereotyped expectations from others that force him to accept his new role identity. He also experiences a polarization with nonusers who label him as someone apart. His reaction to this alienation is to counterlabel the rest of the world as "square."

7. Such polarization divides the perceived world of the user into two groups, "we" and "they," markedly strengthening the in-group solidarity.

8. The social isolation and the stigma incurred by identification with the deviant group leads to self-justification of the new position in society. This is accomplished by adopting the counterideology readily available in the jargon of the new subculture. New values are espoused and the old world is rejected so that reversal of the process becomes difficult once this set of mutually reinforcing mechanisms comes into play after the watershed of labeling is crossed.

MEDICAL SCHOOL SOCIALIZATION

Recruitment and selection for medical school already lays the groundwork for the professional socialization process by creating a rather homogeneous group, which facilitates the development of the student subculture (Colombotos, 1969). In spite of federal scholarship programs and efforts to broaden the social and ethnic composition of medical school classes, students actually admitted represent a very limited cross section of the American population. In the class of 1974–1975, for example, 48% of student's fathers were professionals and 73% had some college education (almost exactly the same percentage as in 1960)—compared with 13% professionals and 20% having some college education in the general population of males of the age to be fathers of college graduates (Purcell, 1976); 14% were physicians, in contrast to 1% of the general population. Sixty-seven percent of the medical students came from families with incomes over $15,000, compared with 40% in the general population; only 5% of the medical student families had an income less than $5000, compared with 13% of the overall population. Apparently the process of family influence on self-selection for professional training described by Hall (1948) 30 years ago still functions today. The one major change in the characteristic of medical school classes since earlier times is the much larger percentage of women—25% in 1978 compared to 11% as recently as 1970 and less than 5% in 1960 (Johnson & Gordon, 1979; Gordon & Dube, 1976).

Sixty percent of medical students come from only 100 of the most elite undergraduate colleges, and this has changed little since 1960. Consequently, the poor high school and college training of most lower-class and minority students makes it unlikely that they will significantly increase their share of admissions vis-à-vis achievement-oriented middle-class students in the near future. Besides these self-selection factors, the large number of applicants compared to available places makes entrance selection an important influence not only in placement itself but also on the type of student electing premedicine in college and on the courses pursued (Baird, 1975). The number of available places in entering medical school classes increased by 33% between 1970 and 1974 as a result of the opening of new medical schools and enlargement of class size. During the same period, however, the number of applicants increased by 66% so that there were 2.9 potential students for every available position compared to 1.9 in 1958 (Gough, 1971). Because of the heavy emphasis on science in the Medical College Admission Test (MCAT) and the heavy weighting of grades in entrance selection, few unconventional students or even nonscience majors apply—or are accepted if they do. In 1974, 85% of the entering students had been biology or physical science or premed majors, while only 15% majored in the social sciences or humanities (Gordon & Johnson, 1977).

In spite of the improved curricula and teaching methods first-year medical students still devour six to eight massive, fact-laden, highly technical textbooks, besides spending from 45 to 50 hours per week in lectures and laboratories. Because of the extremely selective admission process, nearly all entering students are idealistic, conscientious, very capable, and highly motivated. They begin their training knowing that hard work will be necessary, requiring great sacrifices of time and energy (both from themselves and their families if they are married). Yet few are really prepared for the experience:

In their quest for mastery of the materials, students found that they "could study twenty-four hours a day and still not get it done." According to one, "First semester was really bad; my whole complete time was occupied; I was eating and sleeping and that was all. My only diversion was to devour a news magazine once a week." Because of these anxieties and the assumptions that underlie them, students worked diligently, and many of them felt guilty when taking time off to relax. Typical students' comments revealed this feeling of guilt: "There are very few times to call your own, when you can relax with a clear conscience. There is so much work, you can never get away from it. I seldom relax when I go to a movie; it worries the heck out of me to think I should be home studying." To be unable to digest much of the material presented is very frustrating for conscientious students. Frequent examinations pressure them to memorize rather than to correlate and reason, and they worry when memorized materials are soon forgotten. "It seems that we go through the materials so quickly and everything is so jumbled up; I'm not getting as much out of it as I had hoped to." One student explained, "The student doesn't have enough time to learn it like he wants to. A lot of the material is crammed in and you just don't get a good foundation.

You feel like you've done this course haphazardly. You look back and see that it hasn't been anyone's fault but your own, but there is no way; you can't give up sleeping." (Coombs & Vincent, 1971)

Despite the new objective of medical schools to prepare the students to continue learning on their own, the persistent allegiance to the scientific approach leads even clinicians to consider mastery of biomedical science as essential. While much of it might never be used, they believe it must be in reserve to deal with possible new problems. Moreover, the almost universal requirement of passing the standard National Board of Medical Examiners' tests leads to instruction geared to meeting its questions. Thus students still are forced to achieve profession-wide standards of technical knowledge, and in the process adopt very uniform attitudes about the "proper" role of physicians in using that knowledge.

Whether intended or not, the first year does serve as a kind of initiation rite into medicine, welding the class into a student subculture (Becker & Geer, 1958), and eventually playing an important role in the formation of a professional identity. The process of mastering the technical knowledge and skills of the basic technology provides a great deal of common experience, common problems, and the learning of a common argot. These first unite medical students into a subculture of their own and later help merge them into the wider medical profession. The initiation ordeal (rite-of-passage) created by the intensity, rigor, frustration, and sequestered, totally preoccupied life style of medical students during their early years plays an important role in this process. As they encounter the initial trauma of being unable to digest the material that they believe they should master, students adopt mechanisms for coping with the situation. Many of these are important for their ability as professionals to deal with similar frustration and feelings of inadequacy later in their careers. One such mechanism is the development of a "tolerance for uncertainty" (Fox, 1957). Physicians often encounter the need to know more for optimal care of a patient than they can possibly know, or is even available to the medical profession as a whole. Yet, they must go ahead and act in the face of this uncertainty. Medical students cramming for exams or being quizzed by faculty are, of course, in a different situation than practitioners facing patients, but the necessity of presenting an imperturbable appearance of assurance in spite of inner uncertainty is common to both situations. The baptism of fire in medical school is an important factor in acquiring it for later.

Sometime during the first or second year students attend their first autopsy. Unlike the experience of the anatomy dissection room, which somehow becomes quite impersonal after the first 15 minutes, the autopsy is never impersonal or mechanical. The mood in the anatomy dissecting room is one of cheerful banter, with no thought that the cadaver was once a living human being. The mood of the postmortem room is quiet, respectful attentiveness and somber discussion clearly centered on the body that is still viewed in many ways as a living patient. Various clinical physicians who helped care for the patient being autopsied appear from time to time to see what is being found. Their hushed, almost downcast demeanor conveys (in a way that no formal training could) the weight of responsibility borne by the medical profession—for every autopsy is felt as a failure to prevent a death. From the discrepancies between the clinical record and the postmortem findings, students also come to realize how difficult it can be to make a correct diagnosis or carry out an effective treatment. They are struck by the extent to which medicine is still a very inexact undertaking. In the light of this revelation, students also come to realize how much they will need the understanding support of their fellow physicians to bear this responsibility (Fox, 1957).

The initiation effect of first-year medical school helps forge a select, in-group identity that persists throughout professional life. After a brief period of individual competitiveness among beginning students (carrying over from their premed days of striving against classmates in order to gain admission to medical school), the first-year students realize that they are all in the same boat—none can really master what is being asked of them and "failure" is only a matter of degree. The commonality of this experience welds them into a subculture in which group norms, justification of their divergence from ordinary rules of behavior, and "redefinition of reality" take place (Becker et al., 1961). They counterreject the rest of the world in the way that they feel the "world" (the faculty) is rejecting them because of their inability. Their isolation because of the taxing schedule and even their stigmatizing odors from the dissecting room and the biochemistry laboratory add to the sense of being a special embattled subculture. They feel rejected even by the upper classmen at the same school. They begin to eat together and apart from the others, study together, and (occasionally) relax together—in the latter case even sharing a feeling of guilt for taking any time off when so much remains to be done. This class comradeship, which starts as a means of self-defense for coping with an intolerable situation, is gradually molded by the common experience of the next 4 to 10 years of training into a sense of professional solidarity against lay outsiders.

This characteristic group cohesiveness has many of the set-apart features of a deviant subculture. It grows from the feeling that "no one can know what it is like who is not experiencing it with me," and extends into the more general feeling that "no one can understand my thinking about these things who has not experienced what I have experienced." At first this defensive group solidarity is primarily directed against the faculty pressure. It helps redefine the learning confrontation from a situation of failure (to meet an impossible demand for work) into a joint struggle for survival by devising methods of coping with faculty expectations (Becker et al., 1963; Coombs & Vincent, 1971). Yet the process of bridging the tension between faculty and student begins very soon. The amount of material to be learned does not diminish in later semesters, but student alienation gradually disappears as the commonality of faculty and student interests grows. The student solidarity remains, but is transformed from antifaculty into antilayman terms.

During the clinical years amalgamation of the student subculture into the general professional subculture is accelerated by several factors. During the preclinical years the class is together almost continuously, and all the students are doing the same thing most of the time. With the beginning of the clinical clerkships of the third and fourth years, the students are scattered throughout different hospital services. The class unity is dispersed, and individual students are instead brought closer together with interns and residents, who clearly identify, as physicians, with the attending staff. Third- and fourth-year students spend a great deal of time on hospital wards between assigned duties waiting for the next thing to be done. Much of this time is spent in informal discussion or "bull sessions," usually about cases or medical problems, with other students and residents. Here they assimilate the culture of the hospital world as well as the practical knowledge and lore of medical care. The parochial class identity of the student clique is rapidly enlarged to include the wider professional group.

A second factor reinforces the assimilation process and sets a new series of mechanisms into motion that intensifies identification with the profession. The watershed of donning the white coat (and entry into the relationship with patients that it symbolizes) speeds up the assumption of professional norms, values, role behavior, and ideology. The labeling initiated by the white coat calls forth the physician stereotype and a set of expectations on the part of patients, hospital staff, house officers, and attending faculty. Even when it is known that they are still students, patients and staff refer to them as "doctor." Patients allow them special access into their physical and personal privacy, hang on their words and expressions for hints about their conditions, and accept their authority in regard to medical matters as if they were fully qualified physicians. In turn patients expect from them, as physicians, that they appear distinguished, act self-assured, kindly but firm, even authoritarian and a bit mysterious (the priest-shaman tradition still influences the image and role of physicians). The student is forced to take on these attributes in patient encounters. The process is exemplified in a report from a third-year student's diary:

To say that the patient "searches your face for clues" is no overstatement. An example—while on OB, when trying to palpate a baby once, I got a little confused and frowned in puzzlement. Sensed at once that the mother saw the frown and was alarmed. So, I reassured her that everything was all right. I have always tried to remember not to do it again . . . (Fox, 1957, p. 227)

During the clinical years residents and attending faculty accept students as junior colleagues and members of the team. They are expected to shoulder part of the workload, take certain responsibilities, and share in the special attitudes and norms their seniors hold about patients and other hospital staff. Medical students on the hospital wards have access to information about patients of which the patients themselves are kept ignorant. Participating in this secrecy by the use of medical jargon in the presence of patients, plus the need to obtain compliance from patients in difficult situations, creates a "we–they" boundary with patients—inevitably entailing polarization and tension. Sharing this tension vis-à-vis patients, the common argot, the unique kinds of experience familiar to all physicians, the weight of responsibility and expectations applied to them by others, all converge to create a strong physician in-group solidarity in which the students participate.

As in any subculture, this professional solidarity brings with it a harshly enforced, group social control and an ideology consonant with the new role behavior, vested interests, and incentive system. This ideology justifies the many unusual kinds of behavior that students are called upon to engage in and reinforces the sense of professional identity and group solidarity. Such solidarity is particularly strong in the hospital setting, where there is continuous intensive interaction between professionals and where physicians and students face patients together in a solid phalanx. Although the intensity of the interaction and the professional unanimity characteristic of the hospital situation decrease in individual practice after residency training is completed, elements of the subculture remain throughout the life of the physician because many mechanisms that sustain it continue to act. Precisely which parts of the role behavior and attitude structure are retained and which are discarded depends on what is reinforced by the organization of practice, as discussed in Chapter 8.

Nonetheless, three characteristic sets of attitudes and behavior emerge almost universally out of the professional socialization process: (1) overconcern with the technical problems of disease and the tendency to downplay the personal aspects of patient care; (2) increasing specialization of knowledge and practice; (3) secretiveness and authority in relationships to patients. These features have been targets for considerable criticism of the medical profession. The technological orientation and tendency toward specialization are important factors in the mismatch of the health care system to the new needs for care created by the prevalence of chronic diseases today. Examining the underlying mechanisms of these physician behavior patterns helps assess the chances of bringing about change.

TECHNOLOGY FOCUS AND DISEASE ORIENTATION VERSUS PATIENT ORIENTATION IN PHYSICIAN BEHAVIOR

Since the end of World War II there has been a growing uneasiness voiced, not only by critics of the medical profession but also by physicians and medical educators, that modern medical education produces physicians who are more interested in the disease process than in their patients as persons. The critics of this so-called disease orientation argue that physicians take too narrow an approach to the therapeutic relationship, concentrating almost entirely on the technical medical problems and too little on the "human" (emotional, personal, and social) problems of the patient. The perceived inordinate disease orientation of physicians has two aspects. One arises from unrealistic patient expectations (Chapters 5 and 12) that are incongruent with the organization of the health care system. The other is a real change in the attitudes and behavior of the medical profession. Both follow from the developments in medical technology in the last 50 years and from shifts in the country's social structure.

The increasingly impersonal nature of today's complex organizational society frequently places people in need of someone who can play the role of confessor, advisor, and general ombudsman. The physician has often become the focus of these unfulfilled needs. Part of the desire to have physicians play this role stems from a romanticized image of the family physician of pre-Flexner days as a kindly community benefactor ready to provide friendly warmth and counseling. Whether or not this was often really the case, the belief plays an important role in the perceptions that society has of physicians today. Previously, the dominant pattern of practice did allow a relationship with patients, even with entire families, that was maintained over many years. As a result, the physician came to know a great deal about the person and was a confidant and counselor in many matters beyond the strictly medical ones. The desire for a more patient-oriented relationship also flows from the cultural tradition of physicians exercising social control of illness behavior by alleviating anxieties and providing succor to the sick.

Patient-oriented care in general practice, insofar as it did exist, has indeed been one of the casualties of the clinical revolution, but for reasons that are inseparable from the success of clinical medicine. An important explanation for the greater patient orientation of physicians in earlier times was simply their therapeutic impotence prior to introduction of the successful methods of diagnosis and treatment. Physicians were more concerned with patients as persons because there was little else that they had to offer. Some alleviation of symptoms, a good "bedside manner," and possibly the restoration of order into a disrupted life were their only stock in trade. For their professional survival, physicians had to cultivate the art of personal concern and family therapy to offer in exchange for their fees. The technological revolution in medicine and the pragmatic ability to intervene successfully in the disease process have had a profound effect on the relationship to patients. The physician's professional interest has understandably shifted from the human problems to applying the new technology in the most effective manner. The effect of this new capability has not been limited to physicians' attitudes. Patients' first concern is also that the care they receive is technically adequate, and only secondarily that their physician is supportive in regard to their personal welfare (Mechanic, 1972).

The amount of time available for a patient's nonmedical problems has decreased greatly because of the time required to do all the technical things that now can (and therefore must) be done in cases of illness. Since 1930 the number of medical services received per capita has more than doubled while the number of physicians per capita had increased only slightly until the last few years (Chapters 8 and 12), thus decreasing the amount of time for each patient. The technical processes themselves have become steadily more impersonal because of their complexity and because of greater reliance on laboratory methods and technicians (e.g., x-ray operators, specially trained therapists, etc.) who carry out diagnostic and therapeutic procedures for the physicians. The patient is much less apt to be seen in the home where personal aspects confront the physician. Today the patient is more frequently hospitalized for complicated care and cut off from personal ties (Chapter 9). The growth of specialty practice, which is also a consequence of technological progress, adds to the disease orientation. Specialists needing referrals are more dependent on the professional opinion of colleagues about their technical competence than on the opinion of patients about their human relations competence (Freidson, 1970a).

Medical educators themselves have recognized the overemphasis on disease and have taken steps in the last 20 years to redress the balance. Clearly medical education (professional socialization) plays a role in transforming the students from their naive humanitarianism to detached objectivity. It would be misleading, however, to assume that medical school is the only factor influencing physician attitudes and behavior. The technological changes have had a profound impact on the nature of medical practice as well as on medical education. These changes in practice necessitate a more disease-oriented, engineering-type approach by physicians. The physician must reason in objective terms about the mechanisms of disease and the proper action because he can only influence the course of disease in that way. This objectifying "engineering" approach was particularly encouraged in the old system of teaching where the student learned only anatomy or only physiology or pathology at any given time, but the new organ-system approach does not basically change the objectifying perspective—it only makes the relationships between the objective knowledge from different disciplines more immediately obvious and relevant for the student. It may even intensify the specialty bias to medical practice, which tends to parallel the organ systems divisions of the new curriculum.

Dealing with patients during the later years of training does not appreciably change this disease-centered perspective. In the teaching hospital situation the scientific disease orientation in regard to medical care remains central. The incentive system and interactive processes of teaching and practice in university affiliated hospitals are such that the student's thinking is kept focused on the disease process and the scientific approach to treating it. The standards used by faculty (and by other students) to measure student performance are scientific correctness in clinical reasoning and virtuosity in "roundsmanship"—that is, coming up with the latest research findings in reference to a case or with esoteric diagnostic possibilities or dexterously sorting out a complex differential diagnosis and physiological analysis of a case. The ability to relate to patients, allay their fears, or give insight to the role of nonmedical factors in the management of cases is seldom grounds for obtaining distinction.

Prior to the adoption of the specific-defect model of disease, physicians were in effect constrained to treat *symptoms* rather than diseases. Symptoms cannot be as easily separated from the patients as disease entities can. Thus the old model necessarily entailed greater concern with the care of the patient as a sick person. Physicians were forced to think about illness as something *happening to patients* because there was no easy way to deal with diseases as real in themselves. The new technology and disease-model have changed the *meaning* of the therapeutic situation and restructured the reality within which physicians act. The new model of diseases—reinforced by the success of the technology based on it—gives diseases a reality of their own that is just as familiar to physicians as the patients. The language used by harassed nurses and house officers in busy hospitals illustrates this reality and familiarity: "We have just admitted a severe myocardial infarction in the ER; get the defibrillator ready." "The gall bladder in Room 103 has spiked a fever; check the wound for infection."

This disease focus does not mean that physicians cannot or do not consider the patient's own needs and problems. The good clinician certainly does. However, in so far as the physician deals with an illness within the framework of his professional training, the logic of diagnosis and treatment forces him to use impersonal categories. The norms and incentives of his professional role define the diagnosis and treatment of *disease* as his *primary goal*. In order to view the patient as an individual with his own needs, fears, and attitudes, the physician must make an effort partially at variance with his professional training, responsibilities, and interests. This effort may even jeopardize his professional judgment and competence in correctly perceiving and treating the disease. The more specialized and the more technically competent the physician is, the greater is the tendency to concentrate on the disease and to depersonalize the patient.

In addition to the practically motivated disease orientation assimilated in learning the technology of modern medicine, a parallel socialization process imbues the student with the value that this is the *right* way to think about the therapeutic situation. Lief and Fox (1963) have described this as "training for detached concern," the acquisition of attitudes and values during medical school that allow the physician to deal with patients in a detached, objective way while retaining an appropriate level of human concern. They see the conversion of student perspective from one of naive humanitarian sympathy to this detached objective concern as a functional necessity of modern medical practice. Physicians must deal with patients both as objects to be technically repaired (i.e., as diseased physiological systems) and as suffering human beings at the same time. This combined empathetic and detached attitude is foreign to the approach taken by most people in dealing with human beings, where compassion is seen in conflict with manipulating people as material objects. Proper balance between the two extremes is a difficult art for the physician to acquire, and it is understandable that the neophyte or the harassed practitioner can easily slip too far in the direction of detachment.

Becker and Geer (1958) have described the same process of acquiring objective attitudes toward patients as the "fate of idealism in medical school." They believe that the student's defense mechanisms for self-preservation, which lead to formation of the student subculture, also produce a cynicism in regard to patients by redefining the patients' problems in terms of the student's learning objectives. A number of studies have demonstrated that there is indeed a marked shift toward callousness from the first to the fourth year of medical school (Christie & Merton, 1958; Nathanson, 1958; Becker et al., 1961). Becker argues (Becker & Geer, 1958a) that the cynicism is in fact just a veneer and usually reverts to a more realistic objectivity as the students begin to practice medicine.*

Because of the crucial role of the disease model in shaping physician thinking, simply restructuring the medical school curriculum is not apt to change the final value and attitude socialization of physicians very profoundly—as desirable as improvements in the medical curriculum are. Fundamental changes in the disease model, technology, and organization of health care would be necessary to accomplish this. For example, differences in organization of practice, with accompanying variation of incentive systems, and in secondary professional socialization lead to marked differences in the behavior of physicians (Chapter 8). Restructuring the organization of practice and its prestige and financial incentive systems may be more important in reshaping physician attitudes and behavior to become more congruent with the needs of post-clinical medicine than changes in medical education. The potential impact on physician behavior of practice organization and incentives needs to be a serious consideration in planning for the coming changes in health care.

Finally, the strong disease orientation of physicians is closely related to what has been termed the "technological imperative" (Fuchs, 1974): the physician's assumption that whatever can be done to establish the exact nature of a disease, or to treat it, *should* be done, unless there are overwhelming factors militating against doing so. This is particularly strong in teaching hospital (or research) settings where there is the rationale of ad-

---

* The functionalist perspective (in sociological theory) assumes that the behavior and attitudes of "detached concern" are molded to meet the physician's role requirements; the interactionist perspective assumes that disease orientation is a student-subcultural defense mechanism and this later converts to a physician-subcultural stance vis-à-vis patients, helping to maintain a realistic (objective) detached orientation. Undoubtedly there is validity in both, and the present authors view them as two complementary aspects of any situation.

vancing science and knowledge. Concern with the disease process can easily distort a physician's view of the appropriate balance between scientific or therapeutic thoroughness and the financial, social, or psychological interest of patients, their families, and society (Katz & Capron, 1975). Medicine has become a very expensive undertaking. The disease orientation of physicians is a major factor in the rising cost of health care because it leads to unnecessary diagnostic procedures and treatments (Chapter 12). The dividing line between what is necessary and what is optional or unnecessary is a very difficult and subjective judgment in many cases (Scheff, 1963). The attitudes and professional habits nurtured by disease orientation can easily be the deciding factor that keeps hopeless patients alive for additional days or weeks of great suffering to themselves and their families simply because it is possible to do so and because no physician feels he is in a position to say it should not be done.

THE RUSH TOWARD SPECIALIZATION

The goal of the Flexner reforms to standardize medical education and train all medical students to deal with the *full spectrum* of diseases as clinician-scientists was outmoded almost immediately. By 1925 the great majority of newly trained physicians aspired to specialty status and limited practice. Less than 10% of physicians practicing in 1923 listed themselves as specialists in the AMA Directory. Of the physicians graduating from medical school between 1915 and 1925 over 35% eventually became full-time specialists, and another 40% gave part-time attention to a specialty (Weiskotten et al., 1961). Today over 80% of those now in practice are listed as specialists by the AMA, and over 90% of recent classes are specialty board certified or pursuing it. This is a very different situation than exists, for instance, in England, where only 30% of practicing physicians are specialists (consultants) (Stevens, 1966). The causes and effects of this radical change in the structure of the American medical profession are important for understanding the dynamics of health care.

A large percentage of students entering medical school still express interest in general practice, but by the time of graduation or completion of internship they almost universally decide to undertake specialty residency training in preparation for limiting their practices. This now well-known trend was first documented by Kendall and Selvin (1957) in a study of medical students from 1952 to 1954. As might be expected, the growth of commitment to board certification and specialty practice continues during internship and residency training. Today, there is renewed interest in primary care because of social pressure and improved financial incentives. But this practice is anticipated in terms of specialty qualification in internal medicine, pediatrics, or family practice with board certification as an assumed step in the training.

A major factor in this shift is the overwhelming mass of knowledge and skills necessary for the practice of medicine today:

As medical knowledge has grown, practicing physicians have found it increasingly essential to limit their attention to more specialized areas of activity. While it was probably possible for a medical student at the turn of the century to graduate knowing virtually "all there was to know" about medicine, it is today absolutely impossible for any one man to possess all the knowledge germane to a field of specialty practice, let alone the entire field of medicine. (Coggeshall, 1965)

The early decision to specialize redefines the learning situation in medical school even if no decision is reached about *which* specialty to enter (Kendall, 1971). It is one of the mechanisms used by students to cope with a seemingly impossible task.

The learning environment in medical schools and teaching hospitals is dominated by specialists and research people. Such physicians replaced practicing generalists as faculty when philanthropic grants to medical schools enabled building laboratory and research facilities and hiring full-time, research-oriented staff. This trend toward specialized faculty was accelerated in the 1930s by the establishment of the specialty boards. These provided a clear criterion of expertise in a field, and medical schools soon demanded specialty board qualification for teaching. After 1940 federal monies started to flow into medical schools from the National Institutes of Health and other sources. These funds were almost entirely in the form of research grants rather than direct teaching subsidies. As a result medical faculties were increasingly dominated by research-oriented specialists whose interests were even narrower than those of the clinically oriented spcialists. Consequently, medical students live in a world populated by highly expert super-specialists role models.

Nevertheless, we should not exaggerate the influence of role models on the student's decision to specialize. Changing the structure of medical education or exposing students to family practitioners during their training may influence some additional students to go into general practice. However, students are also influenced by the world outside medical school from which they have come (e.g., the values and attitudes prevalent on college campuses) and into which they will go to practice (Funkenstein, 1971). The shift toward specialty training in medical school is probably as much a consequence of *anticipatory* socialization, learning what problems and opportunities exist in practice, as acquiring the attitudes and values of the medical school subculture. Most studies of professional socialization have focused narrowly on the process of medical education and have not examined the problem in the larger context of medical practice and financial incentives.

The hard reality is that specialists have a much better position than generalists (Wolfe & Badgley, 1972). Specialists earn higher incomes, work shorter hours, see fewer patients with more varied and interesting problems, which they have more time to explore in depth. They have much higher prestige than generalists, and this prestige perception is not limited to colleagues—patients are equally aware of it and clearly want specialist care. However much they nostalgically bemoan the passing of the family practitioner, given the choice, patients overwhelmingly select specialists in preference to generalists. Another factor is the increasing importance of the hospital in medical practice because of the need for the complex diagnostic and therapeutic equipment available only there. Medical students are aware that hospital staff appointments are increasingly restricted to board-certified specialists. Without such appointments high quality practice is impossible (Bucher & Strauss, 1960).

The road to success in medicine is specialization, and the fact is not lost on today's student physicians. They are only responding (in anticipation) to the same forces that acted on physicians already in practice in the 1930s. When the prestige and importance of specialty practice began to grow, physicians moved from general practice to specialization informally by building their reputations and gaining referrals in order to limit their practices. Physicians and medical students alike respond to the professional incentive system, and this is largely determined by how the technology and practice of medicine are organized and financed. The attitudes and behavior acquired in medical school are more a mirror of the forces acting on the profession as a whole than the ultimate cause of the trend toward specialization. The larger world of specialty practice and (residency) training beyond medical school is discussed in Chapter 8.

PROFESSIONAL AUTHORITY BEHAVIOR

Professional socialization also gives rise to a third constellation of attitudes and role behavior, resolute authority behavior in relation to patients and the institutions of health care, so-called professional dominance (Freidson, 1970a). Although each new physician acquires the essential demeanor and dominating skills in the course of medical education, as with other physician attitudes, the ultimate causes of authority behavior lie in the structure of the profession and its relationship to the rest of society. Freidson (1970, 1970a) has pointed out the importance of professional authority in obtaining patient compliance, maintaining professional autonomy, and assuring dominance over the technology of medicine. It plays an equally important role in relieving patient anxiety by transferring responsibility for decisions to the physician.

Unlike the disease orientation and specialization, professional authority itself is not generally considered a problematic feature of physician behavior. Yet it is a major component of many problems related to health care that are the subject of criticism, for example, breakdown in physician-patient communication, professional secretiveness, the loss of trust in physicians manifested by increasing malpractice litigation, and the need for regulation of medical practice to maintain quality of care. One probable reason that professional authority is not generally viewed as a problem is its traditional anxiety relieving, social-control function in the healing role (Chapter 3). It became a problem only because of its impact on the demand, cost, and importance of the technology physicians dominate (Dunnell & Cartwright, 1972).

Development of authority behavior in medical students takes place hand-in-hand with learning how to deal technically with patients' problems. Medical students learn early in their careers to assume a dominant stance in patient encounters by emulating the behavior of their faculty and house officer role models. Development of professional authority behavior is intensified by the student subculture for dealing with uncertainty and its later incorporation of professional group ideology. Nevertheless, there is a quantum jump in authority demeanor when students first don the white coat symbolic of professional office. This evokes the stereotypic expectations of patients who react with culturally learned and situationally reinforced attitudes of subordination. Any lapse in authority stance by the student is met with patient reactions that nudge him back to the anticipated role performance (Fox, 1957).

Like new members of any subculture, the first acting out of the self-confident authority role is largely an assumed "front," which tends to be exaggerated and self-conscious (Goffman, 1959). The self-assured posture for dealing with uncertainty is then amplified throughout professional life by the expectation of competence from patients and from others with whom physicians interact. Additional reinforcement occurs because the behavior works effectively in controlling the situation and enforcing the unilateral decisions physicians often must make in the face of uncertainty. The role of self-confident decision-maker soon ceases to be play acting and becomes part of the physician's professional identity.

Learning authority behavior is aided by the structural situation in teaching hospitals where the student is part of a collective front of physicians facing a single, fearful patient (Miller, 1970). During the formative period of professional attitudes, medical students are confronted with patients who are in a position of submissive acquiescence to their orders. In bed, in strange, awe-inspiring surroundings out of their control, patients are deprived of the usual social supports and identity-confirming props. In this situation they almost universally project a posture of obedience, which physicians come to expect. Throughout medical practice the physician-patient interaction situation continues to be structured so that the physician is in the dominant position. The patient is made to feel that submissive behavior is natural and proper, even though it would be considered highly unnatural, bizarre, or even deviant in any other setting. Emerson (1970) describes this process of "restructuring reality" in gynecological examinations, a rather extreme form of the authority-dependent relationship. The stage is set by the props and trappings of the physician's office, which cue patients as to their expected role because of the cultural associations with these symbols. The physician uses stereotyped posturing and language placing patients in a subordinate position and reassuring them that what is happening is necessary and proper. Nurses and other members of the cast reaffirm the propriety of the situation and support the authority of the physician.

The techniques and mechanisms that support professional authority in the individual physician-patient interaction mirror broader social forces which legitimate it: (1) the culturally mandated social-control role of the physician; (2) public willingness to submit to the physician's authority in exchange for the benefit of his knowledge and skills because of his acknowledged effectiveness in dealing with disease; and (3) the legally and socially sanctioned guild power that controls access to the technology and institutions of health care.

Physicians occupy a culturally defined role embodying the ancient social-control function of enforcing proper illness behavior. The power of this cultural mandate, though modified by the new technology of medicine and the changing structure of society, has remained a major source of physician authority and patient control (Parsons, 1952, 1958). Much of the physician's legal and moral authority is a result of this normative function. It is buttressed by control of the mysterious knowledge and ritual of treatment also included in the cultural expectations. Thus, unlike most consulting professionals, physicians still constitute a priesthood of society. The power of that priestly mantle is invoked in each patient interaction to define the patient's status and appropriate behavior in regard to illness.

The cultural mandate gives physicians special access to privileged information about patients and license to subject them to things that are often poorly understood and terrifying. This access to the patient's personal history and body adds an additional intimidating power to the authority of the cultural role. The physician's role also entails high social status and prestige that carry their own authority. These are backed up by symbols of wealth and success, such as an impressive office, expensive cars and clothing, and a familiar demeanor with other men of high rank and prestige in the community (Rosenblatt & Suchman, 1966).

The second source of physician authority derives from patient demand for the benefit of professional competence in skills that are much desired. Power to influence the patient's behavior and overcome resistance to medical advice evolves from the tacit bargaining or exchange relationship between patient and physician. In a sense the consulting relation implies to the client: "If you want my services, you must accept my authority in advising and treating you; if not, you will have to go elsewhere for treatment." This implicit threat to withhold services is almost never used directly as a sanction to gain patient compliance, since that would be openly unethical practice.* But the desire for a physician's services creates a dependency that gives him great authority.

The physician's exercise of authority created by the dependency of the consulting relationship depends on the balance between how much the patient wants a particular physician's services and how willing and able the patient is to turn to alternative sources—other physicians or other institutions. This is a question of availability and of the costs involved, time, money, and the emotional investment of establishing new relationships. Most patients are thankful for any satisfactory access to the medical care system. They are seldom willing to gamble on starting over and have little choice but to accept the advice of a physician. Comparison shopping is not a real option in medical care.

The potential authority of the individual physician increases proportionately as the reputation of clinical medicine grows collectively. It also increases as access to physicians in the area becomes more difficult and as medical care is increasingly provided in organized settings (such as hospitals or clinics) where the patient has little opportunity to turn to other physicians by his own choice. The degree of dependency in the consulting relationship is also affected by the structure of the practice situation. The physician in solo practice has less control over his patients. He is more apt to acquiesce to their demands and less apt to feel constrained by professionally approved standards of care because he is more dependent on the patient than on his colleagues for his livelihood. The physician in group practice or referral practice, on the other hand, is more dependent on his colleagues' approval and is less responsive to his patients (Freidson, 1961).†

The third source of physician authority derives from licensure and specialty-board certification. Licensure actually represents two elements of public endorsement of physician authority. It is testament that the physician possesses the expertise to make medical decisions about the patient and carry out treatment. It is also indirect legal acknowledgement that the medical profession is the only group empowered to occupy the culturally sanctioned priestly healing role with the mandate to define proper illness behavior. Licensure adds official endorsement to the authority of the cultural role. It makes any member of the medical profession also a quasi-functionary of the state. The license to practice medicine does not entail any direct legal authority over patients except in certain public health matters. Yet it

---

* Freidson (1970a) has argued that the reason for the professional ideology of "free choice of physicians" is the need to protect the source of leverage to gain patient compliance. The major rhetorical use for the doctrine of "free choice" today, however, is not to enhance their authority over patients—this is seldom a problem for the physicians who are apt to be making such policy statements—but rather to fight the closed panel group practice of medicine, which denies a part of the patient market to individually practicing physicians in that geographic region.

† This is undoubtedly a factor in the behavior of physicians and in the authority relationship to patients, but it is only one dimension of the complex constellation of behavioral influences acting on different structures of practice to be explored in Chapter 8.

implies that the state certifies the judgement and skills of this physician—and medicine in general—as competent, therefore not to be questioned by the patient.

The other source of authority in licensure derives from the monopoly gatekeeper position it gives to the profession in regard to the use of medical technology. Physicians collectively have a legal monopoly over the practice of medicine and hence over access to medical services in general, hospitals, most drugs, diagnostic facilities, and so on. Each physician holds the sanction not only of potentially withholding his own services, but also of preventing access, at least temporarily, to all other medical services.

FUNCTIONS AND DYSFUNCTIONS OF PROFESSIONAL AUTHORITY

The authority role of the physician is a necessary part of the therapeutic relationship for (1) reassuring patients in the face of illness anxiety and (2) obtaining client compliance in the consulting situation. A major function of physicians continues to be alleviating patient anxiety and controlling their illness behavior. The confident, authoritative demeanor of the physician is an important component of the treatment—even when there is something very concrete that can be done for the disease itself. Great physicians of history have rightly pointed this out. Sir William Osler, one of the founders of modern scientific medicine at Johns Hopkins, described the situation poignantly in his essay, *Aequanimitas*:

In the first place, in the physician or surgeon no quality takes rank with imperturbability, and I propose for a few minutes to direct your attention to this essential bodily virtue. Perhaps I may be able to give those of you, in whom it has not developed during the critical scenes of the past month, a hint or two of its importance, possibly a suggestion for its attainment. Imperturbability means coolness and presence of mind under all circumstances, calmness amid storm, clearness of judgement in moments of grave peril, immobility, impassiveness, or, to use an old and expressive word, *phlegma*. It is the quality which is most appreciated by the laity though often misunderstood by them; and the physician who has the misfortune to be without it, who *betrays indecision* and worry, and who shows that he is flustered and flurried in ordinary emergencies, loses rapidly the confidence of his patients. (Osler, 1919, my emphasis)

The second major function of physician authority behavior is to obtain patient compliance in order to carry out effective treatment (Freidson, 1970a). The professional-client relationship always involves potential tension in regard to control. Although the patient presumably consults the physician voluntarily to obtain advice and treatment, there is often resistance to the advice or refusal of the treatment offered because of fears, denial of the seriousness of the situation, conflicting pressures, and so on. If the physician is not able to overcome this resistance, he fails as a consultant. Unlike the situation between professionals, physicians in the consulting role cannot expect to convince patients by appealing to scientific evidence (accepted by the profession) since patients seldom have the knowledge to make such decisions rationally. Patients must be persuaded by indirect means that it is in their best interest to follow the advice. The simplest and most general way is through a convincing air of authority on the part of the physician (Hollender, 1958).

As necessary as these positive functions of the physician's authority are, important negative effects also arise out of the same behavior. One is the tendency toward secrecy and the consequent breakdown of communication between physician and patient. The need to create the air of confidence in the face of uncertainty often inclines physicians not to disclose any more than necessary about a patient's illness, giving an impression that decisions are made on the basis of more certainty than is actually the case. While this secretiveness arises in part from the physician's posture for dealing with uncertainty, it also stems from the tendency of any subculture to be protective about internal affairs. There is always fear that such things might not be sympathetically or properly understood by nonmembers (Coser, 1958).

To justify their secretiveness and authoritarian pronouncements, instead of the painstaking explanation necessary to allow patients to participate in the decision-making, physicians have numerous explanations. They often assert that patients are not capable of dealing with the uncertainty and the possible dire outcomes that might profoundly affect their lives. "Physicians have spent years learning to make such decisions objectively in the face of uncertainty by acting on the basis of probability," they argue openly or tacitly. "How can patients be expected to deal with such probabilistic decision-making without prior training and when it involves them so personally?" "Moreover," they contend, "patients *do not want to know* the truth about such things." Most physicians have ready examples of instances of self-deceit by patients in the face of threatening facts. Practitioners also argue that it would be technically impossible to include patients in much of the decision-making. No physician could possibly find the time required to discuss the probabilities in detail with patients, and deal with their anxieties, before a decision could be reached (Hulka et al., 1970).

Yet, secrecy can destroy communication with patients at times when it would be most important, for instance, when a patient is suffering from terminal illness or refusing to cooperate with a physician's recommendation where it would be crucial to understand why the patient is reticent (Reeder, 1972; Svarstad, 1976). In chronic illness the authority behavior of physicians can intensify patient dependency, instead of encouraging them to deal with disability and illness on their own (Graham, 1963). Failure of communication is often accentuated in circumstances where the social distance is greater, such as in treating lower-class patients (Walsh & Elling, 1968; Chapter 9).

Use of professional authority to obtain compliance tends to routinize responses to patients in medical situations that might call for more individualized approaches. This occurs in any role-typical behavior, but it has more serious implications where it masks the inherent uncertainty of the therapeutic situation (Koran, 1975). Such routinized role responses may even lull physicians about the risks of some medical uncertainties. In the face of ambivalence physicians often revert to rigidity and conservatism. They may be unreceptive to change in new situations when there is need for reevaluation of the potential advantages and disadvantages of possible actions (Ben-David, 1958).

Physician defensiveness and secrecy is often accentuated by a growing patient ambivalence in their expectations about the physician-patient relationship. As physicians perform a more strictly technical role, the physician-patient relationship becomes a more limited transaction where a given service is purchased. Despite their desire for relief from anxiety through reliance on the physician's authority, patients justifiably feel that they have the right to know what they are buying, both the physician's qualifications and the basis on which important decisions are being made (Belsky & Gross, 1975). Secretiveness and reliance on authority to enforce decisions probably constitute a major reason for the rapid growth of malpractice litigation in recent years. When unrealistic expectations about the infallibility of medicine are not met, breakdown in communication can aggravate the sense of being deceived (Peterson, 1973). This leads many patients to seek an outlet for their frustration through the courts. The increasing number of malpractice suits, in turn, has intensified physicians' inclinations to close ranks and revert to so-called defensive medicine, carrying out procedures and consultations more as protection against possible malpractice suits than because they are actually indicated medically (Defensive Medicine Project, 1971; Hershey, 1972).

Physicians often withhold from the public information about professional affairs and the behavior of other physicians that might be damaging to the image of the profession as a whole (Benham & Benham, 1975). Such behavior is characteristic of all in-groups, but it can lead to silence in the face of professional incompetence or misconduct (Hyde & Wolff, 1954). Professional secrecy and authority attitudes make social control over physician behavior difficult, whether from inside or outside of the profession. Professional ideology about the necessity of autonomy and collegial responsibility for self-discipline has hardened opposition to any form of external interference in medical affairs. Physicians have been quite successful in resisting any incursion of nonphysician influence in policing the quality of care or determining the appropriateness of utilization decisions.

The immense authority that individual physicians and the organized medical profession have acquired over such highly valued technology, however, is starting to be challenged in order to protect the members of society dependent upon it. This reaction is similar to monopoly-controlled industries (Thompson, 1967), where public demands for government regulation grow when the dependence on them becomes too threatening. Congress has already enacted Medicare amendments establishing Professional Standards Review Organizations (PSROs) to police hospital admission practices and length of stay. This kind of regulation of practice is likely to increase. Just as Clemenceau said of modern warfare and the generals, modern medicine had become too important and too expensive to be left entirely to the control of physicians. The evolving policies and strategies for regulating the structure and practice of medicine are dealt with further in Chapters 10, 12, and 13.

REFERENCES

Baird, Leonard L., "The Characteristics of Medical Students and Their Views of the First Year," *Journal of Medical Education,* **50**(December):1092–1099, 1975.

Banta, David H., "Abraham Flexner—A Reappraisal," *Sociology and Medicine,* **5**:655–661, 1971.

Becker, Howard S., *Outsiders: Studies in the Sociology of Deviance,* New York: Free Press, 1963.

Becker, Howard, and Geer, Blanche, "Student Culture In Medical School," *Harvard Education Review,* **28**(Winter):70–80, 1958.

Becker, Howard, and Geer, Blanche, "The Fate of Idealism in Medical School," *American Sociological Review,* **23**:50–56, 1958a.

Becker, Howard, Geer, Blanche, Hughes, Everett, and Strauss, Anshelm, *Boys in White,* Chicago: University of Chicago Press, 1961.

Becker, Howard, Geer, Blanche, and Miller, Stephen, "Medical Education," in Freeman, H., et al., Eds., *Handbook of Medical Sociology,* Englewood Cliffs, N.J.: Prentice-Hall, 1972.

Belsky, M., and Gross, L., *Beyond the Medical Mystique: How to Choose and Use Your Doctor,* New York: Arbor House, 1975.

Ben-David, J., "The Professional Role of the Physician in Bureaucratized Medicine, A Study in Role Conflict," *Human Relations,* **11**:255–274, 1958.

Benham, Lee, and Benham, Alexandra, "Regulating Through the Professions: A Perspective on Information Control," *Journal of Law and Economics,* 433–435, October, 1975.

Bloom, Samuel, "The Sociology of Medical Education," *Milbank Memorial Fund Quarterly,* **43**(November):143–184, 1965.

Bucher, Rue, and Strauss, Anshelm, "Professions in Process," *American Journal of Sociology,* **66**:325–334, 1960.

Burrow, James G., *AMA: Voice of American Medicine,* Baltimore: Johns Hopkins University Press, 1963.

Christie, Richard, and Merton, Robert K., "Procedures for the Sociological Study of the Values Climate of Medical Schools," *Journal of Medical Education,* **33**(October, Part 2):125–153, 1958.

Coggeshall, Lowell T., *Planning for Medical Progress Through Education,* Washington, D.C.: Association of American Medical Colleges, 1965.

Colombotos, John, "Social Origins and Ideology of Physicians: A Study of the Effects of Early Socialization," *Journal of Health and Social Behavior,* 10:16–29, 1969.

Coombs, Robert and Vincent, Clark E., *Psychosocial Aspects of Medical Training,* Springfield, Ill.: Thomas, 1971.

Coser, Rose, "Authority and Decision-Making in a Hospital: A Comparative Analysis," *American Sociological Review,* 23:56–63, 1958.

Defensive Medicine Project, "The Medical Malpractice Threat: A Study of Defensive Medicine," *Duke Law Journal,* 1971(December):939–993, 1971.

Dunnell, Karen, and Cartwright, Ann, *Medicine Takers, Prescribers and Hoarders,* London: Routledge & Kegan Paul, 1972.

Emerson, Joan, "Behavior in Private Places: Sustaining Definitions of Reality in Gynecological Examinations," in Dreitzel, Hans P., *Recent Sociology #2,* New York: Macmillan, 1970.

Fein, Rashi, and Weber, Gerald I., *Financing Medical Education,* New York: McGraw-Hill, 1971.

Flexner, Abraham, *Medical Education in the United States and Canada,* New York: The Carnegie Foundation for the Advancement of Learning, 1910.

Fox, Renee C., "Training for Uncertainty," in Merton, R. K. et al., *The Student Physician,* New York: Columbia University Press, 1957.

Fox, Renee C., *Experiment Perilous: Physicians and Patients Facing the Unknown,* New York: Free Press, 1959.

Freidson, Eliot, *Patients' Views of Medical Practice,* New York: Russell Sage Foundation, 1961.

Freidson, Eliot, *Profession of Medicine,* New York: Dodd, Mead, 1970.

Freidson, Eliot, *Professional Dominance: The Social Structure of Medical Care,* New York: Atherton Press, 1970a.

Freymann, John Jr., *The American Health Care System: Its Genesis and Trajectory,* New York: Medcom Press, 1974.

Fuchs, Victor R., *Who Shall Live?: Health, Economics, and Social Choice,* New York: Basic Books, 1974.

Funkenstein, Daniel H., "Medical Students, Medical Schools, and Society during Three Eras," in Coombs, Robert H. and Clark, Vincent E., Eds., *Psychosocial Aspects of Medical Training,* Springfield, Ill.: Thomas, 1971.

Goffman, Erving, *The Presentation of Self in Everyday Life,* Garden City, N.Y.: Doubleday, 1959.

Gordon, Travis L., and Dube, W. F., "Datagram: Medical Student Enrollment, 1971–72 through 1975–76," *Journal of Medical Education,* 51(February): 144–146, 1976.

Gordon, Travis L., and Johnson, Davis G., "Study of U.S. Medical School Applicants, 1975–76," *Journal of Medical Education,* 52(September):708, 1977.

Gough, Harrison G., "The Recruitment and Selection of Medical Students," in Coombs, Robert H. and Clark, Vincent E., Eds., *Psychosocial Aspects of Medical Training,* Springfield, Ill.: Thomas, 1971.

Gove, Walter R., Ed., *The Labelling of Deviance: Evaluating a Perspective,* New York: Halsted, 1975.

Graham, Saxon, "Social Factors in Relation to Chronic Illness," in Freeman, Howard E., Levine, Sol, and Reeder, Leo, Eds., *Handbook of Medical Sociology,* Englewood Cliffs, N.J.: Prentice-Hall, 1963.

Hall, Oswald, "The Stages of Medical Career," *American Journal of Sociology,* **53**:327–336, 1948.

Hershey, Nathan, "The Defensive Practice of Medicine: Myth or Reality," *Milbank Memorial Fund Quarterly,* **50**(January):69–98, 1972.

Hofstadter, Richard, *The Age of Reform,* New York: Random House, 1955.

Hollender, Marc H., *The Psychology of Medical Practice,* Philadelphia: Saunders, 1958.

Hughes, Edward F. X., "Halsted and American Surgery," *Surgery,* **75**(February):169–177, 1974.

Hughes, Everett C., "Professions," in Lynn, Kenneth, Ed., *The Professions in America,* Boston: Beacon Press, 1965.

Hulka, Barbara S., Cassel, John C., Kupper, Lawrence L., and Burdette, James A., "Communication, Compliance, and Concordance between Physicians and Patients with Prescribed Medications," *American Journal of Public Health,* **66**:847–853, 1976.

Hyde, David R., and Wolff, Payson, "The American Medical Association: Power, Purpose, and Politics in Organized Medicine," *Yale Law Journal,* **63**:938–1022, 1954.

Johnson, Davis G., and Gordon, Travis L., "Datagram: Medical School Enrollment, 1974–75 through 1978–79," *Journal of Medical Education,* **54**(5):431–433, 1979.

Katz, Jay, and Capron, Alexander M., *Catastrophic Diseases: Who Decides What?,* New York: Russell Sage Foundation, 1975.

Kendall, Patricia L., "Medical Specialization: Trends and Contributing Factors," in Coombs, Robert H. and Clark, Vincent E., Eds., *Psychosocial Aspects of Medical Training,* Springfield, Ill.: Thomas, 1971.

Kendall, Patricia L., and Selvin, Hanan C., "Tendencies Toward Specialization in Medical Training," in Merton, R. K. et al., *The Student Physician,* New York: Columbia University Press, 1957.

Koran, L., "The Reliability of Clinical Methods, Data and Judgments," *New England Journal of Medicine,* **293**:642, 695, 1975.

Lanthem, Willoughby, and Newberry, Anne, *Community Medicine: Teaching, Research and Health Care,* New York: Appleton-Century-Crofts, 1970.

Lief, Harold, and Fox, Renee, "Training for Detached Concern," in Lief, H., Lief, V. F., and Lief, N., Eds., *The Psychological Basis of Medical Practice,* New York: Harper & Row, 1963.

Lippard, Vernon W., *A Half-Century of American Medical Education: 1920–1970,* New York: Josiah Macy, Jr. Foundation, 1971.

McKeown, Thomas, *The Modern Rise of Population,* London: Edward Arnold, 1976a.

McKeown, Thomas, *The Role of Medicine: Dream, Mirage or Nemesis,* London: Nuffield Provincial Hospitals Trust, 1976b.

Mechanic, David, *Public Expectations and Health Care: Essays on the Changing Organization of Health Services,* New York: Wiley-Interscience, 1972.

Merton, Robert K., Reader, George, and Kendall, Patricia, *The Student-Physician,* Cambridge: Harvard University Press, 1957.

Miller, Stephen, *Prescription for Leadership: Training for the Medical Elite,* Chicago: Aldine, 1970.

Nathanson, Constance A., "Learning the Doctor's Role: A Study of First- and Fourth-Year Medical Student Attitudes," unpublished master's thesis, University of Chicago, 1958.

Osler, Sir William, *The Student Life, and Other Essays,* London, 1919.

Parsons, Talcott, *The Social System,* New York: Free Press, 1951.

Parsons, Talcott, and Fox, Renee, "Illness Therapy and The Modern Urban American Family," *Journal of Social Issues,* **8**(4):2–3, 31–44, 1952.

Parsons, Talcott, "Definitions of Health and Illness in the Light of American Values and Social Structure," in Jaco, E., Ed., *Patients, Physicians, and Illness,* New York: Free Press, 1958.

Parsons, Talcott, "Professions," in *International Encyclopedia of the Social Sciences,* New York: Macmillan, 1963.

Peterson, James L., "Consumers' Knowledge of and Attitudes toward Medical Malpractice," in *Report of the Secretary's Commission on Medical Malpractice,* Washington, D.C.: USDHEW Publications No. 73-88 and 73-89, 1973.

Purcell, Elizabeth F., *Recent Trends in Medical Education,* New York: Josiah Macy, Jr. Foundation, 1976.

Reeder, Leo G., "The Patient-Client as a Consumer: Some Observations on the Changing Professional-Client Relationship," *Journal of Health and Social Behavior,* 13:406–12, 1972.

Rosen, George, "Some Substantive Limiting Conditions in Communication Between Health Officers and Medical Practitioners," *American Journal of Public Health,* 51:1805–1816, 1961.

Rosenblatt, Daniel, and Suchman, Edward A., "Awareness of Physician's Social Status Within an Urban Community," *Journal of Health and Human Behavior,* 7(3):146–153, 1966.

Scheff, Thomas, "Decision Rules, Types of Error, and Their Consequences in Medical Diagnosis," *Behavioral Science,* 8:97–107, 1963.

Schumacher, Charles F., "The 1960 Medical School Graduate: His Biographical History," *Journal of Medical Education,* 36(May):398–406, 1961.

Shryock, Richard H., *The Unique Influence of the Johns Hopkins University on American Medicine,* Copenhagen: Munksgaard, 1953.

Shryock, Richard H., *Medical Licensing in America,* 1650–1965, Baltimore: Johns Hopkins University Press, 1967.

Stevens, Rosemary, *Medical Practice in Modern England: The Impact of Specialization and State Medicine,* New Haven: Yale University Press, 1966.

Stevens, Rosemary, *American Medicine and the Public Interest,* New Haven: Yale University Press, 1971.

Strickland, Stephen P., *U.S. Health Care: What's Wrong and What's Right,* New York: Universe, 1972.

Stickland, Stephen P., *Politics, Science, & Dread Disease: A Short History of United States States Medical Research Policy,* Cambridge: Harvard University Press, 1972a.

Svarstad, Bonnie L., "Physician-Patient Communication and Patient Communication and Patient Conformity with Medical Advice," in Mechanic, David, Ed., *The Growth of Bureaucratic Medicine,* New York: Wiley-Interscience, 1976, 220–238.

Thompson, James D., *Organization in Action,* New York: McGraw-Hill, 1967.

Walsh, James, and Elling, Ray, "Professionalism and the Poor—Structural Effects and Professional Behavior," *Journal of Health and Social Behavior,* 9:16–28, 1968.

Weiskotten, Herman G., Wiggins, Walter S., Altenderfer, Marion E., Gooch, Marjorie, Tipner, Anne, "Changes in Professional Careers of Physicians. An Analysis of a Resurvey of Physicians Who were Graduated from Medical Colleges in 1935, 1940 and 1945," *Journal of Medical Education,* 36(November):1565–1586, 1961.

Wise, Harold, Beckhard, Richard Rubin, Irwin, and Kyte, Arleen, *Making Health Teams Work,* Cambridge: Ballinger, 1974.

Wolfe, S., and Badgley, R. F., "The Family Doctor," *The Milbank Memorial Fund Quarterly,* 50(April, Part 2):1–20, 1972.

CHAPTER SEVEN

Hospitals as Organizations and Social Systems

Until the end of the last century hospitals were largely custodial backwaters of medical care in this country, but during the last 70 years they have moved into a very central role within the health care system. The new dominant role of hospitals is illustrated by the sheer amount of medical care provided there. About 1 person in every 8 was hospitalized for something in 1978, compared to about 1 in 30 in 1930. This led to a cost of $76 billion for hospital services in 1978 or 40% of the total national expenditures for health care, compared with $0.5 billion, less than 20% of health expenditures in 1929. Since 1966 the average annual growth rate has been almost 16%, nearly twice the growth rate of the gross national product. In terms of budget and amount of services delivered, hospitals have become the dominant element of the health care system.

For many, hospitals have become the symbol of the growth in medicine's ability to intervene effectively against disease. Their roles in research, teaching, and the implementation of new medical developments have made hospitals seem the bearers of the fruits of medicine to their communities. This improved image has raised public expectations regarding the benefits to be had from modern medical care in general and from the hospital in particular. Communities, in fact, tend to see their hospitals as synonymous with the availability of medical care. Threats to close a community hospital can generate political action from a broad cross section—young and old, black and white, rich and poor—something that few other issues can muster.

On the other hand, hospitals have also become the focus of much of the criticism as dissatisfaction with the health system and agitation for reform have mounted in recent years (Sheatsley, 1957). This is partly a consequence of their visibility, which makes them easier targets than individual physicians. But hospitals are also very centrally involved in the problems of health care. They play a key role in the runaway costs. Economists note that the consumer price index (CPI) component for hospital care has been rising twice as fast as the overall CPI for the last 15 years, and much faster than other items in the health component. They often conclude that hospitals are the main cause of inflation in the health budget. In Chapter 12, we see that the price index alone gives a distorted picture of the nature of hospital cost escalation. Nevertheless, careful analysis shows that hospitals are indeed major contributors to the cost problem.

Many blame hospitals for much of the present depersonalization of medical care. A good deal of this is just a natural consequence of the growing technological nature of medicine. Nonetheless, the increasing portion of care provided in institutional settings adds to the problem by reducing the opportunity for a patient to develop a continuing relationship with a single physician. Hospitals are also accused of lacking responsiveness to the populations they serve, and conflicts frequently develop between them and their surrounding communities. This is particularly true of many older, often prestigious, institutions located in inner-city neighborhoods, which originally served social classes and ethnic groups quite different from the current residents of their outpatient catchment areas. Conflict arises partly out of dissatisfaction with the amenities and quality of care in the outpatient departments that these communities have come to depend on. Almost as frequently the conflict is over plans for hospital expansion that threaten to destroy more of the dwindling low-income housing in the neighborhood. Communities agitate for more say in hospital policy, particularly decisions concerning hospital jobs, which have come to be the major source of unskilled employment in many low-income, inner-city areas (Dornblaser, 1970).

Though some of these issues seem to have very little to do with health care per se, they illustrate the degree to which hospitals have become major institutions in their communities, affecting them in many ways. As large organizations, hospitals create vested interests in the jobs they are able to provide, the market they represent, and the influence their members are able to exert. These organizational interests do not always coincide with the interests of their constituents, even of those potential patients whom they were established to serve. This has led to the line of criticism that hospitals have become the centers of "health care empires" (Ehrenreich & Ehrenreich, 1971) pursuing their own goals at the expense of the communities around them and serving only the aggrandizement of their top administrators and medical staffs. This situation is described as a kind of conspiracy of the rich and powerful against the poor—which is a misunderstanding of the nature of social forces acting in organizations. Nevertheless, the fact that such an image exists and that conflicts between hospitals and their communities are increasing points to problems in the role of modern hospitals with serious implications for health care (Blankenship & Elling, 1962; Elling & Halebsky, 1961). This becomes obvious in the difficulties of areawide comprehensive health care planning. Hospitals have vested interests that differ from other groups involved in health planning. Conflicts arise out of these differences and the struggles for prerogatives in the delivery of specialized services, expansion, research, and so on. These conflicts constitute serious barriers to rationalizing the health care system in any large city.

HOSPITALS AS FORMAL ORGANIZATIONS

Hospitals belong to the class of social systems that sociologists call "formal" (or "complex") organizations, and considerable insight can be gained to their nature and problems by applying what is known generally about such organizations. Formal organizations consist of facilities and structured social relationships between their members designed to allow them to accomplish certain objectives as a group. The systematic nature of these relationships makes an organization into something more than the simple sum of its parts. Organizations impose purposefully structured interactions between people. As a result, the roles and relationships within the organization mold the behavior of members into something other than these same people have outside the organization. The relative stability of these interactions and relationships over time and the replaceability of one person by another in positions within the organization, give such systems a life of their own, above and beyond the people who make them up at any given time.

Hospitals have presented confusion for organizational theory because they do not fit any of the typical patterns of organizational structure found in the more widely studied examples from business, industry, and government (Georgopoulos & Matejko, 1967). Investigators have remarked about the multiplicity of goals, power structures, and authority relationships, as well as the conflicting functional requirements. They need flexible, professional discretion because of the frequent emergency situations and human service element of care. Yet they also require efficient, reliable, predictable performance because of the life and death implications of actions taken and the number of personnel and resources that must be coordinated.

Remarkable changes have occurred historically in the organization of hospitals (Perrow, 1963; Rosen, 1963). The mixture of objectives and organizational structures found today is the result of accretion from these historical changes in the technology and power structure (Heydebrand, 1973; Coser 1958). The historical changes are, in turn, consequences of the developments in medical care technology traced in Chapters 4 and 5. This heterogeneity of organizational structure is one of the underlying causes of the high costs and many of the other problems found in today's hospitals. We shall therefore examine the structural evolution of hospital organization, technology, and personnel in relation to changes in their "task environments,"* especially in public expectations and social mandate. As with the

---

* The "task environment" of an organization is defined as that part of the total social and economic environment with which it regularly interacts functionally (Thompson, 1967). The task environment of an automobile factory consists of the suppliers of steel,

history of disease in society, idealized stages are used to illuminate the forces at work rather than attempting to portray any one institution with empirical accuracy. A case study of the changing goals and power relationships in a moderate-sized (300-bed), prestigious hospital summarizes these stages:

Put briefly, an era of trustee control, emphasizing capital investments and community acceptance of hospitals, is followed by a period of control by doctors based on the increasing complexity and importance of their skills. At present there is a trend toward domination by the administration because of the mounting complexity of hospital activities and the increasing contact with health agencies proliferating outside the hospital. Obviously, not all hospitals will go through this sequence or go through it in this order. The sequence is an "ideal type" based on the assumption that in most cases the predicted relationship between the independent and dependent technology and community needs will generally dictate changes in the power structure, but particular historical circumstances may delay changes or produce "premature" ones. (Perrow, 1963)

HOSPITALS AS CUSTODIAL AND CONFINEMENT INSTITUTIONS

During the nineteenth century, most hospitals in the United States were still primarily custodial institutions for the insane, tubercular, and so on. They were operated by local governments or by religious orders to provide care and sustenance to the indigent, homeless, and outcasts who had nowhere else to turn. While providing welfare in this way, they also served the latent function of keeping "undesirables" off the streets. To do this, hospitals exercised considerable coercion to control their inmates. This was most obvious with mental institutions, which were little different from prisons. However, almost as firm if more subtle kinds of coercion were exercised

---

tires and other parts, the labor market for obtaining the various skilled workers, the capital investment market for obtaining financing, the auto market in which it must sell its products and therefore the competing producers of cars, the various public regulatory agencies establishing standards and limitations on its products and activities, and finally public opinion about autos and about the automotive industry that influences its potential sales, sales techniques, design of cars, and many other policy decisions.

The task environment of a hospital consists of the community from which patients arrive for care; the labor market for the various professional and nonprofessional skills needed to operate it; professional users of hospital facilities who are not members of the organization, such as physicians who use laboratories and other facilities; medical schools that use the hospital for teaching and research; government; private insurance carriers; philanthropic agencies and banks that supply financing; the surrounding communities with which the hospital must compete for space and interact in regard to demands for services and jobs; other hospitals with which it must compete for staff, prestige, patients, and financing; regulatory and planning agencies that set limits on the activities and policy of hospitals; and public opinion that influences many of the other relationships as well as its own board of trustees in setting hospital policy.

in general hospitals where compliance with harsh regimens was demanded in exchange for the home of last resort which they offered (Abel-Smith, 1964). Thus nineteenth-century hospitals served as quasi-governmental "commonweal organizations."* They carried out the public function of defining the conditions for which a person should be removed from the community by hospital confinement and enforcing the treatment defined as "proper" for that condition.†

Hospitals in this period had two major dependencies with which to cope: (1) financial support and (2) obtaining the public mandate to legitimatize their policy making and enforcement function in these matters. Both problems were solved by their membership in parent bodies—the religious orders or local governments that had the explicit or tacit public sanction to carry out such social policy functions as part of the moral and general welfare tradition. In the case of government operated hospitals, public health laws usually existed but provided only the vaguest definition of the policy to be carried out by public hospitals. In both religious and government hospitals the directors and staff were left tremendous discretion in making the day-to-day decisions for dealing with individuals under their care. Thus, in exchange for taking on the unpleasant responsibility of caring for and restraining certain social undesirables (who could be designated within the "disease" concept) these organizations were given both financial support and the mandate to set and carry out social policy in the area.

In general hospitals the profound changes in medical technology have led to a series of modifications of the basic organizational structure resulting in their modern complexity. The social policy-making and enforcement mandate in regard to patients has never ceased to exist, however, even in general hospitals. This tacit mandate helps to explain the coercive role they continue to play in regard to patients. It is particularly evident in publicly supported hospitals where the patients tend to be indigent, powerless, and still considered by society as "undesirable." The paternalistic authoritarian attitude among hospital staff at all levels still stems from this persisting mandate (real or assumed) to exercise some degree of police power over those who have been labeled as "sick" enough to need hospital care— whether this is provided at public expense or not.

---

* Blau and Scott (1962) have defined "commonweal organizations" as agencies whose function is making and enforcing cultural, moral, or social policy for the overall "good of the society as a whole." Churches, political parties, law enforcement agencies, and governments are organizations of this kind. Among organizations of this type there is often a division of labor between those primarily concerned with social policy making and those with policy enforcement. The extreme of this division is between legislatures and prisons, with courts and police departments lying in between to make up a total system of law making and enforcement. In other areas of social concern, however, such as morality and health, the separation between policy making and enforcement is nowhere near so clear.
† A few hospitals in the United States went beyond this coercive custodial, commonweal organization, copying the voluntary hospital model already existing in Europe, but they represented only a tiny, though pathbreaking fraction prior to 1880.

THE VOLUNTARY HOSPITAL MOVEMENT IN AMERICA

The voluntary hospital movement did not take hold in this country in the eighteenth and early nineteenth centuries as it did in Europe. Because of the younger, less urbanized population, the stronger laissez faire tradition, and the lack of any widespread medical tradition of clinical research, there was no concerted effort to found voluntary hospitals here until it was clear that medicine could make a difference in the outcome of diseases. This is not to say that the medical profession did not flourish here. There were probably more physicians per capita in the United States in 1880 than in any other country in the world. But the public effort to establish hospitals providing high-quality care came only after it was obvious that middle-class patients could also benefit by being treated in hospitals (Churchill, 1949).

When the effort to establish voluntary hospitals did appear in this country, it came with amazing speed. In 1873 there were only 149 hospitals in the entire United States (0.5 beds per 1000 population), one-third of them in New York alone, and more than another third in Massachusetts, Illinois, and Pennsylvania. Probably not more than 10 of these could have been considered "voluntary" hospitals in the modern sense of caring for both indigent and paying patients and being governed by a board of trustees representing responsibility to the public interest and the interest of its patients. Most were merely prisons for the insane. By 1909 when the next survey of hospitals was conducted, over 6000 were found in the country (if government and special hospitals are included as in the 1873 census, cf. Corwin, 1946). Three thousand of these were general care hospitals, the vast majority being "voluntary" in the modern sense—even if they were often under religious organization sponsorship.

Founding 3000 hospitals in 36 years necessitated more than a considerable construction effort. It required, in effect, creating a new social institution in the United States, establishing its legitimacy, and developing the organizational structure to make it function. The process began in the old hospitals of the Eastern Seaboard cities and was an outgrowth of the change in their primary goal from custodial care (and confinement) to cure. This change of goals was made possible by the development of the new clinical technology described in Chapter 4. The discovery of anaesthesia and aseptic techniques in surgery enabled effective treatment of many surgical diseases that had previously doomed patients afflicted by them. The development of bacteriological techniques eventually led to the possibility of cure for many infectious diseases or at least supportive care of infectious patients in hospitals without endangering others. Under these circumstances, spontaneous recovery could take place in many more cases than before. The introduction of new training and effective organization of nursing services allowed utilizing the new medical knowledge and skills in hospitals, broadening the range of diseases that could be effectively treated.

To realize these objectives it was necessary to create an effective organizational structure to operate hospitals within which the knowledge and techniques could be put to work. Knowledge, skills, techniques, and equipment alone are not a "technology" until they are organized effectively for achieving specific goals. Successful technology always involves appropriate human organization as well. Knowledge of engineering, design, steelworking, and the necessary machines are not the technology of an automobile factory until they are organized into a functioning production line. Likewise, the knowledge, skills, equipment, and techniques of scientific medicine were not the technology of a modern hospital until effective organizations were created within which they could function.

In order to convert custodial hospitals into organizations successfully incorporating the new medical science into functioning technologies (or to found similar new hospitals once the model had been established), a number of problems had to be overcome. In the first period these centered around two needs: (1) providing adequate budgets to pay for the much costlier equipment and personnel; (2) changing the public image of hospitals to conform with the new goals so that patients would use them, especially middle-class patients who could pay for their care and help support the more costly services. The cost of equipping the new breed of hospitals was of a different order of magnitude. Sterile operating rooms had to be built and maintained. Adequate nursing staffs, poorly paid as they were, still necessitated a much larger budget than the few orderlies in the past. In the (then) rich large cities municipal budgets for public hospitals and philanthropy for private ones could go a long way toward financing this in the early years of hospital modernization. However, the philanthropic money had to be procured for hospitals in the face of competition from the many other demands being made on it. To convince potential benefactors that this was a worthy place to put their money for the public good (and for lasting monuments to their fame), it was necessary to create an improved public image. This required public recognition of the new goals of providing services to the entire community, not just to the indigent. It also necessitated creating a well functioning organization for translating the new scientific knowledge and techniques into effective treatment.

Rising expectations in regard to medicine prepared the middle class to reconsider hospitals as places for treatment. Nevertheless, a new image of respectability and competence was needed to overcome the fears and revulsion associated with hospitals for centuries. Paying middle-class patients were needed to provide the high budgets necessary to run hospitals according to the new model. Even if sufficient philanthropic monies could be raised to rebuild or create the new hospitals, it was much more difficult to obtain charitable funds for continuing operating budgets than for the initial "bricks and mortar" (Vladeck, 1976). Paying patients demanded not only respectability and effectively functioning organizations; they also wanted amenities commensurate with the price.

During this period the boards of trustees were in the critical position to deal with these new needs of hospitals. The prestige of prominent, capable, trustees from the community facilitated the transition from the custodial organizations of the past into modern voluntary general hospitals. They proclaimed the new goals as policy and provided the image of respectability to give them credibility. They waged successful campaigns to erase the public image of hospitals as places of last resort for the indigent. They raised the money needed for construction and operation. They supplied the managerial expertise to build effectively working organizations for carrying out the new functions. Trustees, who were business leaders and other public figures in the community, frequently took an active personal part in the operation of the hospital, carrying out administrative reorganization themselves to make it function effectively. As Perrow (1963) reports:

There is no doubt that the affairs of the hospital were dominated by the trustees during this period. Annual reports and other documents make it clear that the serious problems were financial support and community acceptance; problems of medical care or administration are not mentioned during this period. One president held office for twenty years, from 1906 until 1927. He and other trustees intervened in most phases of the operation, making daily tours and firing people on the spot, ordering work to be done here and there, and often having the expenses charged to themselves directly. They borrowed money under their own names to meet pressing bills. It was "their" organization. . . . For the trustees, one may conjecture, the hospital was less a medical institution than a symbol of their contribution of time, money, and effort to community welfare.

Thus the changing technology of medicine and the associated changes in public opinion went hand-in-hand with the reorganizational work of the trustees. Because of similar problems and circumstances, these developments were duplicated throughout the country.

This success in moral leadership by hospital trustees was not accomplished without conflicts and compromises that were to have long-term consequences for the organization of health care in this country. One recurring tension was between the goals of philanthropy and the demands of private patients. This conflict led to divisions between the care of the indigent and of those able to pay, creating the two-class system of institutional health care that still plagues us. The dilemma facing hospital trustees was difficult. On the one hand, they were committed to building a strong charitable public service institution. The basis for raising funds was philanthropy, not business investment. It was necessary to show contributors that the money would be used for the "deserving poor." On the other hand, they also needed to improve the image of the hospitals in order to attract more philanthropic contributions and paying patients. That image could only improve significantly if the clientele expanded to include middle-class patients. The trustees were also committed to raise the quality of hospital care. Similarly, high quality care was only likely if the facilities were also patronized by the middle class. The services of the best trained and respected physicians could only be obtained if there was an opportunity to use the hospital for admitting their private patients as well. Paying patients demanded better amenities and the assurance of not being forced to mix with the indigent patients.

This led to a standard solution of "separate but equal" facilities, which of course were always far from equal. Private (paying) patients were treated by their own physicians on a fee-for-service basis in private or semiprivate rooms, often with private duty nurses. Charity patients were treated on open wards with 10 to 30 beds in a large room screened off from each other by temporary curtains and cared for by interns fresh from medical school. Interns were supervised by so-called visiting physicians who gave their time in exchange for the privilege of admitting their own patients to the private services. This meant that the quality of the charity care was dependent on the public service commitment and interest of the physicians involved.

Despite the danger of slipshod care with little accountability, the visiting physician system often worked remarkably well in the better hospitals because of the teaching and research going on. In this period of rapid change in medical science and the introduction of new techniques, such hospitals were the major transmitters of new knowledge and skills to the physicians already in practice. There was an active exchange of information among colleagues on ward rounds and in clinical conferences for teaching medical students and interns. This made the voluntary hospitals—with their charity wards—the chief arrangement for continuing education in medicine. The best physicians flocked there and sought attending physician positions on the staffs. Prestige, referrals, and the opportunity of achieving speciality status by obtaining sufficient professional recognition, all came to hinge on status within the attending ranks of a reputable voluntary hospital (Hall, 1948; see also Chapter 8). In such hospitals the technical quality of care given by the visiting physicians to charity patients was often excellent—perhaps even better than that given to private patients since it was being watched more closely by their colleagues in the teaching process. On the other hand, charity patients often suffered the inconvenience and indignities of overly intensive investigation and frequent use as "demonstration material" for teaching. In later periods, with the growth of residency programs, the direct care of ward patients in voluntary hospitals was left more completely to the resident physicians, but there was also a stricter supervisory hierarchy.

In outpatient clinics the development took a somewhat different course. Dispensaries providing ambulatory care for indigent patients had been founded in large cities throughout the nineteenth century, and their number grew apace with the founding of voluntary hospitals in the 1880 to 1920 period (Davis, 1918, 1927). Many of the early dispensaries were independent of hospitals and often amounted to little more than glorified charity pharmacies where indigent patients could have prescriptions filled after seeing private physicians. Yet more and more they came to be associated with the new voluntary hospitals as outpatient departments. They were staffed by the attending physicians of those institutions as part of the system of advancement through the ranks of the hospital staff hierarchy. Outpatient care was less prestigious and less dramatic than inpatient care. It offered less opportunity to learn from interesting cases and gain recognition that could lead to referrals and specialty status. However, a period of service in the outpatient department was usually required of new attending physicians as a probationary period before they were allowed visiting privileges on the inpatient services. Thus, despite the rather lowly status of service in the outpatient departments, there was an abundant supply of young physicians eager to serve. Outpatient service also provided new physicians an opportunity to recruit patients for budding private office practices if they were in fact able to pay for their care (Hall, 1948).

As the reputation of the voluntary hospitals rose during this period, increasing numbers of potential paying patients appeared at the outpatient departments in the hope of obtaining higher quality care than could be expected from the poorly trained, pre-Flexner private physicians who still crowded the cities (Rosenberg, 1974).* These clinics might have become hospital based group practices had not two countermovements intervened: (1) Local physicians threatened by the competition of the prestigious hospitals lobbied through their local medical societies for so-called dispensary laws which restricted the degree to which hospitals could do this. The medical societies' ethics committees declared any such "corporate practice of medicine" unethical (Rosner & Thernstrom, 1974). (2) In the next historical period physician domination of voluntary hospitals brought a shift in goals with an emphasis on inpatient care and away from high quality medicine in outpatient departments. Thus, unlike inpatient services, the outpatient clinics of voluntary hospitals were restricted to providing second-class medicine for the poor. Ambulatory care for the middle class was provided almost entirely in the offices of private physicians.

HOSPITALS BECOME THE PHYSICIANS' WORKSHOPS

In the second quarter of this century the situation in American hospitals again changed radically. By 1945 the real control of voluntary hospitals had gradually shifted from the boards of trustees to the medical staffs. Concomitantly, their primary goal had changed from providing essential medical

---

* Hospitals where this was happening began to screen patients with a "means test," and charge sliding fees.

services for all to providing the highest quality and most sophisticated care possible to those able to pay. Physicians originally had little or no official role in the governance of voluntary hospitals. Technically they were not even members of these organizations. As only part-time "attending" or "visiting" physicians, they were simply allowed to make use of the facilities while contributing their skills to the public good. This hospital service was, to be sure, part of the physician's professional obligation. Yet in most cases it was undertaken primarily to gain experience and professional recognition in order to further a private practice outside the hospital—where the physician's true interest lay.

A number of factors contributed to the remarkable change of the physician's position in the hospital. There was an order-of-magnitude increase in the rate of the new developments in technological sophistication of medical science. This was paralleled by rising expectations and demand for hospital care by private patients and escalating costs of providing care. The greater expertise and technology orientation of the new generation of physicians trained in the post-Flexner medical schools added to their dominance in hospitals. Another factor was the economic response, health insurance, that was evoked by the rising importance and cost of medical care. The internal dynamics of the rapidly growing hospitals driven by their own emerging vested interests molded these forces together into a mutually reinforcing pattern that led to the institutional evolution of the modern hospital.

By 1930 a growing cadre of well trained, scientifically oriented young physicians was being turned out from the post-Flexner medical schools. They were eager to build personal empires in which they could emulate the medical environments of the teaching hospitals where they had had their training. The new costly technology of medical practice also gave physicians the upper hand over hospital trustees in gaining prerogatives to use the facilities to their own advantage. The trustees had been able to maintain control as long as the hospital's function was largely charitable and the cost of charity patients could be met by philanthropy. By 1930 hospitals were being patronized by large numbers of paying patients. The improved scientific medicine, which lay behind the now respectable image of hospitals, had increased costs tremendously. Philanthropy was no longer an adequate source of support. Most general hospitals had to pay their way by charging private patients at a rate that would not only meet the full cost of their own services, but also partially subsidize services for those who could not afford to pay. Physicians controlled the flow of paying patients.

This new financial situation had the ironic effect of making so-called nonprofit hospitals into a highly competitive, but self-feeding, "growth industry." To provide the high quality services demanded by paying patients, larger investments were required by the hospitals and a larger staff of professional personnel had to be maintained. Fixed costs were high, whether or not facilities and services were utilized—but income was produced only by utilization for which patients could be charged. Pressure grew to utilize the facilities maximally in order to support them. This led to general expansion because many high cost facilities, like operating rooms and laboratories, could serve many patients for little more cost than was needed to serve only a few patients. The bed expansion required further investment costs, and the need for more paying patients to fill the beds at higher prices. This cycle was fed by its own dynamics and by the increasing demand for hospital services growing out of the rising prestige of medical science. Two results ensued that had major impacts on the power balance within the hospital.

First, the escalating costs of hospitalization, and the potential catastrophic consequences for the patient as well as for the hospital if they could not be paid, nurtured the development of hospital insurance (Chapters 11 and 12). This occurred at the instigation of the growing but financially strapped hospitals as well as at the urging of patients (Somers & Somers, 1962). With hospital insurance schemes widely operating, hospitals became *less* dependent on the fund raising capabilities of their trustees. They became *more* dependent on their physicians for a steady supply of patients whose bills would be paid by hospital insurance. Because most insurance reimbursed hospitals on the basis of costs incurred, this provided essentially open-ended financing and produced one of the most rapid long-term expansions of a major economic sector in American history (Chapter 12).

Second, the growing dependency on paying patients and the role of technological sophistication in determining the hospital's public image led to major changes in the balance of power, the functions and goals, and the organizational structure of hospitals. Physicians gained the critical position of controlling the principal sources of financing and prestige—just as had the trustees in the earlier period. Theirs became the dominant voice on the joint administrative committees that in effect supplanted the trustees in making policy. Physicians also gained hegemony in a more subtle way. The perspective of top hospital administrators (and to some extent of trustees) became almost identical with that of their physicians, because hospital vested interests became (for a period) nearly synonymous with physician interests (Thompson & McEwen, 1958). Prestigious and influential staff physicians could attract the most patients, which allowed the hospital to expand and afford more complex equipment and extensive services. Conversely, what attracted prestigious physicians was the prestige of the hospital, which was determined largely by the sophistication of the equipment and facilities and by the amount of research and teaching.

Thus, even without explicit pressure from the medical staff, administrative committees making policy decisions about hospital expansion, equipment, personnel, and so on, chose what provided the most prestigious setting for physicians. Large hospitals throughout the country improved their scientific research potential. The quality of private care facilities was upgraded, and amenities were added for physicians and patients that gave the atmosphere of sophisticated scientific medicine. Competition among hospitals for prestige, though an important stimulus for improving the quality of care, also made it impossible to coordinate areawide planning to eliminate unnecessary duplication of services. It still remains a major cause of inefficient use of expensive equipment and services like sophisticated X-ray diagnosis and therapy or open-heart surgery.

In addition to their policy influence, physicians also attained a dominant position in *operational* control. The new operational authority was most evident in medical emergencies or in the surgical operating room. Under these circumstances the physician took quasi-military command of the hospital personnel involved in that patient's care. The physician had the acknowledged authority to overrule any procedural rules, and to mobilize any resources that he declared necessary for the well-being of the patient. Such declarations were made solely on the basis of his individual clinical judgment. Because of the possible life-or-death significance, it was necessary for each member of the hospital staff to carry out procedures expected by the physician with competence and absolute adherence to his orders (Georgopoulos and Mann, 1962).

For hospital staff to be disciplined to act instantly and unquestioningly in accord with the physician's intentions, the emergency authority was kept active as a latent relationship between physicians and other members of the hospital staff—nurses in particular. It permeated all day-to-day interactions of physicians with hospital personnel, reinforcing the air of charismatic authority that the physician was accustomed to evoking even when it was unnecessary. Wilson (1959) describes this relationship:

The high tide of the doctor-dominated hospital, perhaps extending from 1900–1950 (although its crest varied by region and type of institution), is preserved in the figure of the great doctor making his ward rounds to the bowing of nurses, the scraping of students, and the worshipful gaze of patients. But this picture of the brigadier inspecting a crack garrison is, like the stereotyped dramatic fiction of Hollywood and ladies' magazines—Dr. Kildare bracing his men (and women) in white—simply an exaggerated telling of the truth that the doctor was not only the central figure in the hospital but a towering one. He gave the orders to nurses, administrators, or whomever, and in his absence the organization ran in deference to precedents he had established or anticipations of those he would establish.

Thus even though the physician had no official place in the line hierarchy of the organization and was theoretically only an outsider using its facilities, he in fact completely usurped direct command. Nurses and technical personnel were his personal troops. They took their orders directly from him and gave them precedence over conflicting rules or orders from the administrative authority. Nurses acted as the physician's proxy in his absence and represented his interests vis-à-vis other hospital staff by simply invoking the dictum "doctor's orders" when necessary. The administrator, nominally in charge of the hospital, was looked upon by physicians as a mere servant to expedite what was needed when it went beyond the immediate jurisdiction of the patient area. Should the administrator resist this incursion into his legitimate domain, the physician could invoke his latent emergency mode of command to obtain concessions. He could use his clinical authority to prevail in matters of nonclinical operation, or to gain professional privileges and prerogatives within the hospital. The implicit threat, voiced as "clinical judgment," was nearly always enough to obtain his way (Wilson, 1963).

During this period it is not surprising that outpatient services deteriorated. These were looked upon by physicians as unpleasant, unprestigious obligations. A concern of the trustees, because of their charitable role and the demand by the surrounding community, these services offered little enticement to the medical profession. The concentration of "interesting" cases and potential for research and teaching lay with inpatient care—as did the major opportunity for reimbursement. Before the institutionalizing of residency programs, physicians often served a kind of apprenticeship in hospital outpatient departments (Hall, 1944). As hospitals became more dependent on physicians, and as residency programs became the accepted route to specialization, there was little leverage to make physicians serve there. Often the only way that outpatient clinics could be maintained at all was to organize them as highly specialized clinics for teaching and research. In such clinics residents in specialty training could select patients with "interesting" pathology and admit them for more intensive inpatient study, providing services to the indigent in the process.

It might seem that residents, like young physicians in previous times, could have manned the outpatient departments as an apprenticeship requirement. Yet as the hospital's need for residents grew parallel to the complexity of medical services, residents were in as strong a bargaining position vis-à-vis the hospital as were staff physicians. The residents wanted to gain intensive clinical experience during their period in the teaching hospital, which meant spending maximal time on inpatient services. As ideals of social responsibility gained ascendancy among younger physicians during the social movements of the late 1960s, there was a reawakening of residents' interest in providing outpatient care for its own sake. It is too soon to tell what the lasting effects of this enthusiasm will be.

ORGANIZATIONAL STRUCTURE OF THE MODERN GENERAL HOSPITAL: PROFESSIONALIZATION OF TECHNICAL STAFF, DEPARTMENTALIZATION, AND ASCENDANCY OF HOSPITAL ADMINISTRATORS

After World War II hospitals changed rapidly again as their size and complexity took another order-of-magnitude leap. During the interwar period of undisputed physician dominance, the growth was primarily of technology that physicians used themselves or was clearly under their direct control in the clinical domain. As the breakthroughs of basic medical sciences from the first half of the century began to pay off in applied bioengineering, however, the increasingly sophisticated nature of this new technology brought an explosion of hospital personnel to operate and maintain it.

Prior to 1945 some technicians, such as for X-ray and laboratory work, were already common on hospital staffs. After the War, however, hospitals soon came to have whole departments for X-ray, clinical pathology and laboratory services, pharmacy, dietetics, physical therapy, anaesthesia, blood banking, social work—and the list continues to grow. With the development of more complex surgery and sophisticated monitoring for cardiac and other critically ill patients, the establishment of intensive care units allowed other technicians and nurses to take over specialized aspects of care. Thus the proliferation of sophisticated technology led to extensive division of labor and delegation of many elements of clinical care formerly carried out only by physicians or by nurses under direct supervision.

The increasing delegation of clinical care made the physician's span of control too limited to supervise and coordinate all patient services. It was impossible for any person, even on a full-time basis, to oversee adequately the complete range of technology operating in a modern hospital. The responsibility for supervision and also coordination had to be delegated. Nurses took over the role of coordinating services for patients, but supervision of technical procedures required new forms of management. The new critical problem for hospitals became the supervision, coordination, and integration of the services and personnel involved in the total care of patients.

In his comparative study of hospitals Heydebrand (1973) outlined four major modes of coordination used in hospitals: (1) professional, (2) departmental, (3) administrative, and (4) hierarchical. This is a useful typology for analyzing how the complexity and control of services is dealt with in modern hospitals. These modes of coordination almost never occur separately, however. They are simply different aspects of the organizational structure found in every hospital with differences in their relative importance from one type of hospital to another. Nor do they signify uniform mechanisms of control—only general categories that take on quite different forms in various groups within a hospital (e.g., physicians, nurses, technicians, administrators), and from one type of hospital to another. We must limit our discussion here to short-term general hospitals.

Professionalism is the most widely occurring and diverse mode of coordination and control found in hospitals. It provides the flexible self-regulation that makes it possible to deal with special situations over a wide range of problems and still have dependable performance with a minimum of supervision. Professionalism is achieved by standardized training in a body of knowledge and skills plus inculcation of norms and values about their application. The norms are maintained by identification with the professional reference group, by interaction with other professionals, and by making advancement within the group contingent upon adherence to the norms. Because of these norms and skills regarding objectives and the means for attaining them, professionalism allows coordination with minimal supervision simply by assigning particular objectives. Professionalism therefore facilitates decentralized decision-making without loss of control. It provides easy lateral integration and coordination of services within the breadth of professional boundaries.

Physicians themselves are the prototype for professionalism. The great breadth of their expertise in former times was the principal means of integrating and coordinating all patient care. Because of this breadth, physician professionalism still remains the principal means of coordination whenever the latent "emergency structure" of the organization is required or in complex therapeutic situations. With the increase in sophistication of medical technology and the division of labor, however, this holistic professionalism breaks down because of the impossible span of control it requires. It is necessary for specialized technicians to assume much of the responsibility for overseeing their own activities. As a result, each group of technicians has pushed for independent professional status and autonomy commensurate with its responsibility (Friedson, 1970). Each developing semiprofession (Wilensky, 1964; Hughes, 1958) began to organize its own training schools, professional associations, and journals in the struggle to secure and consolidate its new-found status.

The professionalism of technicians, however, is quite different from that of physicians. Physicians command a broad scope of knowledge and skills and possess a corresponding sweeping social mandate, which makes it possible for them to integrate the entire range of patient care. Professionalism of technicians, on the other hand, is limited to a narrow area of expertise. This allows them to operate independently only within well-prescribed guidelines and under the ultimate supervision of a physician with legal and social responsibility for the total care of patients. Thus, the professionalization of technicians relieves physicians of supervising certain patient care activities directly, but it by no means allows technicians to practice or organize independently as physicians do. The organization of professionalized technicians in hospitals can never be like that of "free professionals," such as physicians. It has the structure of a service bureaucracy where professionals at the service interface are allowed discretion in interpreting policy rules but are also expected to recognize the limitations of this discretion and refer problems that fall outside that range to someone further up the hierarchy.

Departmentalization has come to be a major means of coordinating services in general hospitals (Heydebrand, 1973). Organizing a group of persons carrying out the same or related functions into a department maximizes internal communication and interaction. Self-supervision and internal coordination of interrelated functions take place automatically or with a minimum of additional hierarchy.* Because of the associated professionalism, where knowledge and experience confer authority, departmentalization in the hospital automatically includes its own hierarchy, allowing more experienced technicians to supervise and coordinate the activities of the less experienced. As the complexity of technician's tasks has increased, physicians have come to specialize in these indirect patient-care areas and head such specialized service departments. This occurred early in radiology and clinical pathology where large departments and laboratories developed rapidly in general hospitals. It is now frequently found in anaesthesiology, physical medicine, and blood banking, and the trend is spreading. Thus departmentalization has led to the mixing of bureaucratic and professional modes of coordination—with physicians themselves increasingly part of the hierarchical structure of hospital service bureaucracies.

While improving control and supervision, however, departmentalization has actually intensified the problem of coordinating patient care. Hospital staffs, once small manageable forces ready to swing into action at the call of physicians and to mobilize all the resources to the momentary problem, have become a maze of independent divisions with their own schedules to meet, their own opinions about what needs to be done, and their own sense of importance. No longer ready to bow to the clinician's every wish, these groups have developed their own vested interests that have to be meshed with those of the rest of the staff—requiring endless interdepartmental negotiations and coordination.

The departmentalization process has not been limited to technical services but has also occurred in clinical medicine itself. The combination of specialization and departmentalization has led to fragmentation of the supervision, coordination, and integration of patient care at the physician level. In large teaching hospitals, and to a lesser extent even in smaller community hospitals, each specialized clinical division has taken on a separate departmental structure. Increasingly these departments include many types of nonphysician personnel (technicians, research staff, support staff, etc.), producing a structure not unlike the situation where physicians head technician departments. In addition, interns, residents, clinical fellows, and junior staff members working for chiefs of clinical divisions form a professional hierarchy of their own (Seeman & Evans, 1961). Thus, even direct patient-care physicians are subject to the bureaucratic mode of coordina-

---

* This is the principle of compositional homogeneity whereby internal administrative needs are reduced by extending the practical span of supervision (Heydebrand, 1973). In production-line technologies, departmentalization serves to simplify control and the assignment of responsibility in the process of rational subdivision of tasks and decision making. In professional service bureaucracies, however, such as the technical departments of hospitals, departmentalization acts more as a means of strengthening professional norms, providing mutual collegial supervision, maximizing solidarity, and enhancing potential for learning from each other—in addition to the obvious efficiency of concentrating the facilities and equipment in one place for interrelated functions.

tion, leaving them less opportunity for individual integration of comprehensive patient care. Hospital physicians are increasingly limited to overall therapeutic policy making and must leave the integration, coordination, and supervision of patient care to the floor nurse. In a sense she has become the new generalist of hospital medicine. She is no longer just the physician's proxy but to a large extent his replacement in this integrative role (Davis, 1966).

As hospitals expanded and medical care became more complex, nursing also had to be reorganized. The kind of personal, one-to-one care that nurses previously provided to patients has been taken over by aides, practical nurses (LPNs), or volunteer workers. Registered Nurses (RNs) are needed to supervise the complex operations of the hospital wards: dispensing more numerous and more potent medications; supervising the horde of other personnel working on the floor; traffic-copping the schedules of appointments for patients with other departments of the hospital; keeping voluminous records of vital importance for the medical care of patients; watching patients in the absence of physicians for signs of possible adverse turns that might call for emergency measures; and being ready to mobilize a full-scale medical assault on any such emergency until a physician can be found to take over. This is a far cry from the bed making, sanitary overseeing, and TLC ("tender loving care") of previous times (Saunders, 1953).

Nurses have become the clinical administrators. Because they are not as highly trained in clinical judgement as physicians, hospital nurses have been organized into an extensive hierarchy for supervision, support, and coordination of this complex new role. Nevertheless, because of the importance of on-the-spot clinical decision-making, the nursing hierarchy places great authority at the decentralized floor nurse level, corresponding in some ways to the professional authority of physicians in the previous period (Mauksch, 1965). This requires greater redundancy of highly trained professionals than would be necessary within most service bureaucracy hierarchies.

Unlike professionalism and departmentalization, which are chiefly concerned with integration and control of patient care activities, *administrative coordination* serves primarily for integration of the hospital as a whole. One administrative function is supervision of backup services such as housekeeping, maintenance, fiscal management, and personnel. These have become major responsibilities in a modern hospital, where the number of employees may run in the thousands and budgets in the multimillions.

A second set of administrative functions involves organization-wide planning, budgeting, fund raising, and negotiation with the hospital's task environment. As hospitals have become major institutions and socioeconomic forces affecting many aspects of the lives of their communities, these negotiations have taken on a highly political nature, like those of other large corporations (Thompson, 1967). Administrators have come to require specialized (professional) training and extensive experience to deal with such responsibilities (Austin, 1975). The growth in magnitude and complexity of administrative functions has also led to the increasing professionalization of hospital administrators. This is evidenced by the rise of professional organizations and training programs and by the increasing mobility of administrators, necessitating identification with the professional group rather than a particular hospital (Heydebrand, 1973).

In addition to these generally recognized administrative functions, the complex division of labor has led to another less recognized function of hospital administrators, the task of coordinating activities between departments. Each department, with its independent professionalization and internal hierarchy, has a semiautonomous existence within the hospital, but it is functionally interdependent with other departments. Coordination must be established through negotiation, allowing departments to have their own internal working arrangements while providing integration of services for the clinical care of patients. Administrators are increasingly preoccupied with this coordinating and negotiating between departments. Thus, the increasing fragmentation of hospitals and growth of specialized, semi-independent departments has added to the problems facing administrators—and increased their power (Litwak, 1961).

Changes in the hospitals' task environments have also necessitated growth of the administrative apparatus. The size of the budgets and the third-party financing (private health insurance and government programs for aged and indigent patients), together with increasing concern over the quality of care, have inevitably led to more outside regulation of hospitals. State and local public health regulatory agencies demand periodic inspection for licensure and auditing of books for rate setting and for public accountability. Accreditation for the training of interns and residents (increasingly essential for hospital operation) requires periodic external quality review as well as standing internal committees for review of discharge records, "tissue" committees to review the appropriateness of surgery, causes of deaths, and so forth. Regional health planning councils and state certificate-of-need legislation (see Chapter 10) require development of master plans and justification of expansion plans, necessitating more joint medical-administrative staff committees.

One of the most important sociodemographic trends in the United States since 1945 has been the marked shift in population growth from the central cities to the surrounding suburban rings, accompanied by a deterioration of the economic base and quality of life in the inner cities. Hospitals (and medical schools) have been left in an increasingly hostile environment where they have to serve as the source of primary medical care and often of jobs for the new urban population (Gaughton, 1975). Local community groups, voicing public discontent over the quality of outpatient care and of other services in the more militant 1960s, demanded the establishment of grievance committees. These committees, which included community members, were formed for the purpose of improving hospital-community relations and to make the hospital more responsive to the needs of the people it served. The unionization of nonprofessional hospital workers has entailed collective bargaining, more extensive personnel departments, and new fringe benefit problems—occasionally even the mobilization of the hospital's professional staff for strikes. These developments have added markedly to the administrative burden of hospitals, requiring increasingly sophisticated political, planning, and organizational skills of administrators, but also enhancing their power in decision-making (Donabedian, 1973).

Administration is the glue that holds an organization together and makes it possible for the functional elements to operate as an effective whole. As the coordination of the units and the resolution of conflicts have become the major operational problems, administrators' influence on organizational decision-making has grown—just as physicians' influence did when the major problem was keeping the beds full, or as the trustees' did when the major problem was image and philanthropic backing from the community (Perrow, 1963, 1965). The rising influence of administrators in hospitals has been less flamboyant, less overt, and less direct, but it is no less real. Since physicians always maintain ultimate control over clinical services, administrators can never assume a position of real dominance like that of physicians in the earlier period. The influence of administrators is exercised by their control over communication, implementation of policy decisions (made by all groups), and use of their negotiating role in conflicts to steer subtly toward goals they desire for the hospital. As with administrators of all dynamic organizations (Downs, 1967), hospital administrators emphasize the goals of solvency, operational strength, and growth more than do trustees who emphasize public service, or the medical staff who emphasize prestige and convenience for the care of their patients.

The fourth mode of coordination in hospitals is *hierarchy* and like the other modes, it is far from a uniform type of structure within hospitals. Hierarchies serve a number of different functions. The relative importance of different functions varies from one department or one situation to another. One function commonly accomplished by hierarchies is the coordination of activities through the repeated subdivision of responsibility for tasks and planning decisions. This is the classical role of hierarchies in production organizations. In hospitals it is found in the backup (support) departments and within the administrative bureaucracy itself—wherever the major problem is coordinating and planning routine services needed to run as an organization.

A second function accomplished by hierarchies is the communication of control through the authority vested in superiors over subordinates. Control hierarchies in hospitals are not uniquely defined, since the superior-subordinate relationship is not always confined to a single department structure or to any other unambiguous line of authority. The clinical line of authority emanating from physicians is largely independent of the administrative line of authority emanating from the hospital director. These two

sources of control may converge from different directions on the same individual and come into conflict. This has been referred to as the "two lines of
authority of hospitals which are one too many" (Smith, 1955). But in addition, each department has its own line of authority that is not directly
ordered within either of these two hospital-wide control hierarchies and
may be crosscut by them under some circumstances. Thus the authority relationship between physicians and other staff members is actually more
complex than the staff/line problem that Smith refers to. The problem of
hospital lines of authority is that they are multiple rather than just double.

Still another function of hierarchies predominates in the professional and
technical departments of hospitals—supervision and problem solving. As
with all professional bureaucracies, there are two directions to this process.
Very general rules are established at the top of the departmental hierarchy
indicating policy for carrying out the functions of the department. Professional discretion is often required in applying these rules to a particular
case.* In the other direction, when new situations arise for which no established rules exist, the hierarchy expedites problem solving by providing
routes of referral whereby more experienced members can advise those who
are less so or establish new policies to deal with the problem. Unlike typical
professional bureaucracies, the rules of each separate departmental hierarchy are amended not only by way of the usual process of testing new decisions within the one hierarchy, but also by negotiation between the different hierarchies (and with physicians) where mutual areas of concern
arise. It also occurs when overall changes in hospital policy are negotiated
at the level of the ruling troika of trustees, medical chiefs of staff, and administrative director. Today the administrative hierarchy also frequently
functions like a professional service bureaucracy, as a problem-solving mechanism through referral.

ROUTINE AND NONROUTINE SERVICES

A final set of coordination problems arises out of the tension between the
routinized service-bureaucracy structure needed to provide dependable, predictable results and the individualized-technology structure that is vital for
the flexible response needed in emergencies and unusual clinical situations.
The tension arises not just out of the disruptive effects of actual emergencies on the ward routines. There is also tension from the functional incongruities between the two coexisting superimposed organizational structures
necessary to deal with the two modes of operation. One structure is the

---

* In a large department there may also be intermediate levels of supervision at which
subpolicies are established for a special subdivision. These subpolicies amount to interpretations of the general departmental policy for a special functional area, and these new
rules in turn require professional interpretation or discretion in applying them to individual cases.

highly differentiated and functionally specific complex service bureaucracy. The other organizational structure, which is usually latent, is based on coordination by direct physician authority and corresponds to the emergency mode. It is the quasi-military organization of command dependent on the clinician's appraisal of the (critical) situation of the moment.

The decreasing span of supervision from physicians (due to specialization) and the increasing complexity of the resources to deal with emergencies, plus the growing bureaucratization of the ward organization, makes the tension between routine and emergency modes of command ever less tolerable. Consequently there is growing pressure to isolate potential emergency situations as much as possible by placing them in intensive care units (ICUs) so as not to disrupt the routine work of the ward. This "routinizes emergencies" by placing them in the hands of those who deal with similar situations all the time, making it possible to delegate much of the care to specially trained nurses. This produces still more specialization and the development of further technology to be used by these specialists, creating new vested interests within the hospital.

Beyond the special units for dealing with predominantly nonroutine situations, the latent dual (emergency/routine) organization has important effects on the hospital as a whole. It is never possible to isolate nonroutine care completely from the routine care units. Consequently the service bureaucracy structure can never be as tightly controlled or as efficient in its routine functions as it could be if it were not also structured for potential emergencies. Each ward must be ready to throw off its routine procedures and accustomed chain of command and fall immediately into another mode of operation that allows disciplined and dependable responses to the ad hoc demands of a momentary field commander. The ever present possibility of such an emergency requires a high degree of flexibility and decentralization (and hence duplication of highly trained professional and policy-making ability). No ordinary service bureaucracy would tolerate the degree of decentralization or excess expertise. The necessary massive functional redundancy is expensive and often counterproductive for the hospital's patient care objectives. This ambiguity of organizational structural types is a major contributor to duplication of facilities and services. Since functional redundancy tends to be utilized whether needed or not, improper utilization and costly overutilization is almost inevitable (Chapter 12).

THE INCREASING DEPENDENCY OF PHYSICIANS
ON HOSPITALS

In addition to being caught up in the bureaucratic structure of hospitals, physicians are becoming generally more dependent professionally on them. First, as modern medicine has come to use more expensive technology in diagnosis and treatment, it is less possible for individual physicians to own the equipment and employ technicians to operate it. Hospitals are the primary place where such facilities are operated, making them available for collective use by the physicians in the area. In recent years private laboratory services have emerged for referral of patients outside of hospitals. Nevertheless, physicians are dependent on hospitals for most specialized services and facilities. Second, as physicians have become more specialized, there is greater need for referral and consultation to provide the full spectrum of professional care needed for more complicated diseases. Since most physicians are not members of group practices where a range of specialists are easily available for consultation, hospitals have become the setting most often used to coordinate supervision of such cases (Gaughton, 1975).

The increasing dependency on hospitals' technological facilities and their organizational setting to coordinate the services of multiple specialists has produced an expensive tendency for unnecessary hospital admissions to carry out diagnostic workups. Hospitals, oriented to their own internal needs, have not made technological services available on an ambulatory basis to the professional community and patients in their areas. They have seldom taken it upon themselves to organize their professional staffs into group practices that might facilitate referral and joint management of patients on an outpatient basis. Consequently it is more convenient to admit patients to the hospital in order to make these services available.

This tendency is compounded by the fact that many patients have insurance that pays for such services as inpatients but not as outpatients (Chapter 12)—even though the same procedures and professional services would be possible on an ambulatory basis at a considerable cost savings. Health policy makers have become increasingly aware of the insurance problem in regard to diagnostic procedures and have pushed for changes in health insurance as a means to remedy it. Yet this does not solve the organizational problem of the availability and convenience of these services on an inpatient versus outpatient basis. Merely modifying insurance policy is not likely to reduce this source of unnecessary hospital utilization significantly.

The problem, in fact, will probably increase as the coordination challenge of postclinical medicine mounts. As noted in Chapter 5, the chronic, complicated diseases of the new era of medical care require early detection, regular surveillance and follow-up, integration of multiple professional services, and behavior modification—all to a degree scarcely dreamed of in previous times. Individual physicians are not equipped organizationally to deal with these problems. With the exception of well-developed, prepaid group practices, such as Kaiser-Permanente, which presently serve less than 3% of the nation's population (Chapter 11), hospitals are the only medical care organizations that fill these needs. Thought must be given to this problem by health policy makers as decisions are required about the community-wide organization of ambulatory medical care. Both the cost of alternative organizational structures for providing such care and the potential conflicting goals and vested interests of hospitals could interfere with their role in its organization.

The growing prominence of hospitals in the delivery of health care has also changed the physician's role, style of practice, and relationship to patients and other physicians. More and more their practice and professional life is caught up in the matrix of hospital relationships. Although physicians arc still predominantly individual practitioners, in the increasing portion of their practice with hospitalized patients even solo office-based physicians are perforce involved in a kind of group practice. Their patients are treated in an organized hospital system where their care is inevitably intertwined with those of other physicians in the hospital. An increasing percentage of physicians are actually practicing as full-time hospital staff members (Chapter 8). Hospitals of any size have interns, residents, and attending physicians who not only take over the care of private patients in emergencies, but also who may well make ward rounds on all patients and follow their records if any teaching is going on. Consultants who are part of the hospital staff also see and examine private patients and participate in their care. The chief of each service has the right, in fact legal responsibility, to review patient records kept by physicians and make recommendations or comments where needed.

Official hospital committees review physicians' discharge records of patients and the pathological reports on surgical cases or deaths that occur in the hospital. Today malpractice suits can be brought against hospitals as well as against individual physicians. This increases the legal need for hospital surveillance over their private physicians and gives them more grounds to say what a physician is or is not qualified to do within their walls. Thus the hospital system encroaches steadily on the physician's care of patients, watching over his shoulder and decreasing the formerly isolated nature of the relationship between physician and patient. Even clinical decision-making, once the sacrosanct domain of each physician in practice, is coming more under the influence of the group process inherent in the hospital setting of medical care (Pellegrino, 1972).

In summary, the development of effective medical technology has led to profound changes in the structure and function of hospitals during the twentieth century. These have important consequences for the cost and organization of medical care. Hospitals were originally custodial commonweal organizations dedicated to providing charity maintenance care to the poor and to removing the undesirable indigent sick from public view. The advent of effective surgery, based on the development of scientific bacteriology, aseptic technique, nursing reform, and safe anesthesia, brought an influx of middle-class patients seeking surgical treatment that could only be provided in this setting. Reorganizing hospitals for this new function required two major steps: (1) The changes in public image to make them acceptable to the middle class, that is, upgrading administration and building modern technical facilities and amenities, which took place under the guidance of the boards of trustees; (2) The conversion of the professional and technical organization from a custodial to curative orientation, which took place under the guidance of physicians as hospitals became their professional workshops. Out of this transition emerged the two-class system of hospital care, one for the poor and one for the paying middle-class and upper-class patients. The transition also produced an intensive technological orientation that was to become a self-feeding impetus toward hospital growth and escalating costs. This was augmented by the establishment of hospital insurance plans during the 1930s and 1940s that removed most cost constraints on implementation of this new technology.

After World War II a new level of sophistication was added to hospital technology as a consequence of medical research and specialty practice. This produced an increasing complexity of hospital organizational structure as many specially trained technicians became necessary to operate the new equipment. Quasi-independent departments emerged that were difficult to control within the overall framework of hospital administration. Because high-quality, sophisticated medical care required the use of this technology, physicians became increasingly dependent on hospitals for the conduct of their practices. One consequence was the widespread movement of medical practice into the hospital-based setting, first in the growth of specialty residency training programs and then in the form of full-time hospital attending staffs (Chapter 8). A second consequence was the uncontrolled escalation of hospital costs because of the mutually reinforcing growth in the use of the expensive new technology, its operating personnel, and the complex new organizational structure (Chapter 12). This structure took on a mixed administrative form that no longer fits any classical pattern for managerial techniques and seems to defy effective control. The internal dynamics of hospitals evolving out of professional incentives and the organizational demands of the new technology produce a self-propelling momentum. This fires hospital growth and directs it toward increasingly specialized, intensive, high-technology, episodic care—a development poorly matched to the increasing need for a continuous spectrum of supportive care, especially for chronic illness (Chapters 5 and 8). The financing and planning problems that have emerged out of these developments are discussed in later chapters.

REFERENCES

Abel-Smith, Brian, *The Hospitals, 1800–1948,* London: Heinemann, 1964.

Austin, D. J., "Emerging Roles and Responsibilities in Health Administration," in *Report of Commission Education for Health Administration,* Vol. 1, Ann Arbor, Mich.: Health Administration Press, 1975.

Blau, Peter, and Scott, W. Richard, *Formal Organizations,* San Francisco: Chandler Press, 1962.

Blankenship, Lloyd V., and Elling, Ray H., "Organizational Support and Community

Power Structure: the Hospital," *Journal of Health and Human Behavior,* 3:257–269, 1962.

Churchill, Edward D., "The Development of the Hospital," in Faxon, Nathaniel W., Ed., *The Hospital in Contemporary Life,* Cambridge: Harvard University Press, 1949.

Coe, Rodney M., *Sociology of Medicine,* New York: McGraw-Hill, 1970.

Corwin, E. H. L., *The American Hospital,* New York: Commonwealth Fund, 1946.

Coser, Rose, "Authority and Decision-Making in a Hospital: A Comparative Analysis," *American Sociological Review,* 23:56–63, 1958.

Davis, Fred, Ed., *The Nursing Profession,* New York: Free Press, 1966.

Davis, Michael M., *Dispensaries: Their Managers and Development,* New York: Macmillan, 1918.

Davis, Michael M., *Clinics, Hospitals and Health Centers,* New York: Harper & Brothers, 1927.

Donabedian, Avedis, *Aspects of Medical Care Administration,* Cambridge, Mass.: Harvard University Press, 1973.

Dornblaser, B. M., "The Social Responsibility of General Hospitals," *Hospital Administration,* Spring: 6, 1970.

Downs, Anthony, *Inside Bureaucracy,* Boston: Little, Brown, 1967.

Ehrenreich, Barbara, and Ehrenreich, John, *The American Health Empire: Power, Profits, and Politics,* New York: Vintage Books, 1971.

Elling, Ray H., and Halebsky, Sandor, "Organizational Differentiation and Support: A conceptual Framework," *Administrative Science Quarterly,* 6:185–209, 1961.

Elling, Ray H., "The Shifting Power Structure in Health," *Milbank Memorial Fund Quarterly,* 46:119–144, 1968.

Freidson, Eliot, *Profession of Medicine,* New York: Dodd, Mead, 1970.

Freyman, Jr., *The American Health Care System: Its Genesis and Trajectory,* New York: Medcom Press, 1974.

Gaughton, J. C., "Role of the Public General Hospital in Community Health," *American Journal of Public Health,* 65:21, 1975.

Georgopoulos, Basil S., and Mann, Floyd C., *The Community General Hospital,* New York: Macmillan, 1962.

Georgopoulos, Basil S., and Matejko, Aleksander, "The American General Hospital as a Complex Social System," *Health Services Research,* Spring: 76–112, 1967.

Georgeopoulos, Basil S., Ed., *Organization Research on Health Institutions,* Ann Arbor: Institute for Social Research, 1972.

Hall, Oswald, "The Informal Organization of Medical Practice in an American City," unpublished Ph.D. dissertation, Chicago: University of Chicago, 1944.

Hall, Oswald, "The Informal Organization of The Medical Profession," *Canadian Journal of Economics and Political Science,* 12:30–44, 1946.

Hall, Oswald, "The Stages of Medical Career," *American Journal of Sociology,* 53:327–336, 1948.

Heydebrand, Wolf V., *Hospital Bureaucracy: A Comparative Study of Organizations,* New York: Dunellen, 1973.

Hughes, Everett C., *Men and Their Work,* New York: Free Press, 1958.

Litwak, Eugene, "Models of Bureaucracy Which Permit Conflict," *American Journal of Sociology,* 67:177–184, 1961.

Mauksch, Hans O., "It Defies All Logic—But a Hospital Does Function," in Skipper, James K. and Leonard, Robert C., *Social Interaction and Patient Care,* Philadelphia: Lippincott, 1965.

Pellegrino, Edmond D., "The Changing Matrix of Clinical Decision Making in the Hospital," in Georgopoulos, Basil, *Organizational Research on Health Institutions,* Ann Arbor: Institute for Social Research, 1972.

Perrow, Charles, "Goals and Power Structures—A Historical Case Study," in Freidson, Eliot, Ed., *The Hospitals in Modern Society,* New York: Free Press, 1963.

Perrow, Charles, "Hospitals: Technology, Structure, and Goals," in March, J., Ed., *Handbook of Organizations,* Chicago: Rand McNally, 1965.

Rosen, George, "The Hospital: Historical Sociology of a Community Institution," in Freidson, Eliot, Ed., *The Hospital in Modern Society,* New York: Free Press, 1963, 1–36.

Rosenberg, E. C., "Social Class and Medical Care in Nineteenth-Century America: The Rise and Fall of the Dispensary," *Journal of the History of Medicine and Allied Sciences,* 29:32, 1974.

Rosner, David, and Thernstrom, Stephen, "The Dispensary and Hospital Abuse Controversy," unpublished Masters' thesis, 1974.

Seeman, Melvin, and Evans, John W., "Stratification and Hospital Care: Part 2, The Objective Criteria of Performance," *American Sociological Review,* 26:193–204, 1961.

Sheatsley, Paul B., "Public Attitudes Towards Hospitals," *Hospitals, Journal of the American Hospital Association,* 31(May 16):47–48, 1957.

Smith, Harvey L., "Two Lines of Authority Are One Too Many," *Modern Hospitals,* 84: 59–64, 1955.

Somers, Herman M., and Somers, Anne R., *Doctors, Patients and Health Insurance,* Washington, D.C.: The Brookings Institution, 1961.

Strickland, Stephen P., *Politics, Science, & Dread Disease: A hort History of United States Medical Research Policy,* Cambridge: Harvard University Press, 1972.

Thompson, James D., *Organization in Action,* New York: McGraw-Hill, 1967.

Thompson, James D., and McEwen, William J., "Organizational Goals and Environment: Goal-Setting As an Interaction Process," *American Sociological Review,* 23:23–31, 1958.

Vladeck, Bruce C., "Why Non-Profits Go Broke," *The Public Interest,* 42(Winter):86–101, 1976.

Wilensky, Harold, "The Professionalization of Everyone?" *American Journal of Sociology,* 70:137–158, 1964.

Wilson, Robert N., "The Physician's Changing Hospital Role," *Human Organization,* 18: 177–183, 1959.

Wilson, Robert N., "The Social Structure of a General Hospital," *The Annals of the American Academy of Political and Social Science,* 346(March):67–76, 1963.

CHAPTER EIGHT

The Changing Structure
of the Medical Profession
and Fragmentation of Practice

As hospitals were changing their structure, function, and internal power relationships during this century, similar changes were also occurring in the organization of the medical profession and medical practice. Some of these changes were parallel to those described for hospitals and occurred for much the same reasons. The improving efficacy of medical technology and raised expectation in regard to medical care increased the demand for physician services and elevated the prestige of the whole profession. In 1925 the first study of occupational prestige ranked physicians behind bankers and college professors (Counts, 1925); by 1947 they tied with state governors; and by 1963 were second only to Supreme Court justices (Hodge et al., 1964).

The profession's improved image made it possible to exercise more influence over patients and medical policy in their communities and to ask higher fees for their services as demand for medical care grew. Some changes in medical practice stemmed directly from the evolution that took place in hospitals. Further changes were due to the more effective organization and increasing influence of the American Medical Association (AMA) as a professional guild striving for greater control of its own domain—both for the improvement of medical practice and for the betterment of its own members. Finally, changes in the profession occurred as consequences of shifts in the demographic characteristics and distribution of the American population, in the method of financing health care, and in government health policy.

As with hospitals, the changes in the medical profession and the organization of practice have not been without problems. Despite the growing prestige of the profession, there are more complaints about the quality of medical care, increasing malpractice suits, and demands for closer surveillance over physician practices. Legislation has been suggested for periodic relicensing examinations and more intensive peer review systems. Consumer groups complain about the impersonalizing of medical care, the lack of continuity of care by a single physician, and the high costs of care. Difficulty is experienced in obtaining services when needed. There are long waiting times for appointments. Many persons, particularly in inner-city poverty areas, are forced to use hospital emergency rooms or outpatient departments for medical services that formerly would have been obtained in physicians' offices. These problems have dominated discussions of possible reform of the health care system in recent years. Yet, they are only symptoms of the profound changes that have taken place in the profession and in the organization of practice that have resulted in the growing mismatch with the needs of post-clinical medicine. Unless the deeper roots of the problem are taken into account, attempted solutions are likely to be ineffective or even counterproductive. Some of these major causes of the present malfunction lie in the evolution of the medical profession and the organization of practice since the turn of the century.

PRE-FLEXNER MEDICAL PRACTICE

In 1900 the population of the United States was still largely rural and in small towns, as was the distribution of physicians. The rapid production of physicians by proprietary medical schools, and even by some university affiliated schools, produced a high physician/population ratio, but the quality of training was, on the average, poor. The combination of minimal training and of sometimes unscrupulous practice, growing out of intense competition for patients, had so depressed the reputation of the profession that little remained of the cloak of professional social mandate. Much of the population was as ready to turn to patent medicine sellers, chiropractors, homeopaths, or other alternative healing groups as they were to consult physicians.

There were also prestigious physicians in 1900, faculty members of the small group of elite, university affiliated medical schools, as well as those who treated the rich and the powerful. Such a practice could accrue to a physician either because of justified professional reputation, his own upper-class origin that provided access to a similar clientele, the sponsorship and partnership of an older physician who already had such a practice, or because of personal charm and social ability. Since so little could be done for patients that made much difference in health outcomes, the major determinants of professional reputation were professional image, social graces, and proper connections. Most members of the profession, however, were relegated to a rather humble position in society. To be sure, their above average education and the opportunity to build up a reservoir of good will over the years for services and sympathy given provided physicians a standing in the community like that of a minister or justice of the peace. In small towns this often made them one of the town elders to whom people turned for advice and aid in regard to matters that, as often as not, had nothing to do with medical affairs. In larger cities the pattern of neighborhood practice was similar with most general practitioners spread fairly uniformly around the city, serving a population in their immediate area and probably of their own ethnic group and social class.

DEVELOPMENT OF THE AMERICAN MEDICAL ASSOCIATION

The American Medical Association (AMA) played a major role in the organizational development of the medical profession in this country during the early decades of this century. The AMA had been founded in 1847 as a professional society dedicated to upgrading medical practice and bettering the profession. Throughout much of the nineteenth century the Association spent most of its limited energies waging an unsuccessful battle against quackery. During the first decade of the present century the AMA became involved politically. Taking a very liberal position, it spearheaded the lobbying effort for the Pure Food and Drug Act of 1905 and the drive for a National Department of Health. It was part of the coalition working for worker's compensation laws in many states (Burrow, 1963). The Association's efforts to promote the upgrading of medical education began in the 1880s and 1890s in alliance with university medical schools and philanthropic organizations like the Carnegie Foundation and were finalized by the Flexner Report of 1910. The second-rate, proprietary medical schools were eliminated during this period (Chapter 6), and uniform admission requirements and standards for curriculum, facilities, and faculty were set. Using the surveillance and accreditation power of its Council on Medical Education, the AMA consolidated the movement to transform medical education into a rigorous preparation for applying the modern medical techniques being developed at that time.

Between 1900 and 1920 while the reforms in medical education were occurring, a profound change also took place within the AMA itself. At the turn of the century the membership of the Association had only been 8400—scarcely 7% of the physicians in the country. Most of the members were from the five eastern states of Massachusetts, New York, Connecticut, Rhode Island, and Pennsylvania. The Association was largely controlled by a small executive committee of medical school affiliated physicians representing the elite of the profession. To further the upgrading of medical knowledge and practice and to build a more powerful political base to lobby for health care reform, a major reorganizational effort was undertaken. Between 1905 and 1910, following the example of successful union organizers, Dr. Joseph McCormack traveled throughout the country as a full-time representative of the AMA to organize constituent county medical societies. These county societies were to act as continuing education organs and increase political strength.

McCormack was extremely successful. By 1915 the AMA's membership had grown to 70,000, and by 1920 to 83,000, 65% of the practicing physicians in the country (Burrow, 1963). In 1910 the governing council was reorganized and a new more workable House of Delegates gave much more opportunity for policy setting to the membership at large. For the first time the AMA could truly speak as the "voice of American medicine." However, the influence of this new larger constituency in the House of Delegates also led to radical changes in the policies that the Association pursued. The established eastern states' medical school elite with its liberal, public interest orientation did not lose its position of influence immediately. Nevertheless, it gradually had to accommodate to the new majority of conservative physicians from the small towns and rural areas who were primarily interested in having the AMA function as a protective guild.

POST-FLEXNER MEDICAL PRACTICE

Between 1920 and 1945 the organization of the profession and the nature of medical practice changed dramatically. Four major trends can be identified: (1) increasing specialization and growing dominance of office-based specialty practice; (2) concentration of physicians into urban areas; (3) development of informal but effective citywide organization of the medical profession, which controlled entry and advancement within the professional system and maintained a fair degree of internal discipline over professional behavior; and (4) development of a unified prestige hierarchy and referral system.

As discussed in Chapter 6, the increasing complexity of medical technology and medical education led inexorably to the rapid growth of specialization in American medicine. Between 1930 and 1945, however, the system of training and accreditation for specialty practice was largely informal and locally controlled—in contrast to the present formal residency training and certification through national specialty examining boards. Specialty status at that time depended primarily on recognition by local professional peer groups. This recognition was simply expressed by their willingness to refer problem cases to the physician who claimed special competence in that area of practice. This system required a network of personal relationships that served both to channel the referrals and confirm the status of the physicians involved.

Specialty practice, particularly when based on such an informal interactive system, requires a higher degree of professional aggregation than existed in the previous (pre-Flexner) period. Prior to 1930 the profession consisted mostly of self-sufficient general practitioners, all potentially in competition for the same patients. Specialists need a much larger population of potential patients to draw from in order to encounter a high enough incidence of diseases in which they are interested (Kendall, 1971). They also need a cluster of other specialists and generalists to provide adequate referrals and to handle the kinds of cases they prefer not to deal with themselves. This informal specialty system led inevitably to a disproportionate concentration of physicians in the large cities. Specialists within the cities concentrated further into certain centrally located areas, maximizing their accessibility to large numbers of patients and to each other. It has long been recognized that increasing specialization leads to greater functional interdependence and the development of regularized work and social relationships to provide for those dependencies (Durkheim, 1893). Such specialization is accompanied by a system of stratification and social control within which rewards and sanctions are manipulated. This was characteristic of the organization of the medical profession that developed in urban areas in the United States between 1920 and 1945 (Hall, 1944).

There were a number of other factors that encouraged the concentration of physicians into cities during this time besides the functional pressures evolving out of specialization. This was the period of rapid urbanization in this country. Urbanization of the general population was accompanied by concentration of profession and service industries in the then thriving cities. Wealth, better educated population, prestige, and amenities of life were all to be had in the cities in greater amounts than in nonurban areas, and physicians understandably followed these trends and incentives (Steele & Rimlinger, 1965). The smaller number of physicians graduating from the more selective post-Flexner medical schools by decreasing the competition made it easier for physicians to locate in urban areas (Dyckman, 1978; Kessel, 1970). The rising public expectations in regard to medical care produced a much greater demand for medical services. In 1930 the average number of physician visits per year per patient was estimated to be 2.5 (Committee on the Cost of Medical Care, 1932). By 1945 the average number of visits had increased to 4.5 per year (U.S. Bureau of Census, 1978), despite the fact that the physician/population ratio had remained essentially unchanged since 1930 (Rayack, 1964, 1967). Decreasing competition, rising demand, and higher fees led to steadily climbing physician incomes (after the initial few years of the Great Depression when they, like the rest of the nation, had suffered severe economic hardships) making it easier for them to practice and enjoy the amenities in larger cities (Dyckman, 1978). With higher incomes, climbing prestige, and urban concentration, physicians were in turn able to move even more easily into specialization (Kendall, 1971). A major negative effect of these changes was the growing scarcity of physicians in rural areas which required residents of many parts of the country to travel long distances in order to obtain medical care (Mountin et al., 1949).

During this period the development of an informal but effective metropolitan organization of the profession led to rigorous internal control and marked stratification within the group. Oswald Hall (1944) described this informal structure in Providence, Rhode Island, in the early 1940s and analyzed the mechanisms by which control and stratification were maintained. The segment of the profession that Hall dubbed the "inner fraternity" was a small group of office-based specialists practicing in a few medical arts buildings in the prestigious East Side residential district (Hall, 1946). They were also within easy access of the business district and downtown hospitals. Solidarity between physicians of this group was created by cross-referral and consultation patterns as well as by joint membership on hospital staffs, committees, shared office space, and so on. On a part-time, so-called "visiting" basis, these same men were chiefs of services at the major voluntary hospitals, or held high ranking staff appointments there. By means of an informal sponsorship system, the inner fraternity in effect controlled the flow of new physicians into the medical care system and their advancement on the hospital staffs (Hall, 1948). This decisively influenced their prestige, potential for receiving referral patients, and hence the type of practice they could expect to establish, for example, whether they could gradually limit their practices to single specialties. Those who stayed at the bottom of the ladder, that is, those who failed to obtain an effective sponsor in order to advance within the hospital staff system, were forced to remain general practitioners (Hall, 1949), depending on a regular clientele in the immediate areas where they practiced.

The mechanisms by which professional stratification was maintained were essentially the same as those leading to professional control of specialization. In fact, during this period—unlike the situation after the institutionalization of residency programs—specialty status, hospital rank, and position in the professional social hierarchy were essentially the same. The social and prestige groupings within the profession corresponded closely to those of the patients they treated, and were based primarily on cultural and social class identity. The rich were cared for by Park Avenue type specialists; the poor by (usually co-ethnic) general practitioners or by the outpatient departments of voluntary and local government hospitals. On the other hand, this stratification was accompanied by a system of referrals and consultations between parts of the profession, and by hospital staff appointments from different ranks in the hierarchy, so that interaction between parts of the hierarchy was frequent. The resulting system of stratification was thus a continuous spectrum from the dominant "inner fraternity" downward (Hall, 1946). Exclusion of the ethnic neighborhood practitioners from the hospital system, however, led to differences in the quality and availability of medical care that various segments of the population received.

At the end of this period the structure of the medical profession and practice in urban areas was reasonably well adapted to the health care needs of society. The pattern of diseases was still predominantly acute. The general practitioner/specialist referral system provided reasonably adequate continuity of care, as well as professional control over the quality of practice in the community. Except for the scarcity of rural physicians, which was already becoming a serious problem, the distribution of physicians provided adequate access to primary and referral care for most patients.

CHANGES IN THE STRUCTURE OF MEDICAL PRACTICE SINCE WORLD WAR II

After World War II American society entered another phase of rapid changes that eventuated in a new period of evolution in the structure of the medical profession and its practice. Some of the changes originated within medicine itself, but others of equal importance were the result of trends in the general social environment. Three trends can be identified that were particularly important in instigating this restructuring of the profession: specialization by way of residency, the growth of hospital influence on practice, and suburbanization of large metropolitan areas. As a result of these trends, the number of physicians in three new types of practice has grown rapidly in the past two decades: (1) full-time, teaching-hospital-based physicians and medical school faculty; (2) inner-city, Medicaid-clinic physicians (usually foreign trained and without hospital affiliations), who serve the new urban poor; (3) suburban, office-based physicians loosely affiliated with community hospitals (Miller, 1977).

Although they played a minor role in the overall makeup of the medical profession in the United States 30 years ago, today these types of practice seem destined to dominate the organization of the profession and control the way health care is provided. Because of the different levels of prestige and competence and because of the different professional organizational systems found in these new prominent groupings, they represent a new envolving system of professional stratification, replacing the old one described by Hall (1944).* Unlike the old system, however, the new groupings of physicians have very little interchange of personnel, knowledge, information, or direct patient referrals. Therefore they tend to divide the profession into mutually isolated sections rather than forming a continuous interacting stratification, as was formerly the case. This has important implications for the quality of care, its continuity for the individual patient, and the availability of services to different parts of the population. It also has important

---

* Of course, the transition to the new physician "stratification" system is nowhere near complete, and some of the old social class and ethnically determined differentiation of the profession continues to exist. In particular, the high prestige medical practice areas have retained a considerable concentration of physicians if the adjoining business or residential districts have retained their high status. However, in cities that have medical schools or hospitals with prestigious residency programs, this group is progressively being excluded from the teaching hospitals where they once had private-patient care privileges and teaching responsibilities (Kendall, 1965). As a result, younger physicians are locating in this type of practice much less rapidly than before. Thus even the "Park Avenue" physicians seem destined not to be replaced in larger cities in the next generation.

implications for the continuing education of practicing physicians and for the most effective use of services. We now turn to a detailed study of these trends, their causes, and effects.

DEVELOPMENT OF RESIDENCY TRAINING AND SPECIALTY BOARDS

The new order-of-magnitude increment in the rate of development of medical technology after 1945 affected the organization of the profession and of practice, as well as hospitals. The increasing corpus of knowledge and skills necessary to provide health care produced a new surge in the growth of professional specialization and subspecialization. Residency training became the mode of entry into specialty status, and national specialty examining boards became the mechanism of legitimation. This route accelerated the process of specialization by enabling direct entry into specialty practice instead of the previous gradual limitation from an established general practice.

Prior to the reforms in medical education, internships in large city hospitals had been a way to gain experience before beginning formal medical training rather than afterwards. This was replaced by the system of postgraduate internships as medical education improved along the lines of the Johns Hopkins-Harvard model toward the end of the century. Internship in a prestigious hospital (there were only a few at that time) was soon looked on as the way to advance rapidly within the profession. It could lead to an appointment to the outpatient clinic and later to the attending staff. Such appointments, by providing association with eminent specialists and the opportunity for professional recognition, made it possible to get referrals and hence to limit one's practice to a specialty. As surgery began to expand rapidly, interns were needed to give anesthesia, perform laboratory tests, and take care of critically sick patients when visiting staff physicians were not available. As the number and size of hospitals expanded with the demand for services, the need for interns also grew rapidly, so that by 1914 almost 80% of all medical school graduates were already taking internships (Stevens, 1971). Soon state boards of health began to make it a requirement for licensure.

Having grown out of the service needs of hospitals rather than as part of medical school programs, internships developed with little concern about the quality of training. Starting in 1912 the AMA Council on Medical Education and then the American College of Surgeons (ACS, founded in 1913) began considering hospital teaching reform. The ACS was more aggressive in hospital inspection and accreditation and gained the upper hand in policy decisions. As a result the AMA suggestion that all internships be affiliated with medical schools was never implemented (Burrow, 1963). Instead internships remained under hospital control, in large part because of the hospitals' concern about meeting needs for professional manpower. The

ACS wanted to make the internship and surgical residency training more practical than the model they had seen in the academic, research-oriented, university hospitals. At Johns Hopkins and Harvard, for example, the objective had been to produce a few very highly trained specialists to become faculty in the leading universities. The ACS opted for the Mayo Clinic model, which consisted of three years of graduate fellowship during which the young physicians were given gradually increasing clinical responsibility to prepare them to *practice* the specialty. Following World War I a joint AMA-ACS investigation of specialty training was undertaken under the direction of the AMA Council on Medical Education. Dominated by specialists, the sentiment of nearly all the participating specialty subcommittees was that the AMA's role should be limited to sponsorship of the specialty advisory committees to develop the standards for graduate training in each specialty. These committees evolved into the separate specialty examining boards in the 1930s (Stevens, 1971).

During the 1920s and 1930s resistance stiffened to any control of specialty training by medical schools or even the AMA Council on Medical Education. Even those who were already specialists saw no need to limit competition by interposing the medical schools as gateways to entry. Since their hold on their specialties as guilds was still very tenuous, specialists feared the potential elitist interference of medical school faculties more than they feared the competition of peers. Public demand for specialist care was growing faster than the number of specialists, so that competition did not seem to be a real threat. Having their hospitals involved in residency training actually increased the demand for the services of established specialists because of the prestige and attention that was attached to them. House officer physicians available to carry part of the load of caring for private patients also made it possible to have more patients and more income. Hospitals also began to find it advantageous to have residency programs. The treatment of complicated cases needed specialty trained house officer physicians available on a full-time basis just as it was necessary to have interns for more routine care. These incentives led to a snowball-like growth of residency training programs and to a rapid increase in the number of specialists (Kendall, 1971).

The founding of the American College of Surgeons (ACS) in 1913 was one of the first important steps toward regulation of specialization and specialty practice in the United States. Around the turn of the century surgery was becoming increasingly important because of the growing potential for effective intervention in many disorders. It also became significant financially for the profession and for hospitals because of the public demand for surgical care. Understandably many fights arose over who should be allowed to perform surgery in hospitals. There were scandals concerning the practice of fee splitting, where the referring physicians received part of the fee collected by the surgeon as a means of encouraging further referrals. Hospitals were reticent or unable to determine who was qualified to use their operating rooms. The ACS was founded to deal with these problems by providing continuing education for surgeons through journal articles and clinical congresses as well as setting standards for surgical training (Stevens, 1971). The College administered an examination of surgical competence as a requirement for membership, but the required level remained rather minimal until the American Board of (General) Surgery was established in 1937. The major impact of the ACS was its role (together with the AMA) in setting hospital accreditation standards for internship and residency training. It was originally hoped that the ACS would assume a strong regulatory role, limiting the practice of surgery to certified specialists as with the Royal College of Surgeons in England. In the face of the egalitarian tradition of American medicine, this role failed to materialize. The founding of the American College of Physicians (ACP) in 1915 had even less of a regulatory affect on the practice of internal medicine.

The first rigorous specialist board examination was the American Board of Ophthalmic Examiners established as a joint undertaking of the AMA Section on Ophthalmalogy, the American Ophthalmic Society, and the American Academy of Ophthalmics and Otolaryngology in 1916. It grew out of a dispute between ophthalmologists (MDs) and optometrists (opticians) over the measurement of refractive errors in fitting eye glasses and was the first real attempt to limit specialty status to qualified practitioners. The two specialty societies agreed to admit only board certified diplomates after 1920. In 1924 the counterpart American Board of Otolaryngology was established. Between 1930 and 1940 thirteen more specialty examining boards were founded, including those for general surgery and internal medicine, followed by a few more specialty groups after World War II— the most recent being the American Board of Family Practice.

Thus, little by little, the entire range of specialties came to be covered by a system of examining boards and corresponding specialty societies. Yet, specialty boards failed to provide anything like an overall regulatory system for specialty practice. In 1933 the Advisory Board of Medical Specialties (ABMS, renamed the American Board of Medical Specialties in 1970) was established as a joint effort of the AMA's Council on Medical Education (CME), the Association of American Medical Colleges (AAMC), and the American Hospital Association (AHA) to coordinate specialty board activities and specialty training—but in fact it had little influence. Each specialty board and society remained quite independent. Each hospital specialty department independently determined the number of residents to be trained— a decision that depended more on the immediate need for manpower in their own department than on any overall specialty manpower policy. Prestigious professional study groups repeatedly suggested that stronger interspecialty regulations be set up and that the medical school supervise the instruction of interns and residents in teaching hospitals. Yet all parties resisted these changes until very recently. Hospitals wanted control of their house officer manpower supply, while specialty boards and societies feared interference or domination by the large major specialties (medicine and general surgery), and the medical schools were loath to take on the additional responsibilities of graduate medical education.

In 1940 the Committee on Graduate Medical Education, formed jointly by the AMA (which by this time had come to be dominated by specialty oriented groups rather than by the general practitioners of the last generation) and the American Hospital Association, strongly recommended formal residency programs as the preferable route to specialty status to replace any remnants of the old system of gradual specialization by part-time hospital appointments. This policy was vigorously pursued, and following World War II residency training programs were established in most major hospitals so that such training was available to any medical school graduate who wanted it.

By the middle 1960s, however, it became obvious that the snowballing growth of residencies and uncontrolled increase in the number of specialists, especially surgery, had gotten out of hand. Hospitals were in open competition with each other for the limited number of American medical school graduates to fill their programs, and large numbers of foreign medical graduates were being recruited to make up the difference between supply and hospital demand. Growing concern about this situation led to convening a series of study committees that produced reports calling for increased supervision of graduate medical education by medical schools and some kind of nationwide regulation of the specialty entry system.

The most influential, the Coggeshall Report (1965) and the Millis Report (1966), recommended and finally set in motion: (1) abandonment of the internship as a separate element of medical education (graduate medical education would essentially be limited to large teaching hospitals that offered the full range of specialty residency training); (2) accreditation of an institution's entire graduate medical education program as a whole, rather than by each individual specialty residency; (3) establishment of a Commission on Graduate Medical Education (CGME)* to plan, coordinate, and set standards for specialty training and institutional accreditation. In 1970 the AMA's CME resolved not to approve any new internships after 1971 unless integrated into complete residency programs and to abolish all such existing internships after 1975. Founding of the American Board of Family Practice and accreditation of combined internship-residencies in that field was to replace the old rotating internships for training GPs. How effective this new attempt at regulation of specialty training and practice will be still remains to be seen. Increased health cost consciousness on the part of the federal government and additional pressure for regulation in the Health

---

* The Liaison Committee on Graduate Medical Education (LCGME) including the AMA, AHA, AAMC, ABMS, and CMSS (Council of Medical Specialty Societies) plus representatives of the federal government and the general public was established in 1972—much like the CGME recommended by the Millis Report.

Manpower Acts of 1971 and 1976 make it likely that a more effective system of controlling specialty training will evolve soon.

INTERNSHIPS AND SPECIALTY RESIDENCY TRAINING

Graduation from medical school marks only the halfway point in medical education and professional socialization for most physicians today. Three to six years of internship and residency lie ahead to qualify for their specialty and subspecialty board examinations. Beginning the internship,* however, does mark a major branching point in the process of socialization. The type of internship has an important influence on further professional socialization (Mumford, 1970). Physicians who eventually become full-time hospital staff, take their residency in a major teaching hospital with specialty training, research, and medical student teaching. The socialization of the teaching hospital physician occurs as a direct line of transmission from one generation of medical school faculty to the next. The setting of undergraduate medical education within the teaching hospital shapes attitudes that are more in accord with the role of the academic physician than of the physician in community practice. Consequently, teaching hospital physicians have the least problematic and ambivalent socialization process as long as they remain within the university hospital system. However, it may ill-prepare them attitudinally and socially if they later take up community office-based practice.

University hospital residents continue to have the highly specialized and prestigious superiors as role models that they had in medical school. The transition is minimal; they move gradually up the hierarchy learning from those above and teaching those below, with the certainty that they will qualify for their specialty boards in due time and take their position among the professional elite (Miller, 1970). Identification is with their hospital-based colleagues and with the leaders of their specialty group wherever they practice and teach. In Merton's (1968) sense, these new physicians become cosmopolitans (Kendall, 1971; Mumford, 1970), seeking national recognition through scientific publication and membership in nationwide societies for their professional advancement.

Involvement in hospital care makes physicians more closely knit as a group but less responsive to patients' attitudes and pressures. Physicians working in a setting with a high degree of professional interaction, such as group practice or hospital practice, tend to be much more sensitive to opinions of colleagues about their medical judgements and professional standards (Freidson, 1970). They are less sensitive to the feelings of patients and

* Today internships have been eliminated in a formal sense by merger with residency programs. Nevertheless the first year of hospital training after medical school still functions as "internship" in regard to professional training and socialization.

less ready to meet their demands and expectations for personal consideration. This interactive influence on professional behavior is even stronger in hospital practice where there is also formal and informal surveillance of each other's work and increased opportunity to learn about the latest technological standards and advances in clinical care. The teaching hospital situation rewards technical brilliance in diagnosis and knowledge of the latest literature, during ward rounds as well as during informal consultations. During residency patients are seen almost exclusively in the hospital setting. Contact between the resident and patients, families, or communities is limited to brief encounters on the wards under stressful conditions. Patients are considered as "teaching material," and though they usually receive excellent technical care, the resident has little chance to relate to them as people. This attitude is accentuated by the pressure of the work load and the close identification of interests with the hospital as the specialists' work domain and the source of professional security, prestige, and income. Thus, hospital training creates incentives that enhance the technical quality of care but decrease the closeness of the physician-patient relationship and lessen responsiveness to the nontechnical needs of patients.

The congruence between socialization and the continuing incentive and organizational system guarantees a smoothly functioning professional subculture in teaching hospitals. The team practice organization of care and the graded hierarchy of responsibility assure the continued orientation toward technical excellence and prestige. This, together with the dependency on the hospital for income and patients, assures the persistence of a specialty, research, and disease orientation rather than a patient orientation. In such hospitals, where referred patients present complex diagnostic and therapeutic problems, these attitudes serve well. In other settings the result is often less satisfactory.

EFFECTS OF SPECIALIZATION

Specialization has had important effects on the organization and delivery of medical services and on the cost of health care. The most obvious impact is the decreasing availability of physicians who provide so-called "primary care." These are physicians who make the first contact with a patient in an episode of illness, no matter what its nature, and either provide the necessary care or investigate the case far enough to make a preliminary diagnosis and refer the patient to the appropriate specialist. In spite of the increasing prevalence of complex diseases where specialist care is necessary, the great majority of medical treatment still falls in the category of primary care. If a particular case requires attention from specialists, it would be advantageous for the primary-care physician to provide coordination, continuity, and general support for the patient in negotiating the complexities of the health care system (Alpert & Charney, 1973; Bodenheimer, 1970).

Formerly primary care was provided almost entirely by general practitioners (GPs). Since 1930 the number of practicing physicians barely kept pace with the growth of the population (until the last decade) and the percentage of physicians electing to be generalists has declined precipitously. Consequently the number of GPs per 100,000 population has dropped markedly in that time. Specialists have had to assume much of the load of primary care. Today adults go directly to internists for much of their general medical care and take their children directly to pediatricians. Similarly, obstetrician-gynecologists have taken over most of maternity care and have absorbed much of the care of diseases of women once handled by generalists. Even if these three groups of specialists are added to the number of practicing generalists, the total number of physicians providing primary care per 100,000 population has still declined markedly. Since the per capita demand for primary care (as well as for other medical services) has increased during the same period (Chapters 5 and 12), a significant shortage of primary-care physicians exists compared with 50 years ago. For the last 10 years the number of medical school graduates has been increasing more rapidly, and from 1960 to 1974 there was a major influx of foreign medical graduates. Nevertheless, the net gain in primary-care physicians has still been minimal.

The shortage of general practitioners is aggravated by a number of factors. For one thing, internists (and obstetrician-gynecologists, and to a lesser extent pediatricians) see relatively fewer patients per week than generalists. In part this is because they are not only providing primary care, but as specialists are also seeing referred cases, which tend to be more complex and require more time. Their standards of training encourage them to be more thorough in pursuing diagnostic and treatment possibilities. They also spend more of their time in the hospital, where they see fewer and more complex cases than in their offices. Finally, because specialists command higher fees, it is possible for them to have adequate incomes while seeing fewer patients. Thus the amount of primary care provided by specialists is appreciably less than given by an equal number of generalists, reducing further the effective equivalent number of primary-care physicians per 100,000 population.

Specialization has also aggravated the accessibility of primary care because of the impact it has had on the distribution of physicians (Robertson, 1970). As noted, prior to World War II specialists tended to locate predominantly in metropolitan areas, where there is a large enough population of potential patients for the variety of cases needed to support a specialized practice. This trend continues even for the internists who are now providing the primary care for a large segment of the population (Miller et al., 1978). The maldistribution of the new specialists contributes to primary care scarcity not only in the rural-metropolitan sense but also increasingly as a problem of accessibility within metropolitan areas. Traditionally, urban office-based specialists were concentrated in a few high-prestige areas near the business district and hospitals and adjacent to the higher income residential sections where many of their patients resided. Generalists, who tended to serve the lower income groups, were scattered about the city in the various neighborhoods they served (Hall, 1944).

Today a growing number of specialists no longer have their practices in private offices, but are instead full-time staff members of hospitals. Although hospital-based physicians continue to care for ambulatory patients (as well as for hospitalized patients), they see more cases by referral to the medical center, and are less readily accessible to patients than are those in office-based practice. The new trend toward full-time hospital-based staff is gradually excluding the remaining urban office-based specialists from the large teaching hospitals where they once had staff affiliation (Kendall, 1965). Many are therefore following their higher-income patients and moving into the suburbs. Younger specialists without full-time hospital staff appointments are likewise predominantly locating their practices in the suburbs and creating a rapid rise in the density of specialists there (Miller et al., 1978). Since the general practitioners in the inner city are not being replaced by a new generation, this leaves the poor in the inner city neighborhoods with little access to office-based physicians for primary care. They are forced to turn to hospital outpatient clinics and emergency rooms for their medical needs.

HOSPITAL-BASED PRACTICE

As noted in Chapter 7, the increase in complexity and cost of technological facilities and the growth of the specialized nonphysician staff needed to operate them have made hospitals the natural place for the centralization and coordination of medical care. Today the hospital is not only the physician's workshop, where care is conveniently provided for sicker patients, but a positive force in its own right around which the organization of care is structured. When complicated cases are referred to a major medical center the hospital as a whole, with its full-time medical staff, takes the responsibility for care (Pellegrino, 1971). Instead of the hospital's being an adjunct to the physician's practice, today the physician is increasingly becoming a cog in the organization of hospital practice (particularly in large urban teaching hospitals where medical research and training of new specialists take place).

An important consequence is the growing number of physicians who practice essentially full-time in a hospital setting. Since physicians have become more dependent on hospitals and the hospitals remain dependent on physicians, there is a strong incentive on both sides to develop closer associations. Hospitals are now legally accountable for activities of physicians within their walls. Their interests are therefore better protected by bringing physicians more formally into the organization. More staff physicians are needed to supervise interns, residents, and other professionals in training.

Convenient and attractive situations are made available on hospital premises for physicians to carry on private and hospital-patient practice side by side, as well as increased financial and nonfinancial incentives for doing so. Health insurance carriers add incentives by allowing hospitals to collect charges on a fee-for-service basis for physician services, from which physicians can be paid a high salary or a percentage after deductions for hospital costs such as offices, nonprofessional personnel, and so on. Hospitals can offer physicians the advantage of many nontaxable fringe benefits, such as retirement plans, educational leaves, and vacation. Such fringe benefits are not easily available to physicians in private office practice.

Physicians today seem more ready to give up the traditional independence of private office practice in order to gain additional control over the hospital environment on which they have become dependent. Because the hospitals continue as the sites for the discovery and transmission of new medical knowledge, the physician affiliated full-time with such an institution is better able to keep abreast of new developments in medical science and clinical practice. In the post-World War II period there was massive growth in health related research grants. Hospitals and medical schools became the recipients of large amounts of money to establish research institutes and carry out clinically related research. This provided hospitals another avenue for paying full-time staff physicians as well as further prestige that could be shared by the physicians working for them.

In 1930 fewer than 5% of (nongovernment) practicing MDs were hospital based. In 1978 the proportion reached 30%, and in major urban centers almost 40% (AMA, 1979). A recent study (Miller et al., 1978) of trends in 16 large metropolitan areas found that the continuing shift to hospital-based practice is widespread and massive. In 1959, on the average, 27% of the physicians in the central city counties were engaged in hospital-based practice. But by 1974 this had increased to 38%. Another 10% of the physicians were engaged in teaching, research, or administration, leaving barely 50% in office-based practice. Even in the suburban counties the percentage of hospital-based physicians increased from 8% in 1959 to 15% in 1974.

The massive growth of residency training in central city teaching hospitals accounts for a large part of the increase in hospital physicians. Interns and residents alone make up 70% of all hospital practitioners. The full-time staff physicians associated with teaching and research programs in hospitals providing residency training comprise a sizable share of the remaining 30%. The fact that such a large portion of hospital physicians are "trainees" does not mean, however, that the growth of hospital practice is an artifact that distorts the actual distribution of physician services. If anything, the reverse distortion is more likely. Interns and residents are the major source of professional manpower for providing services in most large urban hospitals. They work longer hours, see more patients, and provide more services than the average physician in private practice (Hughes, 1973, 1975). They provide readily available, professional labor which is essential for large hospitals to meet their service commitments. Increasingly, even hospitals without residency programs (and therefore no longer any interns) are finding it necessary to hire full-time staff physicians to man their emergency rooms and be available for urgent inpatient problems. This is particularly so with suburban hospitals as they have grown in recent years and as their care becomes increasingly sophisticated.

Teaching-hospital physicians, whether residents or staff, are a marked contrast to the solo office-based practitioner who represented the traditional stereotype of the physician. Hospital-based physicians depend directly on their institutions for at least part of their income and virtually all of their patients. Patients are referred directly to the hospital or to particular physicians because of their position there. Practice takes place on a team basis, which results in great interdependence among physicians and close identification with the organization in which they practice (Roemer & Friedman, 1971). Consequently there is much more emphasis on the technical aspects and scientific quality of care than on responsiveness to patients. Advancement in status and salary within the teaching-hospital hierarchy, and hence in the profession, depends on technical virtuosity, astuteness in the diagnosis and analysis of difficult cases, and national recognition within the chosen subspecialty group by means of research and publication. This is intensified by the geographic mobility of faculty members, which is similar to that found in other university faculties. Consequently the subculture of teaching-hospital physicians is cosmopolitan, prestige motivated, and colleague oriented (Mumford, 1970; Miller, 1970).

The dependency of the staff physician on the hospital produces a strong vested interest in the system of high-technology intensive, specialty care, which is largely hospital based. Combined with the growing dependency of teaching hospitals on government funding for research and faculty support, this leads to a situation that could be important in future health policy formulation and planning. In a departure from the traditional ideology of physicians in private practice, teaching-hospital physicians have come to accept a stronger government role in the financing and even organizing of health services, as long as professional control is maintained over the technical aspects of care and research (Colombotos et al., 1975). They have nothing to fear, since their dominant position in the system is assured no matter what form of financing and organization of care exists.

It is not only in inpatient care that the shift to hospital-based practice is being felt. Today hospital outpatient departments, emergency rooms, and other institutionally based clinics supply about 30% of the ambulatory care in metropolitan areas (as opposed to only about 10% as recently as 20 years ago; Piore et al., 1971). For inner-city poverty areas the portion may be as high as 80 to 90%. Outpatient departments were not designed for this purpose, having been intended for a more limited role of providing care to the truly indigent or acting as ultraspecialized referral clinics. Since the hospital clinics were often established primarily for teaching and research, they were not designed to provide the kind of massive service to their surrounding communities that is now being demanded of them (Beloff, 1968). The result is that, although the technical and professional quality is usually beyond reproach, the total effectiveness and satisfaction from the point of view of the patients leaves much to be desired (Burns, 1974). Services are organized for the convenience of the hospital and the professionals rather than for the patients forced to use them. Amenities are lacking, and care is fragmented because there is seldom a continuing primary personal physician. As a result patients are unable to negotiate the system to obtain the care potentially available, and the continuity of their care is often lost where follow-up would be necessary (Aday, 1975). The services are not responsive to individual needs, cultural differences, and community problems because there is no real institutional accountability or responsibility to the patients or the community served (Belloc & Fox, 1972). Thus, one of the effects of increased hospital-based practice and concurrent loss of inner-city, office-based, primary-care physicians is the perpetuation of a two-class system of health care. Those living in the suburbs or affluent urban neighborhoods receive office-based, attentive specialist care. Those living in most inner-city areas are forced to use impersonal and organizationally unsatisfactory hospital-based clinics (Alpert et al. 1969; Jonas, 1973; Knowles, 1965).

Faced with long waiting times, inconvenient hours, and difficulties in negotiating the hospital clinic system, more patients simply appear at the emergency room (ER) at their own convenience (Acton, 1973; Leveson, 1970; Ford, 1976). ERs have in effect become walk-in clinics for all ailments, trivial and serious, in a mixture that often requires expert triage decisions to expedite the true emergencies (Satin & Duhl, 1972). A recent study of New York City ERs showed that half of the patients seen were not really emergency or even urgent cases (Jonas et al., 1976). This crowds and disrupts the use of the ER for its intended purpose and often leads to inferior care, or at least to less considerate treatment by the harassed ER physicians. It produces further fragmentation of care since the ERs often have staffs and record systems different from the regular clinics. In spite of the assembly-line atmosphere of hospital clinics and emergency rooms, the cost of providing care in these settings is considerably higher than in physicians' offices. This is a consequence of the inefficient organization of services; the high utilization of expensive, readily available laboratory tests; and the high personnel-to-patient ratio. Moreover, patients seen in hospital clinics are more apt to be admitted for expensive in-hospital care than are those seen in private physicians' offices (Leveson, 1973; Miller, 1973).

INNER-CITY OFFICE-BASED PHYSICIANS AND THE INFLUX OF FOREIGN MEDICAL SCHOOL GRADUATES

In the central city the physicians are rapidly dividing into two completely separate groups—teaching-hospital specialists and neighborhood practitioners (Miller, 1977). The teaching-hospital group traditionally extended into the community as part-time attending (visiting) physicians who had admitting privileges on the hospital's private services in exchange for teaching and providing of services in the outpatient department. As the residency system and the number of full-time positions in the hospital have grown, however, there is increasing restriction of these part-time attendings, who are usually older and less research oriented (Kendall, 1965). This intensifies the mutual isolation of hospital-based and office-based physicians in the inner city, even for the once prestigious but now shrinking group of "Park Avenue" physicians, but more particularly for a newly growing group of physicians—the so-called Medicaid physicians.

Side by side geographically, but in no professional contact with hospital-based physicians, this new group of physicians practices in the deteriorating neighborhoods that have come to surround most university-affiliated hospitals. These physicians often have no hospital privileges at all or have them only at one of the small, outmoded hospitals left behind in the middle-class flight to the suburbs. Until the 1965 Medicaid legislation, inner-city neighborhood physicians were mostly older men who had practiced all their lives in these areas, usually serving a particular ethnic group (Elesh & Schollert, 1972; Marden, 1977). As these groups migrated to the suburbs, many of those physicians followed their patients (Rees, 1967). Those too old to start over are finishing out their years in the neighborhoods grown foreign to them. If present trends continue, this group will not be replaced in the next generation. The age distribution of physicians who have their primary offices in poverty areas indicates that the older ethnic neighborhood doctor described by Hall (1944) is a vanishing breed even in urban working-class ethnic communities (Miller, 1973; Miller et al., 1978; Reibstein & Stevenson, 1974).

More recently, however, as Medicaid has again made private medical care financially feasible in these areas, these older physicians are being joined by increasing numbers of foreign-trained physicians (Haug & Stevens, 1973; Holahan, 1975) whose chances for a successful practice in the suburbs are poor. As entrepreneurial opportunists they are making handsome incomes in so-called Medicaid centers (*New York Times*, 1976). These newcomer physicians establish several part-time offices in poor areas in groups that include dentists, podiatrists, chiropractors, and pharmacists, often with their own commercial laboratory facilities. By cross-referral, excessive use of laboratory and prescription services, and seeing patients at a rapid rate, they are able to build up large charges even at the low rates often paid by Medicaid fee schedules. Patients with complicated or time-consuming problems are sent to the nearest hospital outpatient department, which is the only specialty referral possibility in these areas. Since there is no interaction between Medicaid physicians and hospital, follow-up or continuity of care for the patient seldom occurs. In the eyes of the local communities Medicaid centers do perform an important service because there are no other sources of medical care except the hospital outpatient departments with their long waits and fragmented, impersonal health care (Goodrich et al., 1972). In the Medicaid clinics patients can get prompt care and find out whether it is necessary to undertake the outpatient department ordeal. Nevertheless, the quality of care is often poor, and the potential for abuse of the payment system is staggering.

Little information is available about the number of office-based physicians practicing in these poverty areas or about their subculture, professional organization, and incentive systems. The number of such (Medicaid) physicians defies accurate assessment because they often have several offices, working in each one only part of the time and giving the best neighborhood as their official address. Nevertheless, judging from the high density of storefront Medicaid centers along the main streets of poverty communities, the number of physicians practicing in this way is considerable.

In spite of the fact that the Medicaid centers or clinics have the appearance of group practices and often list a half dozen MDs on their gaudy advertising sign boards, their professional organization is essentially solo and fee-for-service. There is usually only one physician on the premises at a time—the other space being occupied by dentists, chiropodists, and other health practitioners. The part-time basis on which they practice in each location implies that they have no regular panel of patients, but only a shifting clientele available because of the restricted choice open to residents of such communities. Thus these physicians have neither the cosmopolitanism, colleague orientation, and prestige motivation of teaching-hospital physicians, nor the localism, guildlike professional solidarity, patient dependence, and community orientation of the older urban ethnic community physician or the suburban office-based physician. They are excluded from the technology of the hospitals essential for the practice of high-quality medicine and from the colleague solidarity or community ties necessary to develop a patient-responsive practice. In effect, the only incentive left open to them is the financial one, and the remaining organizational principle for professional activity is commercial (Miller, 1977).

SUBURBANIZATION OF MEDICAL PRACTICE

One of the most important sociodemographic trends in post-World War II America has been the shift in population growth from the central cities into the surrounding suburban rings, accompanied by a marked deterioration of the economic base and quality of life in the inner cities. Partly as a result of this general sociodemographic shift of the middle class out of the central city, and partly as a result of increasing exclusion from privileges at the large urban teaching hospitals (Kendall, 1965), office-based physicians have relocated away from the urban centers, or at least fewer new physicians have located there in recent years. For example, between 1959 and 1973 the number of office-based physicians in the New York City suburbs increased by 30%, outpacing even the growth rate of the general population in these counties so that their density increased by 15%. With the increase in hospital-based physicians included, the total physician density in the suburbs grew by 56%. During the same period there was a 25% loss of office-based physicians within the New York City limits. A study of trends in 15 large standard metropolitan statistical areas (SMSAs) from 1959 to 1974 (Miller et al., 1978) demonstrates that the density of office physicians has grown rapidly in large, older Northeastern metropolitan suburban counties. In New York and Philadelphia the density of office specialists in the suburbs now exceeds that of their central cities. The trend is also present but less marked in large metropolitan areas of the South and West.

Suburban office practice today has many of the characteristics of the inner-city office-based practice described by Hall (1944) 30 years ago. However, it is less integrated professionally because it is geographically more diffuse and lacks the hierarchical structure of hospital appointments and consultation patterns that were found formerly. Nearly all suburban office physicians have admitting privileges at the local community hospital, but cases are mostly routine and uncomplicated, requiring less physician supervision and interaction than in teaching hospitals.* Since they also are not obligated to contribute time for teaching or working in the clinics, these physicians have less structured professional interaction with their colleagues in the hospital setting. Community physicians can seldom limit their practice entirely to a single subspecialty, even if they are board certified, because of the more scattered pattern of practice and less opportunity for referral work in the suburbs. This decreases identification with the national subspecialty peer group and evokes solidarity with local colleagues of all specialties, more on a "guild" basis rather than because of technical interdependency (Freidson, 1970, 1970a).

The community physician's income is nearly always on a fee-for-service basis, and this creates much greater patient dependence on the part of the physician (Freidson, 1961; Roemer, 1962). In order to develop a stable clientele, physicians in solo, fee-for-service practice must conform to patients' expectations and pressures, at times even at the expense of the technical quality of care. Physicians in this setting tend to prescribe more freely ("to give the patient a feeling he is getting something for his visit"), to recommend more frequent return visits (which are usually shorter), and to postpone or avoid more complex, diagnostic testing as well as routine preventive care. Furthermore, the financial incentives and constraints embodied in the usual health care insurance schemes, as well as the patient pressure, lead to more frequent hospitalization and surgery (Luft, 1978; Bunker, 1970). Thus it is not only the poor who are adversely affected by the over-

---

* Only in teaching hospitals are there ordinarily large numbers of complicated cases, which are infrequent in the general population, since they are concentrated there by referral.

specialization and maldistribution of physicians—the rich may very well suffer from too much specialized medical care, especially too much surgery (Stroman, 1979: Hughes, 1972).

Community physicians may be well trained and desirous of maintaining high technical standards of care, but they neither receive the constant new information and stimulation found in the teaching hospital nor do they have an incentive system that motivates them to keep abreast of the latest medical knowledge. Their livelihoods and professional advancement depend not on research and teaching prestige, but on the good will of their fellow physicians and of their patients. They receive patients not by referral based on their position in the hospital, but because of personal reputation within the community. Among patients this reputation derives from the physician's responsiveness, concern, professional image, and, more and more today, from sheer availability. Among fellow community physicians this reputation is based to some extent on technical competence but more importantly on following the norms of the local professional group, including reciprocity in referral and return of patients and solidarity vis-à-vis the lay public (Freidson, 1970).

The subculture of the community office-based physician is predominantly "local" (Merton, 1968a), financially or socially motivated, and patient oriented, with norms that emphasize the practical daily concerns of the practice of medicine. The dependency of the physician on patient, immediate community, and the local colleague group leads to an ideology that strongly opposes any government initiative or power in the financing and organizing of health care—in contrast to the attitudes of most teaching-hospital physicians (Strickland, 1972; Colombotos, 1968, 1969, 1971). These guild perspectives are mirrored in the county medical societies' and AMA House of Delegates' stands against national health insurance, Medicare, Professional Standards Review Organizations (PSROs), and the like (Hyde & Wolff, 1954).

REFERENCES

Abrams, Herbert K., "Neighborhood Health Centers," *American Journal of Public Health,* 61:2236–2239, 1971.

Acton, Jan, "Demand for Health Care Among the Urban Poor with Special Emphasis on the Role of Time," Memorandum R-1151—DEO/NYC, Rand Corp., April, 1973.

Aday, Lu Ann, "Economic and Noneconomic Barriers to the Use of Needed Medical Services," *Medical Care,* 13:447–456, 1975.

Alpert, Joel J., Kosa, J., Haggerty, R. J., Robertson, L., and Heagarty, M. C., "The Types of Families that Use an Emergency Clinic," *Medical Care,* 7:55–61, 1969.

Alpert, Joel J., and Charney, F., *The Education of Physicians for Primary Care,* Washington, D.C.: USDHEW Publication No. (HRA) 74–3113, Autumn, 1973.

American Medical Association, *Profile of Medical Practice,* Chicago: American Medical Association, 1979.

Belloc, Nedra B., and Fox, Renee, "Role Strains of a Health Care Team in a Poverty Community," *Social Science and Medicine*, 6:697, 1972.

Beloff, Jerome S., "Adapting the Hospital Emergency Service Organization to Patient Needs," *Hospitals, Journal of American Hospital Association*, 42(April 16): 65–69, 1968.

Bodenheimer, Thomas S., "Patterns of American Ambulatory Care," *Inquiry*, 6(September): 26–37, 1970.

Bunker, John P., "Surgical Manpower—A Comparison of Operations in the U.S. and in England and Wales," *New England Journal of Medicine*, **282**:135–144, 1970.

Burns, Evelyn M., *Health Services for Tomorrow*, New York: Dunnellen, 1974.

Burrow, James G., *AMA: Voice of American Medicine*, Baltimore: Johns Hopkins University Press, 1963.

Coggeshall, Lowell T., *Planning for Medical Progress Through Education*, Washington, D.C.: Association of American Medical Colleges, 1965.

Colombotos, John, "Physicians, Attitudes Toward Medicare," *Medical Care*, 6:320–331, 1968.

Colombotos, John, "Physicians and Medicare: A Before-After Study of the Effects of Legislation on Attitudes," *American Sociological Review*, **34**:318–334, 1969.

Colombotos, John, "Physicians' Responses to Changes in Health Care: Some Projections," *Inquiry*, 8(March): 20–26, 1971.

Colombotos, John, Kirchner, Corinne, and Millman, Michael, "Physicians View National Health Insurance—a National Study," *Medical Care*, **13**:369–396, 1975.

Committee on the Costs of Medical Care, *Medical Care for the American People*, Chicago: University of Chicago Press (Reprinted, USDHEW, 1970), 1932.

Counts, George S., "The Social Status of Occupations: A Problem in Vocational Guidance," *The School Review*, **33**(January):16–27, 1925.

Durkheim, Emile, *The Division of Labor in Society* (1893; translator, George Simpson), New York: Free Press, 1933.

Dyckman, Zackary U., *A Study of Physician Fees*, Washington, D.C.: Council on Wage and Price Stability, 1978.

Elesh, David, and Schollaert, Paul T., "Race and Urban Medicine: Factors Affecting the Distribution of Physicians in Chicago," *Journal of Health & Social Behavior*, **13**: 236–250, 1972.

Fein, Rashi, *The Doctor Shortage*, Washington, D.C.: Brookings Institution, 1967.

Ford, Amasa B., *Urban Health in America*, London: Oxford University Press, 1976.

Freidson, Eliot, *Patients' Views of Medical Practice*, New York: Russell Sage Foundation, 1961.

Freidson, Eliot, *Profession of Medicine*, New York: Dodd, Mead, 1970.

Freidson, Eliot, *Professional Dominance: The Social Structure of Medical Care*, New York: Atherton, 1970a.

Freyman, Jr., *The American Health Care System: Its Genesis and Trajectory*, New York: Medcom Press, 1974.

Goodrich, Charles H., Olendzki, Margaret C., and Crocetti, Anna-Marie, "Hospital-based Comprehensive Care: Is It a Failure? *Medical Care*, **10**:363, 1972.

Hall, Oswald, "The Informal Organization of Medical Practice in an American City," unpublished Ph.D. dissertation, Chicago: University of Chicago, 1944.

Hall, Oswald, "The Informal Organization of The Medical Profession," *Canadian Journal of Economics and Political Science*, **12**:30–44, 1946.

Hall, Oswald, "The Stages of Medical Career," *American Journal of Sociology*, **53**:327–336, 1948.

Hall, Oswald, "Types of Medical Careers," *American Journal of Sociology,* **55**:243–253, 1949.

Hambleton, John W., "Main Currents in the Analysis of Physician Location," Working Paper No. 8, Madison: Health Economics Research Center, University of Wisconsin, 1971.

Haug, J. N., and Stevens, Rosemary, "Foreign Medical Graduates in the United States, in 1963," *Inquiry,* **10**(March): 1973, 1973.

Hodge, Robert W., Siegel, Paul M., and Rossi, Peter H., "Occupational Prestige in the United States, 1925–63," *American Journal of Sociology,* **70**:286–302, 1966.

Holahan, J., "Physician Availability, Medical Care Reimbursement, and Delivery of Physician Services: Some Evidence from the Medicaid Program," *Journal of Human Resources,* **10**(Fall):3, 1975.

Hughes, Edward F. X., Fuchs, Victor, Jacoby, John, and Lewit, Eugene, "Surgical Work Loads in a Community Practice, *Surgery,* **70**(March):315–327, 1972.

Hughes, Edward F. X., Lewit, Eugene, and Rand, Elizabeth, "Operative Work Loads in One Hospital's General Surgical Residency Program," *New England Journal of Medicine,* **289**:660–666, 1973.

Hughes, Edward F. X., Lewit, Eugene, and Lorenzo, Frederick, "Time Utilization of a Population of General Surgeons in Community Practice," Department of Community Medicine, Mt. Sinai School of Medicine, **77**(3):371, 1975.

Hyde, David R., and Wolff, Payson, "The American Medical Association: Power, Purpose, and Politics in Organized Medicine," *Yale Law Journal,* **63**:938–1022, 1954.

Jonas, Steven, "Some Thoughts on Primary Care: Problems in Implementation," *International Journal of Health Services,* **3**:177, 1973.

Jonas, Steven, Flesh, R., Brooks, R., and Wasserthal-Smollen, S., "Monitoring Utilization of Municipal Hospital Emergency Department," *Hospital Topics,* **54**:43, 1976.

Kendall, Patricia, "The Relationship Between Medical Educators and Medical Practitioners," *Journal of Medical Education,* **40**(1):137–245, 1965.

Kendall, Patricia L., "Medical Specialization: Trends and Contributing Factors," in Coombs, R. H., and Clark, V. E., Eds., *Psychosocial Aspects of Medical Training,* Springfield, Ill.: Thomas, 1971.

Kessel, Reuben A., "The A.M.A. and the Supply of Physicians," *Law and Contemporary Problems,* **35**(Spring):267–283, 1970.

Knowles, John H., "The Role of the Hospital: The Ambulatory Clinic," *Bulletin of the New York Academy of Medicine,* **41**(2nd Series):68, 1965.

Krizay, J., and Wilson, A., *The Patient as Consumer,* Lexington, Mass.: Heath, 1974.

Leveson, Irving, "Demand for Neighborhood Medical Care," *Inquiry,* **7**(December):17–24, 1970.

Leveson, Irving, *Influence of Outpatient Clinic Utilization in New York City,* New York: NYC Health Services Administration, mimeo, 1973.

Lewis, Charles E., Fein, Rashi, and Mechanic, David, *A Right to Health: The Problem of Access to Primary Medical Care,* New York: Wiley-Interscience, 1976.

Luft, Harold S., "How do Health Maintenance Organizations Achieve Their 'Savings'?" *New England Journal of Medicine,* **298**:1336–1343, 1978.

Marden, Parker G., "A Demographic and Ecological Analysis of the Distribution of Physicians in Metropolitan America," *American Journal of Sociology,* **72**:290–300, 1966.

McWhinney, I. R., "Family Medicine in Perspective," *New England Journal of Medicine,* **293**:175(letters in response, *NEJM,* **293**:781, 1975), 1975.

Mechanic, David, *Public Expectations and Health Care: Essays on the Changing Organization of Health Services,* New York: Wiley-Interscience, 1972.

Mechanic, David, *Politics, Medicine, and Social Science,* New York: Wiley-Interscience, 1974.

Mechanic, David, *The Growth of Bureaucratic Medicine: An Inquiry into the Dynamics of Patient Behavior and the Organization of Medical Care,* New York: Wiley-Interscience, 1976.

Merton, Robert K., "Patterns of Influence: Local and Cosmopolitan Influentials," in Merton, R. K., *Social Theory and Social Structure,* New York: Free Press, 1968.

Miller, Alfred E., *Distribution and Utilization of Health Services in New York City,* New York: NYC Comprehensive Health Planning Agency, mimeo, 1973.

Miller, Alfred E., "The Changing Structure of the Medical Profession in Urban and Suburban Settings," *Social Science and Medicine,* 11:233–243, 1977.

Miller, Alfred E., Miller, Maria G., and Adelman, Jonathan, "The Changing Urban-Suburban Distribution of Medical Practice in Large American Metropolitan Areas," *Medical Care,* 16:799, 1978.

Miller, Stephen, *Prescription for Leadership: Training for the Medical Elite,* Chicago: Aldine, 1970.

Millis, John S., *The Graduate Education of Physicians: The Report of the Citizens Commission,* Chicago: American Medical Association, 1966.

Millis, John S., *A Rational Policy for Medical Education and Its Financing,* New York: National Fund for Medical Education, 1971.

Mountin, J. W., Pennell, E. H., and Brockett, G., "Location and Movement of Physicians—Changes in Urban and Rural Totals," *Public Health Reports,* 60:173, 1945.

Mumford, Emily, *Interns: From Students to Physicians,* Cambridge: Harvard University Press, 1970.

New York Times, "The Problem of Incompetent Doctors," Series of five articles, January 26–30, 1976.

Parker, Alberta W., "The Dimensions of Primary Care: Blueprints for Change," in Andreopoulos, Spyros, Ed., *Primary Care: Where Medicine Fails,* New York: Wiley, 1974, pp. 15–80.

Pellegrino, Edmond D., "The Changing Matrix of Clinical Decision Making in the Hospital," in Georgopoulos, Basil, *Organizational Research on Health Institutions,* Ann Arbor: Institute for Social Research, 1972.

Perrott, George S., *The Federal Employees Health Benefits Program,* Washington: USDHEW, May, 1971.

Petersdorf, R. G., "Internal Medicine and Family Practice," *New England Journal of Medicine,* 293:326, 1975.

Petersdorf, R. G., "Issues in Primary Care: The Academic Perspective," *Journal of Medical Education,* 50(December, Part 2):5–13, 1975.

Piore, Nora, Lewis, Deborah, and Seeliger, J., *A Statistical Profile of Hospital Outpatient Services in the United States: Present Scope and Potential Role,* New York: Association for the Aid of Crippled Children, 1971.

Rayack, Elton, *Professional Power and American Medicine: The Economics of the American Medical Association,* Cleveland: World, 1967.

Rayack, Elton, "The American Medical Association and the Supply of Physicians: a Study of the Internal Contradictions in the Conception of Professionalism," *Medical Care,* 2:244–253, 1964.

Rees, Philip H., "Movement and Distribution of Physicians in Metropolitan Chicago," working paper No. 1.12, Chicago Regional Hospital Study, 1–20, June, 1967.

Reibstein, Regina, and Stevenson, Gelvin L., "A Study of Physicians Mobility in New York City—1960–1970," New York: New York City Department of Health, mimeo, 1974.

Reinhardt, Uwe E., "Proposed Changes in the Organization of Health Care Delivery: An Overview and Critique," *Milbank Memorial Fund Quarterly*, 51(Spring):169–222, 1973.

Reinhardt, Uwe E., *Physician Productivity and the Demand for Health Manpower*, Cambridge, Mass.: Ballinger, 1975.

Robertson, Leon S., "On the Intraurban Ecology of Primary Care Physicians," *Social Science and Medicine*, 4:227–238, 1970.

Roemer, Milton I., "On Paying the Doctor and the Implications of Different Methods," *Journal of Health and Human Behavior*, 3(Spring):4–14, 1962.

Roemer, Milton I., and Friedman, Jay W., *Doctors in Hospitals: Medical Staff Organizations and Hospital Performance*, Baltimore: John Hopkins University Press, 1971.

Satin, D. G., and Duhl, F. J., "Help?: The Hospital Emergency Unit as Community Physician," *Medical Care*, 10:248, 1972.

Sloan, Frank, "Lifetime Earnings and Physicians' Choice of Specialty," *Industrial and Labor Relations Review*, 24(October):47–56, 1970.

Stevens, Rosemary, *American Medicine and the Public Interest*, New Haven: Yale University Press, 1971.

Stevens, Rosemary, Goodman, L., Mick, S., and Darge, J., "Physician Migration Reexamined," *Science*, 190:439–442, 1975.

Strauss, Anselm L., "Medical Organization, Medical Care and Lower Income Groups," *Social Science and Medicine*, 3:143–177, 1969.

Strauss, Anselm L., *Where Medicine Fails—Medical Ghettos*, Chicago: Transaction Books-Aldine, 1967.

Strickland, Stephen P., *U.S. Health Care: What's Wrong and What's Right*, New York: Universe, 1972.

Strickland, Stephen P., *Politics, Science, & Dread Disease: A Short History of United States Medical Research Policy*, Cambridge: Harvard University Press, 1972a.

Stroman, Duane T., *The Quick Knife: Unnecessary Surgery, U.S.A.*, Port Washington, N.Y.: Kennikat Press, 1979.

Sun Valley Forum on National Health, "Medical Cure and Medical Care," *Milbank Memorial Fund Quarterly*, 50(4, Part 2):entire issue, 1972.

U.S. Bureau of Census, *Statistical Abstract of the United States*, Washington: U.S. Department of Commerce, 1978.

U.S. House of Representatives, Interstate and Foreign Commerce Committee, Subcommittee on Oversight and Investigations, "Getting Ready for National Health Insurance: Unnecessary Surgery," Hearings, July 15–18/September 3, Washington, D.C.: G.P.O., Serial 94–37, 183–190, 1975.

Whitaker, Leighton, "Social Reform and the Comprehensive Community Mental Health Center—The Model Cities Experience, Part II," *American Journal of Public Health*, 62:216, 1792.

White, Kerr L., "Organization and Delivery of Personal Health Services: Public Policy Issues," *Milbank Memorial Fund Quarterly*, 46:225, 1968.

White, Kerr L., "Life and Death and Medicine," *Scientific American*, September 1973, p. 23.

White, Kerr L., "Health and Health Care: Personal and Public Issues," Michael M. Davis Lecture, May 29, 1974, University of Chicago School of Business, Center for Health Administration, Chicago.

White, Kerr L., Greenberg, B. G., and Williams, T. F., "The Ecology of Medical Care," *New England Journal of Medicine,* **265**:885–892, 1961.

Williams, K. N., and Lockett, B. A., "Migration of Foreign Physicians to the United States: The Perspective of Health Manpower Planning," *International Journal of Health Services,* **4**:213, 1974.

Wilson, F. A., and Neuhauser, D., *Health Services in the United States,* Cambridge, Mass.: Ballinger, 1974.

Wolfe, S., and Badgley, R. F., "The Family Doctor," *The Milbank Memorial Fund Quarterly,* **50**(April, Part 2):1–20, 1972.

Yerby, Alonzo, "The Disadvantaged and Health Care," *Public Welfare,* **24**(January):73–77, 1966.

Zwick, D. I., "Some Accomplishments and Findings of Neighborhood Health Center," in Zola, I. K., and McKinlay, J. B., Eds., *Organizational Issues in the Delivery of Health Services,* New York: Prodist, 1974.

CHAPTER NINE

Illness Behavior and Public Attitudes Toward Sickness

The behavior of patients is influenced and organized very differently from that of other participants in the health sector. As a result it is much more diverse. Unlike being a physician or other provider of health care, being a patient is usually not a continuous or primary role and does not serve as a basis for a person's ongoing identity. Being sick is ordinarily considered an episode or interruption of normal life activities. It is viewed as an undesirable, temporary status to be put aside as quickly as possible to return to one's normal roles. The sick role is actively rejected as a part of a person's identity. Thus the patient is *ipso facto* in an unstable, vulnerable position. From nearly every aspect patients' relationships to their sick roles are fundamentally different from those of providers of health care.

Health care providers, like persons in most ongoing, identity-constituting roles, have attitudes and behavior patterns systematically fitted to their social institutions and to the organizations necessary to operate their specialized technology. They belong to a subculture embodying the norms, values, and ideology defining the proper attitudes and behavior for carrying out their roles. They interact with others in such a way that expectations, incentives, and sanctions consistently reinforce this behavior. This congruent constellation of influences leads to predictable responses in most situations and provides constant positive reaffirmation of professional identity so that self-doubt or alienation from one's role is seldom a problem. The forces influencing provider behavior are consistent and mutually reinforcing because they are integrated into the social institution of medicine built around a unified stable source, the central technology of the profession. Most social roles are similarly stable and internally consistent because they are reinforced by being well integrated into some social institution, such as the family. Persons conform to these roles because the norms and values of the institution are in accord with and protect the interests of the members. Even deviant roles are usually supported by membership in a corresponding subculture that provides a sense of identity and reinforcement by participation in a set of special activities, common argot, and counterideology. These justify the mode of life regardless of its differences from the accepted norms and institutions of society.

Patients, on the contrary, do not belong to a social institution providing uniform, stable, or consistent behavioral direction for them, as patients. They have no ongoing organization, no social structure of their own that can support patterns of behavior fitting their own interests and needs. They have no subculture (as patients) to supply the norms, values, and incentives for a consistent set of responses; no ideology to reaffirm their identity or support the appropriateness of their attitudes and actions. Patients are at the mercy of multiple, often conflicting outside forces converging on them from many sources and directions.

Unlike most temporary, nonidentity-constituting roles, such as "being a customer in a department store" or "being a rush-hour-traffic driver," "being sick" is neither elective, instrumental, nor trivial. It is not simply used as a means to obtain other ends, nor can it be treated with detached "role distance" as something not really affecting the core of one's identity. If the illness is serious—more than a slight inconvenience imposed on normal roles—being sick is *existential*. The anxiety, disability, and potential threat to continuation of normal, identity-constituting roles make sickness too important to be taken with distance and objectivity. It cannot be treated as something separate from the self, something merely being acted out for the moment.

With most temporary roles the expected behavior is clearly prescribed by the ongoing (guest) institution and simply played out by the person entering it on the temporary basis. Service organizations, for instance, determine the behavior of clients; clients conform in order to get what they want from the organization. When a person is sick, however, he is often unwilling to accept unquestioningly all the behavior expected of him by health care organizations; nor is his family, work group, or community ready to let him act independently in his illness behavior, as they would in his customer behavior. The potential effects of illness are too important and anxiety provoking to all concerned. Each social group, each organization, each culture has norms, attitudes, beliefs, and expectations toward illness of various sorts that are enforced through group sanctions. Since the norms and attitudes of various parties involved may arise from different belief systems or be focused on quite different objectives, conflicting pressures frequently come to bear on the patient.

First, the patient always faces at least an inner conflict about how seriously to take being ill. On the one hand, he feels bad and wants to use the prerogatives of the sick role to be relieved of his normal duties in order to rest and get better. On the other hand, he rejects the identity of being sick as something foreign and threatening to him. This conflict may be intensified or the equilibrium shifted in one direction or the other depending on: how serious he perceives the situation to be; how much he stands to lose by abdicating his normal roles; what norms of duty versus prudence he applies to himself and what norms he believes other persons who are significant in his life apply to him; and finally what secondary gains, such as sympathy and special privileges, he might obtain.

Second, the same dilemmas are mirrored in the expectations and pressures employed by family, friends, fellow workers, and community. Illness with its need for help and the concern about its possible seriousness evokes sympathy, permissiveness, and even urging of the patient to assume the sick role. At the same time, anxiety about the potential seriousness together with resentment because of the extra load imposed can lead to denial of the seriousness and pressure on the patient to continue in the normal role as long as possible. Because of potential ambivalence over how to react to someone who is sick, most groups have well-established norms about how to deal with various degrees of illness or particular symptoms. Nonetheless, application of these norms to a particular case may still be ambiguous, leaving the basic conflict open. In addition, various persons and groups that the patient interacts with may have quite different norms for the same case. Thus the patient may find himself confronted with different expectations from different sides.

Third, as soon as contact is made with the health care system, a new set of dilemmas arises. Physicians perceive illness in the framework of an objective disease model. They see the situation in terms of what they can and should do to treat the disease according to professional standards. The patient perceives the situation in terms of the potential meaning for his own life and his other responsibilities (Mechanic, 1978). A patient consulting a health professional, therefore, faces the quandary of whose perspective to accept. The medical interpretation of his situation is sanctioned by society as "rational." Yet, his own interpretation of the situation is more influenced by his subjective anxieties and concerns and takes into account many important personal factors not considered in the medical judgements and advice. If the patient comes from a tradition that holds a world view at variance with the scientific belief of the medical profession, the possibility of disagreement with health care providers will be magnified. Even those patients who share the scientific world view may adhere to certain folk medicine beliefs that may consciously or subconsciously buttress attitudes and behavior against the advice of the physician.

Fourth, even within our accepted tradition of medicine, there is a two-fold relationship of patients to physicians (Chapter 3) that can lead to conflicting demands, attitudes, and behavior. On the one hand, the physician possesses certain technical knowledge and skills, which the patient seeks as a client to facilitate regaining his health. On the other hand, the priestly tradition of medicine establishes the physician as an agent of society who directs the prescribed behavior in time of sickness, provides psychological and social support for the patient, and relieves him of some of the anxiety of being sick. In the priestly role the physician can remove the burden of decision from the patient, ameliorate anxiety by making him feel taken up in good hands, and providing other psychological support.

The patient frequently faces the dilemma of choosing between the two physician functions that tend to exclude each other (Chapter 6). On the one hand as a critical and rational consumer of technical services, he wants to relate to the physician by seeking and encouraging the most skilled and specialized technical competence, if necessary at the expense of "bedside manner." On the other hand, weakened by illness and burdened by anxiety, the patient wants solace for his anxiety, unshouldering of the difficult decisions presented by illness, and reassurance that necessary arrangements will be made. In exchange he is often ready to give the physician complete discretion and to abandon any pretext of being a critical consumer or equal participant in the decision making. Frequently the patient vacillates between these two poles of expectation and demands in his relation to a physician and the health care system.

Finally, the patient is at least partly removed from the customary roles that affirm his identity. At the same time he rejects the (temporary) role thrust upon him and sees even his own behavior as foreign. This self-alienation is enhanced by the subtle rejection of his state and his illness behavior by other members of his social group and by the conflict of influences shaping his attitudes and behavior. The alienation compounded by the discomfort, weakened state, and unforeseen problems of illness produces an anxiety typical of being caught by mysterious forces outside of one's control.

To a degree these problems have always been characteristic of illness. Being sick is inherently fraught with anxiety and rejection, both by patient and associates, so that alienation and conflicts occur. In most previous societies, however, the situation was assuaged because the institution of healing was itself more integrated into the social and moral order of the community. The behavior of patients and of the physician, even if mysterious and terrifying, was familiar and accepted. This situation made it possible to *share* in the process and to receive support for the otherwise deviant behavior patterns necessitated by the circumstances. As noted in Chapter 3, in primitive societies the ritual of treatment was closely integrated into the moral order by the priestly role of the physician. The healing art was strongly supportive of patient and family and often succeeded in converting the anxiety and potentially alienating deviance of illness into a positive force reaffirming the moral values of the society. This gave the patient a positive role in his community that often helped reconstitute social support for his position.

Even in modern societies before the scientific revolution in medicine, the roles of physician and patient were reasonably well integrated into the social structure of the community. For all its problems, being ill still allowed a person to continue as part of society. Sickness was accepted as a normal part of living. It took place within the supportive structure of the family. The physician came into the community to treat illness. Only in the most medically or socially difficult situation was the patient removed from these normal social props. The physician himself remained a central figure in community life, maintaining much of the old priestly relationship with the moral order of the community. Thus he could serve as a social expediter to secure the support needs for the patient and sanction the changed situation so that the rejection and alienation were minimized.

Since the scientific and technological revolution in medicine, the situation of the patient has changed radically. Despite the greater potential for being helped technically by health care, many of these changes have increased the degree of conflict and alienation entailed in the sick role: The increasingly technological orientation of medical practice has removed it from the community system and the family. Healing arts are practiced in the hospital or in the physician's office behind closed doors. The patient is more frequently removed from his familiar supportive settings. Illness is played out in strange terrifying surroundings just when the patient most needs reaffirmation of his identity. The more serious the illness, the more likely the patient is to be extracted from his natural setting and from public view and thus to be more vulnerable to the conflicting forces impinging on him. Dying takes place in the hospital, and increasingly the entire phenomenon of sickness tends to be excluded from the community and treated as something that is entirely the province of the health care system—allowing society to close its eyes to the fact. At the same time the complex, technological structure of health care isolates it as a closed system increasingly out of functional contact with the society it serves. Thus being a patient more and more means being segregated from normal society.

Formerly the physician, having little to offer technically to the treatment of patients, was obliged to maintain his position by aiding patients and families in overcoming anxiety and arranging supportive care. Today the physician's interest and time are absorbed in the technical aspects of care. As a result families are thrown onto their own resources and initiative in coping with the social problems of illness. Understandably they are more frequently ready to allow the health care system, wherever possible, to substitute the easily available technological resources of care for the difficult to obtain social support. Changed demography and social structure with increasing urbanization, mobility, loss of the extended family, smaller living quarters, and less time spent in family affairs—all decrease the ability and readiness to carry out the care of the sick in the family setting. The rising expectations in regard to health care generated by the success of scientific medicine provides a natural focus for the desire of families and communities to find some place to transfer the responsibility for "care" of the sick. On the other hand, the traditional health care system, increasingly focused on high-technology, episodic, *cure*-oriented treatment, is no more willing or able to cope with the *care* of the sick than are families. Either whole new organizations, such as nursing homes or hospices, have to be created to provide the "care" elements of health care, or else patients are simply left to struggle with the competing pressures as best they can.

Added to these problems is the increasing prevalence of chronic illness and disability, for which the health care system is poorly matched to care. The patient is left to flounder in the social and health care systems with decreasing accommodation for his situation and lack of necessary support services and continuity of care. As a result chronic illness accentuates the factors that increase the patient's alienation, loss of identity and rejection from his normal place in society. This development has important implications for health care organization and planning. We return to the subject in a special section later in the chapter after examining the general principles of patient behavior.

Given the multiplicity of dilemmas, ambiguities, and conflicting pressures converging on the patient's situation, it is hardly surprising that his behavior is often inconsistent and may seem enigmatic to providers of care. Patients are accused of behaving irrationally when in fact they are merely marching to a different drummer or trying to march to several at the same time. If the health care system is to provide more effective services to patients, these dilemmas and conflicts must be taken into account.

Health services and social medicine researchers have long been aware of certain conflicts and strains in the patient's role. The problems of health-seeking and illness behavior among the poor and minority groups have been investigated extensively because of their nonconformity with the expectations of health professionals in using health services, following advice, and so on. In the 1960s researchers became interested in the conflicts experienced by minority group patients because of the attitudes of middle-class health professionals and the difficulties in obtaining adequate care because of the bureaucratic organization of the system. This body of research and critical analysis has tended to leave the impression that these problems are limited to the poor or minority groups. Yet, the problems and contrasts highlighted for these special patients in fact only dramatize the pervasive difficulties facing nearly all persons in the patient role. Though less obvious for middle-class persons—and better dealt with by them because they are more able to manipulate the system to their advantage—there are deep-seated conflicts inherent in modern society for almost anyone who is seriously ill.

THE STAGES OF ILLNESS

During an episode of illness a patient passes through a number of stages with different psychological states and social interactions that shape his actions. In each stage a different set of factors influences his behavior, differ-

Table 9.1   Stages of Illness

Illness Behavior	
Presick-role behavior	
Symptom experience	Realization that "something is wrong"
Illness validation	Consultation with family or other laymen
Sick-role behavior	
Becoming a patient	Consultation with a health professional who takes over control of treatment
Hospitalization	Health care system takes over control of all patient activities
Rehabilitation	Medical rehabilitation and reentry into normal life
Chronic illness	Adaptation and social organization leading to an ongoing sick role
Preventive and health behavior	
	Habits and activities affecting the health status and/or conscious activities for preventing disease by use of preventive services or change of life style

SOURCE: Suchman, 1965a; Kasl and Cobb, 1966; Mechanic, 1978; Freidson, 1970; and Haggerty, Roghman, and Pless, 1975.

ent kinds of decisions are required, different social relationships are entered, and different roles are assumed.*

ILLNESS BEHAVIOR†

Illness behavior begins with the experience of symptoms and proceeds to seeking help if the symptoms seem significant. It may involve taking on the

* The definition of "stages of illness" originated in health-services studies based on the traditional division of the health care system into diagnostic, curative, rehabilitative, and preventive services. Health professionals involved in these various activity areas of practice are faced with quite different problems of organizing services and influencing patients. As research objectives have changed, many different classification schemes for the stages of illness have been proposed, leading to considerable confusion about which to use. The process or career of any illness is a continuum, and the stages described by different researchers are arbitrary. Different patients may pass through quite different sequences of decisions and different constellations of social relationships in various episodes of illness, while they use different types of health services. The classification shown in Table 9.1 is a useful system of reference for our analysis, but makes no claim to be definitive.

† Because of the difference in perspectives of health professionals and patients, the convention has been adopted by sociologists of referring to the process as "disease" when considered from the viewpoint of the physician (i.e., in terms of diagnosis, causal, and therapeutic categories), and as "illness" when considered from the viewpoint of the patient. The behavior of the patient in response to his disease is therefore termed "illness behavior" (Mechanic, 1968).

"sick role," consulting a health professional, receiving care from the health system, and ordinarily ends with the return to normal activities when the illness passes. If the disease is not reversible or leaves a residual dysfunction, the sick role may become a chronic adaptation to the new circumstances of life. Many potentially conflicting factors influence the patient's behavior during this process, creating confusion, anxiety, and inappropriate use of health services. The conflicts arise not only among the *influences* from different sources, but also between the various *mechanisms* that shape all human behavior generally. There are at least three sets of influences operating through different mechanisms that must be considered in examining patient behavior:

1. The conscious or psychological determinants of behavior involve factors that affect how a patient *perceives* and *evaluates* his illness. In deciding what to do he must balance the perceived *risks* and the possible *benefits* of various options for action against the direct and indirect *costs*— economic, personal, and social (Rosenstock, 1966).

2. All social and cultural groups have certain *norms* about the "proper" behavior in various illness situations. These constitute so-called "sick roles," or social customs, that are applied more or less automatically when persons find themselves with certain kinds or degrees of illness. Social group and cultural norms also provide basic attitudes toward the system of care and therefore shape the nature of interaction with it.

3. Interacting with other persons and organizations such as their families, physicians, clinics or hospitals, patients encounter various *expectations* and are urged to behave in certain ways. If these expectations are not met, various *sanctions* are usually available to bring added pressure for compliance.

These same three sets of behavioral mechanisms are also involved in shaping the actions of health care providers (and other persons). However, the multiplicity of control is usually not so apparent because the different sets of influences are ordinarily congruent as a result of their integration around the central technology and organization of medicine. Thus, the various behavioral influences reinforce each other to produce a consistent overall pattern. For example, physicians *perceive* a decision situation in terms of the technological means at their disposal to remedy it. They are *motivated* to this action by the values espoused as health professionals, as well as by the prestige and financial gains entailed in carrying out this treatment and by their vested interests in the uses of such technology. The *norms* of professional behavior that they learned as medical students and that have been reinforced over the years as physicians prescribe appropriate action in almost any conceivable patient-care situation. These norms are congruent with the technological basis of determining what action to take. Those norms obviate the need to go through the processes of rational decision making in terms of the appropriate motivations and objectives in each case. The *organizational* situation of medical practice where interaction with patients and other health professionals takes place also provides consistent reaffirmation of the appropriateness of their behavior because it meets the expectations and approval of the others.

This is *not* the case for patient behavior. The influences acting through the different mechanisms of control are often in conflict with each other. Patient behavior lacks the unified framework found for physicians, and is therefore ambivalent, less predictable, less controllable and tends to produce dissatisfaction in contacts with the health care system. We must examine these mechanisms and conflicts in more detail during the various stages of illness.

The first step in the process of becoming a patient is becoming aware that "something is wrong"—perceiving a symptom. Symptoms serve as cues in reaching the decision that help is needed and therefore play a central role in influencing patient behavior. Severe symptoms, especially pain, fever, bleeding, or shortness of breath, can be sufficient in themselves to instigate seeking care (Suchman, 1965a). In diseases of slow onset, however, there may simply be an abnormal sign, such as weakness, some change in bodily function, weight loss, unusual bleeding, persistent cough, a new skin growth, or even a physician's finding or an abnormal laboratory report from a routine screening procedure. Perception of such a condition *as* a symptom involves more than just being aware of it; it entails *evaluation* of the situation leading to the realization that "something may be wrong with me." Recognizing some condition as *abnormal* depends on individual and social standards as to what is "normal." Acknowledging an abnormal condition as a symptom depends on the patient's knowledge or fear (expectations) of *potential consequences* (Apple, 1960).

In this seemingly straightforward, rational perceiving and interpreting of symptoms, the patient is already operating under conflicting influences converging to shape his behavior. On the one hand, his discomfort, disability, and fear govern his reaction to symptoms. But on the other hand, social class and cultural norms dictate what is abnormal or tolerable as discomfort or disability, and what the "proper" response is (Lorber, 1967). The meaning of a situation depends on the perceiver's expectations regarding it. Many of the expectations are socially determined by the norms of the cultural group and by interpersonal interactive processes. The meaning (and therefore perception) of a symptom is a function of at least:

1. The visibility, severity, and rapidity of onset of the symptoms and the immediate functional impairment
2. How tolerable they are as measured against the individual, social class, and cultural norms
3. The understanding, knowledge, and fear of the potential significance of the symptoms for his life

4. The significance of the dysfunction in reference to the individual's social milieu

5. The potential personal, social, and economic cost or possible benefits of being sick and seeking care (Mechanic, 1978; Suchman, 1965)

6. The emotional response of fear or anxiety that the discomfort and its interpretation evoke

These aspects are interlinked in the perception of and response to any symptom. For instance, emotional anxiety or rational fears of the significance can markedly intensify (or mask) pain, as Beecher (1959) has shown by the varying amount of morphine (or even of a placebo) required to relieve pain from comparable injury under different circumstances.

Becoming aware of a symptom is only one step on the way to becoming ill and taking on the patient role. Some symptoms may be tolerated for years without doing anything—even when a person "knows something should be done about it." Before making a decision to seek care, a patient has to weigh the potential risk of the illness and the potential benefit of treatment against the possible cost to himself—economic, personal, and social. This evaluation is heavily influenced by the patient's knowledge and beliefs about the nature of the disease potentially involved and about the efficacy of medical care (Becker, 1974; Baumann, 1961).

In a classic study Koos (1954) demonstrated the wide social-class variations in the assessment of situations requiring medical attention (cf. Kuntz et al., 1975). Lower-class patients tend to ignore all but the most serious and incapacitating symptoms. Less severe symptoms are not looked upon as indicative of "real illness" with potential implications and are tolerated because of the economic costs of having them tended to. Upper-class patients are more apt to have some scientific knowledge of the causes and symptoms of serious disease and are willing to accept certain immediate costs in the hope of preventing more serious future difficulties (Zborowski, 1952; Zola, 1966). On the other hand, there is growing evidence against the once prevalent belief that lower-class persons are less likely to seek medical attention early in an illness because they are "less concerned about health matters" (McKinlay & Dutton, 1974). Such delay is often a case of other competing priorities of existence being more urgent for lower-class patients.

The down-ranking of symptoms in relation to other needs may be accentuated if they threaten to disrupt social routines, particularly job routines. Persons involved in heavy physical work are more apt to disregard certain bodily pains such as backaches as a natural consequence of life, and therefore to be less inclined to seek help. There is a greater inclination for the poor and blue-collar classes to resort first to self-medication and to think of the body and its ailments in simple mechanistic terms. Symptoms are seen as something to be "flushed out, unblocked, or cleansed as the need arises" (Freidson, 1970). Rosenblatt and Suchman have suggested that, for the poor:

The body can be seen as simply another class of objects to be worn out but not repaired. It is as though the white collar class think of the body as a machine to be preserved and kept in perfect functioning condition, whether through pros- thetic devices, rehabilitation, cosmetic surgery, or perpetual treatment, whereas blue collar groups think of the body as having a limited span of utility; to be enjoyed in youth and then to suffer with and to endure stoically with age and decrepitude. (Quoted in McKinlay, 1975)

Similarly, the poor tend to consider repeated episodes of illness as the same and therefore not requiring new medical consultation. Often an old prescription is simply reused. Women who have been through one preg- nancy delay prenatal care in subsequent ones until very late in the gesta- tion period (McKinlay, 1975).

Another set of factors influencing the interpretation of symptoms and the decision to seek care involve some aspect of "stress." Stress may heighten the sensitivity to symptoms or produce an increased awareness of symptoms that might otherwise be ignored, increasing the likelihood that action will be taken (McKinlay & Dutton, 1974). When the normal "well" role is un- satisfactory or stressful, the individual may retreat into the "sick" role as a means of avoiding that stress or a sense of failure in fulfilling socially de- fined roles (Twaddle, 1969; Cole & LeJeune, 1972). A large portion of pa- tients presenting physical complaints may be disguising a need for help pri marily for psychological problems or stress (Kasl & Cobb, 1964, 1966; Stoekle et al., 1963). "Interpersonal crisis," and "social interference," can act as trig- gers for patients' decisions to seek medical care (Zola, 1964). Lower-class groups, especially, tend to express psychological distress in physiological terms (Crandell and Dohrenwend, 1967). On the other hand, for upper- income persons the importance of the work role, even under very stressful conditions, may be a deterrent to seeking help (Robinson, 1971).

Between the initial perception of symptoms and the entry into profes- sional medical care there may be a series of steps that Freidson (1970) has named the "lay referral system." Public opinion in nearly all social groups today accepts the efficacy of modern medical technology for dealing with serious illnesses. The prestige and well publicized successes of modern medi- cine have convinced most people of its value—whether or not they understand the details of how it works or precisely what is involved in most treatment or prevention. Members of the middle class have in general been educated to turn immediately to the medical profession as the appropriate source for help. They accept the professional theory of disease as part of their own rationalistic approach to the world.

Other segments of our society, especially members of the lower class and of certain ethnic groups, are not so ready to accept the attitudes and tech- niques of the medical profession. Although they use the standard medical system as a last resort in serious illness, such patients are less likely to turn to it immediately for help in a time of illness. Moreover, they are less likely to know how to make appropriate use of the health care system and negotiate the numerous barriers that lie in the way of those from the lower class who attempt to obtain care. Instead of consulting a physician immediately in the case of illness, the person usually turns first to the immediate family or circle of friends. This entails getting verification that one is "really ill"—therefore legitimizing the sick role—and obtaining suggestions about what should be done. In many cases this family consultation will eventuate in using folk remedies, patent medicines, or simply going to bed to wait it out.

Healing traditions from earlier periods of a society are often carried in ethnic cultures, families, and communities as "folk medicine." In most cases folk medicine has become simply a set of rules of thumb for dealing with illnesses short of resorting to the professional health care system. In some cases it constitutes a conflicting set of influences, creating dilemmas for the patient who may also want standard medical advice. The further the values and attitudes of a culture are from those of the Western scientific tradition, the greater the role of such folk medical remedies tends to be. In some ethnic groups the beliefs and practices become a true parallel system of medicine, as with the Botanicas and spiritualists among Puerto Ricans. Even in the most Westernized middle-class group, some elements of folk medicine provide norms for dealing with minor health problems and can create conflicting forces influencing the behavior of patients.

In certain cultures and social groups there will be a whole hierarchy of persons occupying roles that perpetuate and employ the traditional knowledge of the culture concerning health and sickness. The further removed the patient's culture and social class are from those of the medical profession and the more cohesive the social structure of his own group, the more likely he is to follow the full route of traditional lay referral instead of immediately consulting a physician (Kadushin, 1964; Suchman, 1964; cf. Geertsen et al., 1976). Thus cultural distance and social cohesion have the effect of decreasing the utilization of medical services and of lengthening the delay in seeking care for potentially serious diseases such as cancer or tuberculosis (Goldsen, 1963).

In general, middle-class patients come from a less extended and less tightly knit family system and feel more secure in making the "self-diagnosis" that an illness is serious, or at least in reaching the decision to seek professional help. Therefore, lay consultation for such patients is apt to be only a cursory confirmation from spouse or friend, followed by an immediate visit to the physician if symptoms persist or are considered at all serious. Middle-class lay consultants are usually more knowledgeable about the health care system and attuned to the professional approach to disease. They will usually urge the patient to seek professional help at an early stage. In any culture strongly accepting the beliefs and attitudes of the medical profession, a cohesive extended family may actually bring pressure to speed consultation with a physician—the opposite effect of a cohesive family in a culture that does not share the beliefs of the medical profession. Anxi-

lationship is often indirectly expressed as a nostalgic sense of loss of the traditional family practitioner and criticism of overspecialization or the overly technological perspective of modern physicians (Chapters 6 and 8). Historically, physicians played a very important role in relieving the anxiety of illness by exerting social control over patient and family through their priestly moral-directive function in society (Chapter 3). This socially sanctioned authority, together with the ritual and magic employed, lent a sacred element to the treatment. This also provided reaffirmation of the patient's identity and sense of belonging, which were frequently damaged by the episode of illness.

Patients continue to need the alleviation of their anxiety and the special psychological and social support once provided by this priestly function (Hollender, 1958). Cultural tradition leads them to expect it from their physicians. The changes in the demographic and social structure of American society have even intensified the inclination to use physicians for personal counseling and general psychological and social support—many times almost as a kind of general-purpose ombudsman. In today's secular society the medical profession remains for many people the only "priesthood" to whom they can still turn for personal guidance and a sense of being taken up under the wing of societally sanctioned, moral authority to set them at peace with their problems. Difficulties that would formerly have been dealt with by (extended) family members or the parish priest are now taken to the physician. Such personal counseling and social support are not easily obtained elsewhere in our highly fragmented and depersonalized modern urban society (Parsons, 1952, 1963).

On the other hand, these personal counseling functions tend to be at odds with the specialized technical role of the physician, which is equally desired by the patient (Hulka et al., 1976; Dunnell & Cartwright, 1972). This leads to ambivalence on the part of patients and in public policy toward the medical profession. The desire for more personalized care and greater availability of primary care has led to demands for the training of more family physicians and decrease in specialization. At the same time there is concern about the cost of overutilization and so-called inappropriate utilization of physician services, such as simply for reassurance or for social problems. Many policy makers argue for insurance co-payments to discourage unnecessary visits and for the use of physician extenders (nurse practitioners and physician assistants) to provide care that does not really require highly technical medical skills.

On the other hand, there is also growing concern about the quality of care, which is usually an indirect way of saying technological competence. Many advocate legislation to require continuing education of physicians, periodic relicensing, peer review of medical records, and requirements of board certification in a specialty to obtain hospital admitting privileges. These pressures tend to push physicians away from the personal-concern role and toward greater preoccupation with the technological function.

Thus there is a fundamental ambivalence in public expectation toward the medical profession that tends to create contradictory policies, increase the cost of care, and lead inevitably to dissatisfaction because of the incongruent demands made on the system. Careful examination of the organization of care in reference to the various objectives is necessary for developing realistic priorities (Chapters 8 and 10).

NEGOTIATING THE HEALTH SERVICES SYSTEM

Loss of family physicians and fragmentation of medical practice have increasingly forced the poor to obtain medical care in organized settings and have increased their difficulty in finding appropriate care at all (Chapter 8). In lower-class communities the lack of availability and poor organization of health care, which usually takes place in impersonal, crowded, uncomfortable clinics (Strauss, 1967), adds greatly to the reluctance to use these services. These organizational settings for health care (especially hospitals and outpatient departments) also create additional factors that influence patient behavior. Such organizational arrangements were originally an outgrowth of provider attitudes and expectations about appropriate patient care. Yet, the bureaucratic procedures have come to have an organizational life of their own, to some extent no longer under the control of either the providers or the patients whom they serve. The specialty clinic organization of outpatient departments fragments and depersonalizes care and forces both patient and professional behavior into the technological mold. This problem of inflexibility at organization-client interfaces is not unique to the health care system. It occurs wherever many clients with little power are served by an organization whose members are more dependent on the organization and each other than on clients. The clients, whose interests are ostensibly the goal of the organization, come to be treated as means to the organization's own internal objectives (Blau & Scott, 1962). As a result the organizational procedures have a powerful influence in shaping the behavior of clients, while clients have little influence over the organization.

The impact of the organization of professional services and the patient's background on his ability to utilize those services has been intensively studied in regard to the poor and certain ethnic subcultures. Three factors have been particularly stressed: (1) The importance of life style, values, norms, and knowledge about health, illness, and the use of the health care system; (2) inflexible professional behavior and unrealistic expectations among health service workers; (3) inflexible bureaucratic structure of clinics and institutions. These factors lead to impersonal care, complexity in negotiating the system to obtain care, and failure of the system to adapt to its clientele or institute practices making it easier to overcome these barriers. Cultural differences between lower-class patients and middle-class physicians lead to lack of understanding on both sides, with consequent failure of communication, hostility, and ineffective treatment (Malone et al., 1962). Suspicion or reticence in regard to the health care system is exacerbated by the fact that patients' and their acquaintances' experiences with medical care professionals and institutions have often been less than satisfactory.

McKinlay (1975) notes that much of the earlier literature on the inability of the poor to get adequate health services in institutional settings alluded to personal and class characteristics that somehow placed the blame on them, such as "neglectful," "irresponsible," "parochial," "distrustful," "ignorant," "culturally deprived." This may have represented an unfair cultural bias on the part of social scientists studying the problem and the fact that the bureaucratic structure of institutional health services is very middle-class oriented. It puts lower-class patients at a decided disadvantage. The basic assumptions of health services (e.g., rationality, future orientation) are consonant with the values and life styles of the middle class. The poor often have a world view and values quite foreign to these assumptions. Because health professionals are generally from the middle class, there is much less status-sensitivity during encounters with middle-class patients, and professional personnel are better able to understand their problems.

Middle-class socialization and education provide skills in manipulating the mechanics of bureaucracy and the ability to verbalize feelings, attitudes, and "need." The poor lack the expertise to negotiate bureaucratic settings, and tend to seek the more personal care of kin and friends, corner druggists, and semiprofessionals. While shielding the poor from the frustration of impersonalized clinics, this tactic also deprives them of care they may need (McKinlay, 1975). The poor tend to be in a constant state of crisis and therefore socially and economically unable to tolerate the methodical, sophisticated clinic structure. Because their situation allows them less opportunity to plan ahead, they are more likely to resort to emergency services and are unlikely to utilize preventive services. Preferential utilization of emergency services by the poor is even found in Great Britain, where the cost of services is not a problem (McKinlay, 1975).

The "social distance" between middle-class health personnel and lower-class patients leads to attitudes and practices that discriminate against the poor. Even today they are treated as charity cases when, for the most part, their fees are paid through such government programs as Medicare and Medicaid. Many studies have documented the condescending attitudes and punitive behavior directed toward lower-class patients treated in outpatient departments and emergency rooms (Straus, 1969). Physicians tend to consider them as "undesirable" and assume that they will follow poor health practices, fail to observe directions and keep appointments, and live in a situation that makes it impossible to establish appropriate health regimens (Roth et al., 1967). These assumptions all too frequently become "self-fulfilling prophecies."

In the outpatient departments and emergency rooms of public (government supported) hospitals, the staff is usually overworked and harassed.

They develop a hardened, negative image of patients from experience with the many alcoholics, fight victims, derelicts, and other social outcasts whom they are called upon to treat. There is resentment if nonemergency or non-urgent cases appear for treatment at off-hours in emergency rooms. This is spoken of as "abusing" the emergency room, and a welfare case is likely to be denigrated for "taking up the valuable time of doctors and nurses any time they damn please" (Roth, 1975, p. 290). Under these circumstances a patient may be given short shrift, superficial diagnosis, and careless treatment. Public-hospital staffs tend to treat all patients as "welfare cases" unless there is strong evidence to the contrary, subjecting them to punitive treatment, arbitrary and peremptory orders, and to questioning about their personal affairs that would be considered impertinent by middle-class patients (Roth, 1975; Strauss, 1967). In private hospitals patients are even more likely to be subjected to questioning about their personal affairs in the attempt to obtain financial information that might lead to their referral to a private physician or that might provide evidence that the patient has some insurance or Medicaid coverage to pay for his care. If no coverage is available, the patient may well be sent to a public hospital for treatment, unless the situation is an extreme emergency.

A major problem in large hospital outpatient clinics is the structure of the clinic, organized to provide episodic treatment for specific ailments. The schedule often makes it difficult for a patient to obtain complete care at one visit to the clinic. Experiments with comprehensive care programs, and particularly with those located in neighborhood health centers, have demonstrated that it is possible to overcome many of the shortcomings of public clinics in providing care for low-income populations. Unfortunately, at present, financial resources are not available to provide them universally for the poor in urban centers, let alone in rural areas, since they are both expensive and difficult to staff with medical personnel.

THE MEANING OF HOSPITALIZATION

There is a generally favorable attitude toward hospitals in this country, which influences patient acceptance of hospitalization and willing compliance with most hospital-imposed behavior. Most patients who are admitted to hospitals get well. The expert knowledge and sophisticated equipment of the modern hospital have given it awe-inspiring prestige in society. In times of illness patients may, in fact, feel relieved by the protection from outside tensions and interference, the cheerful environment containing familiar artifacts for their comfort (TVs, books, etc.), and the concern displayed by hospital staff for their emotional as well as physical condition. At the same time, if hospitalization is necessary in the course of an illness, a quantum increase in dependency of the sick person and in the loss of normal personal identity occurs. Being hospitalized, even for a short time, is a profound psychological experience. As King describes it:

To the uninitiated the world of the hospital is a strange, an exciting, and yet a forbidding place, full of sights, sounds, and smells that are not comparable to everyday experiences outside. Even for the patient who has been in a hospital before, there is a distinct break with familiar things as he steps or is carried through the door. Here is the world of sickness in which the patient must become immersed; here are different values, unusual routines; here is a host of strangers who will take liberties with the body that would be unthinkable elsewhere. Here is where emergency rules action, where pain is commonplace, where behavior ranges from heroism to disintegration, where some of the great dramas of life are acted out. (King, 1962, p. 349)

Besides the pain, fear, and disruption of being removed from one's family, friends, job, and other normal activities, adjusting to the strange practices, unfamiliar routines, and threatening situations of a hospital can have severe effects on patients. In the world from which he has just come, the patient was a master in his own home, respected at his job, recognized in his community. Ties with this outside world are cut, and many symbols of his normal identity are removed. On arriving in the hospital, the patient's clothes are taken away for the convenience and standardization of certain procedures. He is given a strange kind of gown to wear, which offers little cover for most of his body, and told to get into bed, even though it is the middle of the day and he may feel quite well. Gone is much of the privacy and propriety with which he is accustomed to shield himself against the intrusion of strangers into his intimate affairs.

The ability of the short-term hospital patient to adapt to this strange new environment is limited by the hospital social structure. Although an ongoing, complex social system exists in all hospital wards, short-term patients are not part of it. This system exists solely for the hospital personnel; patients are at best mere passive observers of ward social life. Formation of an effective patient community, which could offset this exclusion, is hindered in short-term institutions by rapid patient turnover, the isolation of patients into single or semiprivate rooms, and the tendency of the sick toward egocentricism and emotional dependency upon the hospital staff.

Consequently, the burden of adapting to hospital life falls largely on the patient's own psychological methods for coping with stress. In a study at a general hospital Coe (1970) noted four ways that patients adjust to hospitalization: withdrawal, aggression, integration (most common in long-term care institutions), or acquiescence (the usual adaptation in short-term hospitals). Patients' attitudes toward physicians and the hospital could be classified as either "instrumental" or "primary." Patients with instrumental orientations saw the physician's task as only to treat illness and considered the hospital simply as the appropriate place for that treatment. This group complied with hospital routines and regulations only in order to get well sooner and return to their normal roles. Patients with primary orientations viewed the doctor as a person to make them happy and the hospital as a place where needs could be gratified and protection obtained. They submitted to hospital rules procedures out of an enjoyment of being cared for and protected within the hospital environment. These attitude types found by Coe correspond to the division between the technical and priestly role of the physician that we have noted in numerous other contexts. Not surprisingly, the latter group tended to develop a more dependent role in the hospital situation, which led to longer stays and greater difficulty in resuming the normal role after discharge.

Hospital staff attitudes often exacerbate this situation rather than countering it. Variation in the ease of handling patients prompts staff to label patients "good" or "bad" according to their manageability. The more aggressive, independent, and inquisitive patients are seen as "bad" since their cooperation is less easily won, while the dependent, compliant, unquestioning patients are identified as "good" and encouraged. Yet this patient-staff interaction may potentiate and prolong dependency, slowing the patient's return to full health and social responsibility. Staff responses can also worsen the situation with aggressive patients by alienating them, leading to breakdown in the communication necessary for effective treatment.

In short-term hospitalization for acute illnesses these problems seldom have serious consequences. For the chronically ill patient, however, with long-term or repeated hospital stays, staff-patient interaction and other institutional influences on patient behavior can become crucial factors in the overall outcome of care. This has to be examined in the broader context of patient behavior in chronic illness.

CHRONIC ILLNESS AND DISABILITY

The conflicts, societal rejection, and self-alienation found even in acute, curable diseases take on new importance in chronic illnesses—where being sick becomes a permanent state. The temporary sick-role norms call for certain behavior on the part of the patient, such as the "motivation to get well," that makes little sense for the permanently disabled whose conditions can be alleviated but not eradicated. The role of the practitioner, whose exclusive knowledge places him in firm control of the therapeutic situation in acute illnesses, also changes in chronic cases. With long-term disabilities and continuing treatment programs, patient awareness and involvement become decisive for the success of therapeutic and rehabilitative regimens.

The special norms for sick persons and their relationships to others play an important role in organizing the function of the family as well as patients during episodes of illness. The norms governing these relationships for acute illnesses are untenable in the chronic situation because they require concessions that are only possible for short-term emergency conditions. Adjustment of illness norms to the long-term situation are a source of strain within the family as a result of the competing needs of the patient and of the family. It may not be possible or necessary for the chronically ill patient

to be excused from his normal societal roles. There can also be conflict between family interests and recommendations emanating from the medical
profession. The chronic sick role cannot be all-pervading, since it is permanent (Kassebaum & Baumann, 1965). The patient's regular pattern of treatment and adjustment to disability must become part of his "normal" way of
life and must not entail the degree of isolation from the "well" population
that characterizes acute, curable, short-term illnesses. If isolation does occur,
the consequences are much more serious in terms of alienation and the degeneration of other relationships.

The societal and personal response to acute illness is very different from
that to chronic illness and permanent disability. Acute illness is looked upon
as something *happening to* a person, an unfortunate but temporary outside
interference with the normal course of things, but not a change in his basic
identity. The self-reinforcing mechanisms, such as "labeling," that contribute to identity transformation in professional socialization (see Chapter 6),
deviance, or chronic illness are usually not brought into play in acute illness, even if the illness is serious.*

Any chronic illness, however, except the most minor and invisible (without disability or unusual demands placed on other persons), sets in motion
mechanisms that do change self-image and social identity. Incorporating the
chronic sick role into one's identity entails many of the same mechanisms of
adult socialization discussed in Chapter 6. One major difference, however,
is that the professional socialization takes place largely within the subculture into which the person is moving—labeling being only a strong rein-
forcer of identification with this reference group. Socialization into the role
of chronic illness usually does *not* take place within a new reference group
or subculture of peers. It occurs instead within a continuing problematic
interaction with family, friends, and other members of society who reinforce the new identity by acting as role complements to the chronically ill
patient. Persons who play these role counterparts undergo complementary
role socialization that is equally a part of the development of the chronic
illness role. In fact, variations in the ways that persons in the counterpart
roles react and develop in relation to the patient may have even more effect
on the final functional outcome than variations in the patient himself. The
family relationships may be the most feasible place to intervene in order to
influence the patient's adaptation to his illness.

"Labeling" or "stigmatization" of the patient is a critical step in the social process of forming the chronic illness role (Gove, 1975). It calls into
play the secondary behavioral influences that produce the social and psychological similarities in the final state of most chronic illnesses. There are

---

* If the patient is in some way held responsible for the onset of the illness, as with venereal
diseases or accidents occurring out of carelessness, a limited form of "stigma" or labeling
may occur (Freidson, 1970). Such moral blame may indeed influence the way that the
patient is treated by health professionals or the patient's family, but it does not in itself
lead to a new, identity-modifying role.

several features of chronic illnesses that can produce stigmatizing societal reactions to patients. The labeling evokes adverse expectations about the patient just as with stereotypical deviant roles. These expectations create a new reality imposed on the patient, which makes it nearly impossible for him to escape from the new role. Thus the label becomes a "self-fulfilling prophecy" (Merton, 1967), inexorably forcing the patient into the role expected by society and gradually converting his self-image into conformity with the expectations (Cooley, 1902; Mead, 1933). This changed self-image is accompanied by the need for self-justifications of the deviant (sick) behavior and a tendency to withdraw from association with normal members of society. These mechanisms intensify the deviant aspects of the chronic illness behavior already present and intensify the social perception of the individual as deviant. Thus labeling sets into motion a complex of positive-feedback mechanisms that increase behavioral divergence from the normal, increase psychological identification with the new way of life, and force adoption of corresponding social relationships.

First, the most common features of chronic disease are disabilities and dependencies that restrict the normal or desired activities of the individual and place burdens on others. Heart disease or crippling accidents can reduce the ability to earn a living or to do one's share of the work involved in life activities. Diabetes can necessitate a different life style, special diets, and so on. Many chronic disorders create the need for assistance in carrying out certain life activities, for special services, or an inordinate share of family resources to pay for treatment. Any such disability can make heavy demands on family members, friends, fellow workers, or others with whom the patient regularly associates. This burden is felt both by the patient and by the others who have to share the inconvenience. The patient is aware of his dependency and of the continuing special privileges that his disability requires. He is grateful for the privileges and help but resentful of the dependency—no matter how lovingly or willingly the privileges and assistance are given. The chronic patient can hardly avoid some feeling of guilt as a result of imposing a seemingly unfair relationship on those persons who mean most to him. At the same time, he resents the situation in which he constantly has to feel guilt and indebtedness. It is a rare case where this resentment does not spill over against the persons to whom he is indebted.

On the other side, family members, friends, and associates intimately involved in the life of a disabled person are bound to have times when they feel the burden is somehow an unfair limitation on their own lives (Graham, 1963). Doubts arise as to how necessary the burdens really are, and resentment comes to be focused on the dependent person rather than on the disease situation. Since they know that it is not the patient's fault, this resentment easily turns into guilt. Family members chastise themselves for having emotions like resentment against someone they love and who places burdens on them through no fault of his own. One natural consequence is to compensate by overprotecting the patient—making him feel even more de-

ment of the health system has reduced its traditional role in the management of patient and family behavior in the face of illness. Health care has been removed from the community so that it is less able to influence the availability of social support and provide justification of the sick role through its moral-directive, priestly function. This mismatch leaves serious unmet needs of a social and psychological nature in addition to the technical needs already noted (Chapter 5).

In families with chronically ill members some mechanism is necessary to to defuse the resentment and guilt that adds social disability and rejection to the physical disability already present. Patients are often prematurely dumped into the long-term care system at a high loss to themselves and their families and a growing economic cost to society. It would be advantageous to reintegrate sickness and its care into society (and into family life). A health care system able to accomplish this would have to provide a much broader continuum of technical and support services structured to fit the needs of patients and family rather than the interests of providers. Thus, for reintegrating patients into society, the health system itself would have to be reintegrated into the community! As rational and straightforward as this sounds, the barriers to accomplishing it are formidable. In Chapter 10 we examine some of the strategies that are being attempted to make the health system more responsive to the needs of patients and society.

REFERENCES

Aiken, Linda H., "Chronic Illness and Responsive Ambulatory Care," in Mechanic David, *The Growth Bureaucratic Medicine,* New York: Wiley-Interscience, 1976.

Antonovsky, Aaron, "Social Class and Illness: A Reconsideration," *Sociological Inquiry,* 37:311–322, 1967.

Apple, Dorian, "How Laymen Define Illness," *Journal of Health and Human Behavior,* 1:219–225, 1960.

Baumann, Barbara, "Diversities in Conceptions of Health and Physical Fitness," *Journal of Health and Human Behavior,* 1:39–46, 1961.

Becker, Marshall H., Ed., *The Health Belief Model and Personal Behavior,* Thorofare, N.J.: Slack, 1974.

Beecher, Henry K., *Measurement of Subjective Response: Quantitative Effects of Drugs,* New York: Oxford University Press, 1959.

Blackwell, Barber, *The Literature of Delay in Seeking Medical Care for Chronic Illnesses,* Society of Public Health Educators, Inc., Health Education Monographs No. 16, 1963.

Blau, Peter, and Scott, W. Richard, *Formal Organizations,* San Francisco: Chandler, 1962.

Bullough, Bonnie, "Poverty, Ethnic Identity and Preventive Health Care," *Journal of Health and Social Behavior,* 13:347–359, 1972.

Callahan, Eileen M., et al., "The 'Sick Role' in Chronic Illness: Some Reactions," *Journal of Chronic Disease,* 19:883–897, 1966.

Chen, Edith, and Cobb, Sidney, "Family Structure in Relation to Health and Disease," *Journal of Chronic Disease,* 12:544–567, 1960.

Cobb, Beatrix, et al., "Patient-Responsible Delay of Treatment in Cancer," *Cancer,* **7:** 920–926, 1954.

Coe, Rodney M., *Sociology of Medicine,* New York: McGraw-Hill, 1970.

Cole, S., and LeJeune, R., "Illness and the Legitimation of Failure," *American Sociological Review,* **37:**347–356, 1972.

Comfort, Alex J., *The Process of Ageing,* New York: Signet, 1964.

Conover, Patrick W., "Social Class and Chronic Illness," *International Journal of Health Services,* **3**(3):357–368, 1973.

Cooley, Charles H., *Human Nature and the Social Order,* New York: reprinted Schocken, 1964, 1902.

Crandell, D. C., and Dohrenwand, B. P., "Some Relations Among Psychiatric Symptoms, Organic Illness and Social Class," *American Journal of Psychiatry,* **123:**1527–1538, 1967.

Dunnell, Karen, and Cartwright, Ann, *Medicine Takers, Prescribers and Hoarders,* London: Routledge & Kegan Paul, 1972.

Dyk, R., and Sutherland, A., "Adaptation of the Spouse and Other Family Members to the Colostomy Patient," *Cancer,* **9:**123–138, 1956.

Feinstein, A., "Symptoms as an Index of Biological Behaviour and Prognosis in Human Cancer," *Nature,* **109:**241, 1966.

Frank, J., "Mind-Body Interactions in Illness and Healing," presented at the May Lectures, "Alternative Futures for Medicine," April 4, 1975, Airlie House, Airlie, Va.

Freidson, Eliot, *Profession of Medicine,* New York: Dodd, Mead, 1970.

Freidson, Eliot, *Professional Dominance: The Social Structure of Medical Care,* New York: Atherton Press, 1970a.

Geertsen, Reed, Klauber, Melville, R., Rindflesh, Mark, Kane, Robert L., and Gray, Robert, "A Re-Examination of Suchman's Views on Social Factors in Health Care Utilization," *Journal of Health and Social Behavior,* **16:**226–237, 1975.

Goffman, Erving, *Stigma: Notes on the Management of Spoiled Identity,* Englewood Cliffs, N.J.: Prentice-Hall, 1963.

Goldsen, R., "Patient Delay in Seeking Cancer Diagnosis: Behavioral Aspects," *Journal of Chronic Disease,* **16:**427–436, 1963.

Gove, Walter R., Ed., *The Labelling of Deviance: Evaluating a Perspective,* New York: Halsted, 1975.

Graham, Saxon, "Social Factors in Relation to Chronic Illness," in Freeman, H., Levine, S., Reeder, L., Eds., *Handbook of Medical Sociology,* Englewood Cliffs, N.J.: Prentice-Hall, 1963, pp. 65–98.

Haggerty, Robert J., Roghmann, Klaus J., and Pless, Ivan, *Child Health and the Community,* New York: Wiley-Interscience, 1975.

Hollender, Marc H., *The Psychology of Medical Practice,* Philadelphia: Saunders, 1958.

Hulka, Barbara S., Cassel, John C., Kupper, Lawrence L., and Burdette, James A., "Communication, Compliance, and Concordance between Physicians and Patients with Prescribed Medications," *American Journal of Public Health,* **66:**847–853, 1976.

Kadushin, Charles, "Social Class and the Experience of Ill Health," *Sociological Inquiry,* **34:**67–80, 1964.

Kasl, Stanislav V., and Cobb, Sidney, "Some Psychological Factors Associated with Illness Behavior and Selected Illnesses," *Journal of Chronic Diseases,* **17:**325–345, 1964.

Kasl, Stanislav V., "Physical and Mental Health Effects of Involuntary Relocation and Institutionalization on the Elderly—A Review," *American Journal of Public Health,* **62:**377–284, 1972.

Kasl, Stanislav, and Cobb, Sidney, "Health Behavior, Illness Behavior and Sick-Role Behavior," *Archives of Environmental Health,* 12:246–266, 531–541, 1966.

Kassebaum, Gene G., and Baumann, Barbara O., "Dimensions of the Sick Role in Chronic Illness," *Journal of Health and Human Behavior,* 6:16–27, 1965.

King, Stanley H., *Perceptions of Illness and Medical Practice,* New York: Russell Sage Foundation, 1962.

Koos, Earl, *The Health of Regionsville: What the People Thought and Did about It,* New York: Columbia University Press, 1954.

Krizay, J., and Wilson, A., *The Patient as Consumer,* Lexington, Mass.: Heath, 1974.

Kunitz, S., et al., "Changing Health Care Opinions in Regionville, 1946–1973," *Medical Care,* 13:549, 1975.

Kutner, Bernard, and Gordon, G., "Seeking Care for Cancer," *Journal of Health and Human Behavior,* 2:171–178, 1961.

Leventhal, Howard, "Fear Communications in the Acceptance of Preventive Health Practices," *Bulletin of the New York Academy of Medicine,* 41:1144–1167, 1965.

Lipman, Aaron, and Sterne, Richard S., "Aging in the United States: Ascription of a Terminal Sick Role," *Sociology and Social Research,* 53:194–203, 1969.

Lorber, Judith, "Deviance as Performance: The Case of Illness," *Social Problems,* 302–310, 1967.

Ludwig, Arnold M., and Farrelly, Frank, "The Code of Chronicity," *Archives of General Psychiatry,* 15(December):562–568, 1966.

Malone, Mary, Berkowitz, Norman H., and Klein, Malcolm W., "Interpersonal Conflict in the Outpatient Department," *American Journal of Nursing,* 62(3):108–112, 1962.

Maxman, Jerrold S., *The Post-Physician Era,* New York: Wiley-Interscience, 1976.

McKinlay, John B., "Some Approaches and Problems in the Study of the Uses of Services: An Overview," *Journal of Health and Social Behavior,* 13:152–155, 1972.

McKinlay, John B., "The Help-Seeking Behavior of the Poor," in Kosa, John and Zola Irving, *Poverty and Health: A Sociological Analysis,* 2nd Ed., Cambridge: Harvard University Press, 1975.

McKinlay, John B., and Dutton, Diana B., "Social-Psychological Factors Affecting Health Service Utilization," in Mushkin, Selma J., Ed., *Consumer Incentives for Health Care,* New York: Prodist, 1974.

Mead, George H., *Mind, Self and Society,* Chicago: University of Chicago Press, 1934.

Mechanic, David, *Public Expectations and Health Care: Essays on the Changing Organization of Health Services,* New York: Wiley-Interscience, 1972.

Mechanic, David, *Politics, Medicine, and Social Science,* New York: Wiley-Interscience, 1974.

Mechanic, David, *The Growth of Bureaucratic Medicine: an Inquiry into the Dynamics of Patient Behavior and the Organization of Medical Care,* New York: Wiley-Interscience, 1976.

Mechanic, David, *Medical Sociology,* 2nd ed., New York: Free Press, 1978.

Merton, Robert K., *Social Theory and Social Structure,* New York: Free Press, 1968.

Moreland Act Commission, *Regulating Nursing Home Care: The Paper Tigers,* Albany, N.Y., October 1975.

Mushkin, Selma J., *Consumer Incentives for Health Care,* New York: Milbank Memorial Fund by Prodist, 1974.

New, Peter K., Ruscio, A. T., Priest, R. P., Petritsi, D., and George, L. A., "The Support Structure of Heart and Stroke Patients: A Study of Significant Others in Patient Rehabilitation," *Social Science and Medicine,* 2:185–200, 1968.

Parsons, Talcott, *The Social System*, New York: Free Press, 1951.

Parsons, Talcott, and Fox, Renee, "Illness Therapy and the Modern Urban American Family," *Journal of Social Issues*, 8(4):2–3, 31–44, 1952.

Parsons, Talcott, "Definitions of Health and Illness in the Light of American Values and Social Structure," in Jaco, E., Ed., *Patients, Physicians, and Illness*, New York: Free Press, 1958.

Parsons, Talcott, "Social Change and Medical Organization in the United States: A Sociological Perspective," *The Annals of the American Academy of Political and Social Science*, 346:21–33, 1963.

Petroni, Frank A., "The Influence of Age, Sex, and Chronicity in Perceived Legitimacy of the Sick Role," *Sociology and Social Research*, 53:180–193, 1969.

Picken, Bruce, and Ireland, George, "Family Patterns of Medical Care Utilization," *Journal of Chronic Diseases*, 22:181–191, 1969.

Reeder, Leo G., "The Patient-Client as a Consumer: Some Observations on the Changing Professional-Client Relationship," *Journal of Health and Social Behavior*, 13:406–412, 1972.

Reif, Laura Jean, "Cardiacs and Normals: The Social Construction of a Disability," Ph.D. dissertation, University of California, San Francisco, 1975.

Rivkin, Marion, "Contextual Effects of Families on Female Response to Illness," unpublished dissertation, Johns Hopkins University, Baltimore, 1972.

Robertson, Leon S., "Factors Associated with Safety Belt Use in 1974 Starter-Interlock Equipped Cars," *Journal of Health and Social Behavior*, 16:173–177, 1975.

Robinson, D., *The Process of Becoming Ill*, London: Routledge & Kegan Paul, 1971.

Rosenblatt, D. A., and Suchman, E. A., "Blue-Collar Attitudes and Information toward Health and Illness," in Shostak, A. B., and Gomberg, W., *Blue Collar World*, Englewood Cliffs, N.J.: Prentice-Hall, 1964.

Rosengren, William R., and Lefton, Mark, *Hospitals and Patients*, New York: Atherton, 1969.

Rosenstock, Irwin M., "What Research in Motivation Suggests for Public Health," *American Journal of Public Health*, 50:295–302, 1960.

Rosenstock, Irwin M., "Why People Use Health Services," *Milbank Memorial Fund Quarterly*, 44(July, Part 2):94–127, 1966.

Rosenstock, Irwin M., "Prevention of Illness and Maintenance of Health," in Kosa, John and Zola Irving, *Poverty and Health: a Sociological Analysis*, 2nd ed., Cambridge: Harvard University Press, 1975.

Rosett, Richard, and Lien-fu, Huang, "The Effect of Health Insurance on the Demand for Medical Care," *Journal of Political Economy*, 81:281, 1973.

Roth, Julius A., "The Treatment of the Sick," in Kosa, John and Zola Irving, *Poverty and Health, a Sociological Analysis*, 2nd ed., Cambridge: Harvard University Press, 1975.

Roth, Julius A., et al., "Who will Treat the Poor?" paper presented at the meeting of the American Sociological Association, 1967.

Rubel, Arthur J., "Concepts of Disease in Mexican-American Culture," *American Anthropologist*, 62:795–814, 1960.

Scheff, Thomas J., *Being Mentally Ill: A Sociological Theory*, Chicago: Aldine, 1966.

Schweitzer, Stuart O., "Consumer Behavior in Preventive Health Services," in Mushkin, Selma, *Consumer Incentives for Health Care*, New York: Prodist, 1974.

Shanas, Ethel, Townsend, P., Wedderburn, D., Friis, H., Milhoj, P., and Stehouwer, J., *Old People in Three Industrial Societies*, New York: Atherton, 1968.

Shulman, D., and Galanter, R., "Reorganizing the Nursing Home Industry: A Proposal," *Health and Society*, **54**:129, 1976.

Simon, John L., and Smith, D. B., "Change in Location of a Student Health Service: A Quasi-Experimental Evaluation of the Effects of Distance on Utilization," *Medical Care*, **11**:59–71, 1973.

Slesinger, Doris P., "The Utilization of Preventive Medical Services by Urban Black Mothers," in David Mechanic, *The Growth of Bureaucratic Medicine*, New York: Wiley-Interscience, 1976.

Solon, J. A., "Medical Care: Its Social and Organizational Aspects: Nursing Homes and Medical Care," *New England Journal of Medicine*, **269**:1067, 1973.

Stoeckle, John D., Davidson, Z., Irving, K., and Davidson, G., "On Going to See the Doctor, the Contributions of the Patient to the Decision to Sick Medical Care," *Journal of Chronic Diseases*, **16**:975–989, 1963.

Stotsky, Bernard A., *The Nursing Home and the Aged Psychiatric Patient*, New York: Appleton, 1970.

Strauss, Anselm L., *Where Medicine Fails—Medical Ghettos*, Chicago: Transaction Books-Aldine Publishing Company, 1967.

Strauss, Anselm L., "Medical Organization, Medical Care and Lower Income Groups," *Social Science and Medicine*, **3**:143–177, 1969.

Strickland, Stephen P., *U.S. Health Care: What's Wrong and What's Right*, New York: Universe, 1972.

Suchman, Edward A., "Sociomedical Variations among Ethnic Groups," *American Journal of Sociology*, **70**:319–331, 1964.

Suchman, Edward A., "Social Patterns of Illness and Medical Care," *Journal of Health and Human Behavior*, **6**:2–16, 1965.

Suchman, Edward A., "Stages of Illness and Medical Care," *Journal of Health and Human Behavior*, **6**:114–128, 1965a.

Susser, Merwyn, "Ethical Components in the Definition of Health," *International Journal of Health Services*, **4**:539, 1974.

Szasz, Thomas S., *The Myth of Mental Illness*, New York: Hoeker-Harper, 1961.

Szasz, Thomas, *The Manufacturer of Madness*, New York: Harper & Row, 1970.

Tagliacozze, Daisy M., and Kenji, Ima, "Knowledge of Illness as a Predictor of Patient Behavior," *Journal of Chronic Diseases*, **22**:765–775, 1969.

Thomas, Edwin J., "Problems of Disability From the Perspective of Role Therapy," *Journal of Health and Human Behavior*, **7**:2–14, 1966.

Twaddle, Andrew C., "Health Decisions and Sick Role Variations: An Exploration," *Journal of Health and Social Behavior*, **10**:105–115, 1969.

U.S. Comptroller General, *Study of Health Facilities Construction Cost*, Washington, D.C.: U.S. General Accounting Office, 1972.

USPHS, *Surgeon General's Report on Smoking*, Washington, D.C.: USDHEW, 1979.

U.S. Senate Special Committee on Aging, Subcommittee on Long-Term Care, *Nursing Home Care in the United States: Failure in Public Policy*, Washington, D.C.: November, 1974.

White, Kerr L., "Health and Health Care: Personal and Public Issues," Michael M. Davis Lecture, May 29, 1974, University of Chicago School of Business, Center for Health Administration, Chicago, 1974.

White, R., *Right to Health: The Evolution of an Idea*, Ames: University of Iowa Press, 1971.

Yerby, Alonzo, "The Disadvantaged and Health Care," *Public Welfare*, 24(January):73–77, 1966.

Zborowski, Mark, "Cultural Components in Responses to Pain," *Journal of Social Issues*, 8:16–30, 1952.

Zola, Irving, "Illness Behavior of the Working Class," in Arthur Shostak and William Gomberg, Eds., *In Blue-Collar World: Studies of the American Worker*, Englewood Cliffs, N.J.: Prentice-Hall, 1964.

Zola, Irving K., "Culture and Symptoms—An Analysis of Patients' Presenting Complaints," *American Sociological Review*, 31:615–630, 1966.

CHAPTER TEN

Strategies for Reform of Health Care Delivery

The high cost of medical care and the failure of the health system to meet the expectations of the public have gradually forced policy makers to turn their attention to many of the problems that we have been considering. While little consideration has yet been given to the fundamental nature of the mismatch between the health system and the needs for care, there is increasing recognition of the effect of: (1) the perverse incentives created by the reimbursement system; (2) the maldistribution and inappropriate nature of manpower, facilities, and services; (3) the way in which availability of facilities, technology, and services generates unnecessary utilization. In recent years these seemingly esoteric, economic, and organizational insights about the health system have become fairly common subjects of discussion in Congressional committees and state legislatures as well as in the Department of Health, Education, and Welfare (DHEW) and state health departments. Wrestling with these difficulties at all levels of health policy formulation has led to a series of legislative and organizational initiatives over the years attempting to deal with some of the more pressing problems. A complete history of such health policy initiatives is beyond the scope of this book. We examine a few representative strategies that are being tried and attempt to appraise their potential impact and effectiveness.

Most strategies for "reforming" the health care delivery system can be grouped into four general types. First, *planning and development* strategies approach the health system as a public service that must ensure that the necessary services are available to the entire population—but not in wasteful excess. Many of the long-standing, special-category, Federal health programs follow this general model. For example, the Maternal and Child Health Program provides subsidies to states to provide low-income mothers with prenatal and child care. This is done by formula grants that match funding to regional need. The Hill-Burton Program, providing subsidies for hospital construction in underserved areas, requires state plans to determine areas of need. Comprehensive Health Planning Agencies and their successor Health Systems Agencies carried this planning and development strategy to the logical conclusion. They are charged with examining the adequacy of the entire range of health services in an area and developing a master plan to meet the needs identified.

Second, *regulatory* strategies view health services as a public utility where the consumers' interests must be protected by oversight and rules. Classical uses of this approach in the health care field have focused on quality regulation, such as licensure of professionals and accreditation of facilities or the certification of drugs and devices for marketing by the Food and Drug Administration (FDA). Newer regulatory initiatives also emphasize quantitative restrictions, such as certification of need for new facilities and utilization review of services. Regulatory strategies now being discussed are potentially much more sweeping, for example, assessment of new (and existing) health technologies, not only for efficacy but also for cost effectiveness, before certifying them for reimbursement or approval by planning agencies.

Third, strategies for *reorganizing* parts of the delivery system to improve efficiency and responsiveness to patient needs have been inaugurated—not only by government programs but also as initiatives from private groups. Prepaid group practices originated with health provider and consumer groups as a market strategy to compete with prevailing fee-for-service care by overcoming the fragmentation and improving the accessibility of services. Their effectiveness has triggered government programs to subsidize their faster development because of the cost savings from their more efficient use of hospital care. Concern in the 1960s with the unsatisfactory record of hospital outpatient departments as ambulatory care facilities instigated the program for neighborhood health centers to improve the organization of services and make them more responsive to their communities.

Fourth, health care *financing* and *insurance* strategies, such as Medicare and Medicaid or the Crippled Children's Program provide subsidies to enable individuals to buy into the system of care as it exists. For this reason such financing programs traditionally have not been considered methods of system reform. However, growing awareness of the impact that financing and reimbursement policies have on organization and professional decisions is leading many to consider modification of financing mechanisms as an important strategy for system reform. National health insurance, and the new reimbursement methods it will entail, is today viewed by many as the ultimate and potentially most potent lever for health system reform—a "national health *plan*" rather than just national health insurance. In the present chapter we examine a few representative initiatives for health system reform in the narrower sense. In Chapter 14 we look at some of the current proposals for national health insurance and their potential for reform of the health system.

In nearly all health care policy areas involving the Federal government there has been a subtle but significant evolution in recent years from a position of subsidy or development to one of attempting to restrain the unbridled escalation of costs. Most policy initiatives began in the 1960s or earlier as attempts to improve existing services or supply new resources to areas of scarcity. However, skyrocketing costs have prodded policy makers to the realization that overabundant facilities and services can precipitate unnecessary utilization. This insight has led to a gradual shift toward planning and regulation for better allocation of presently available resources— and even to explicit strategies for limiting unneeded facilities and services.

The Hill-Burton program began as a mechanism to subsidize more hospital beds in underserved (primarily rural) areas. It eventuated in planning councils whose goal was to *limit* construction of additional hospital beds by requiring certification of need before such construction. Comprehensive Health Planning was first envisaged as a means of providing optimal health care services to communities. It has gradually evolved into a system of agencies whose primary mission is to hold down costs by scrutinizing the need for each new program or service proposed for the area. Federal health technology policy following World War II was to subsidize the rapid development of new modalities of care through research grants and underwriting of development costs. In the 1980s we are moving toward more cautious development and dissemination of new technologies until their benefits are clearly demonstrated. Health manpower policy in the 1960s established new professional schools and subsidized existing ones to enlarge their class sizes in order to make more health professionals (especially physicians) available. In the 1980s we are cutting back on educational subsidies, placing restrictions on grants to require better geographic and specialty distribution of graduates, and moving toward limiting the availability of residency training in overabundant specialties.

In the 1960s Federal ambulatory care policy was to support the development of neighborhood health centers as a means of bringing additional services to underserved areas. Prepaid group practice, initially developed in the private sector, was also first intended primarily to improve the quality and availability of care. Today Federal policy encourages health maintenance organization (HMOs), including prepaid group practices, primarily as a means of controlling utilization of hospital services and reducing costs. Medicare and Medicaid began as attempts to bring the aged and the poor into the mainstream of American medicine by simply paying their health insurance costs out of public monies. As costs have climbed, amendments to the Act have mandated utilization review and other forms of cost containment. National health insurance was originally seen primarily as a means of making high quality health care available to the entire population regardless of one's ability to pay. Today national health insurance is increasingly seen as a means of getting control of the health system in order to put a lid on runaway costs. Thus in general "system reform," once viewed as a means of improving services, is now increasingly meant to improve efficiency and manipulate incentive structure in order to reduce costs.

REGIONAL HEALTH PLANNING

Many health system problems are the result of resource allocation controlled by professional interests or the momentum of technology and organizations rather than rational planning or other methods of matching services to needs. Maldistribution of resources, gaps and duplications in services, difficulty in access to care, unnecessary utilization and costs due to excess capacity, all mirror the lack of coordination between the multiple decision centers in our pluralistic health system. Given the absence of effective market forces to make resource allocation responsive to consumer needs, providers have distributed themselves in accord with their own interests and have effectively avoided external coordination efforts.

Despite the large share of funding from Federal sources, which has evolved in the last few decades, little fiscal leverage has been exerted for more rational distribution and organization of services because the channels through which it is funneled into the system are equally uncoordinated. The lion's share today comes from the Medicare and Medicaid programs, which simply use the traditional, uncontrolled, third-party reimbursement channels. Much of the remainder flows through special-category program grants (such as maternal and child health or community mental health), which feed multiple blocks of money (controlled by different programs) into the same area with little coordination. The irrational distribution of services and the uncontrolled subsidy and growth of the health care system have increasingly come to the public awareness as costs have grown. Today policy makers have come to realize that the deficiency of coordination and planning is itself a major problem.

Awareness of the distributional and coordination problems goes back at least to the Committee on the Cost of Medical Care (1932). Many pieces of Federal and state health legislation have addressed the problem over the years with little lasting success. In 1946 Congress passed the Hill-Burton (Hospital Survey and Construction) Act to provide matching funds for constructing hospital beds in underserved (primarily rural) areas. The law stipulated that state health facilities plans be developed to determine the areas of need as a requisite for funding (Stebbins & Williams, 1972). This proposal was modeled after the New York State regional hospital planning council program, begun in 1939. Later amendments to the Act provided funding for remodeling, replacement, and improvement of hospital facilities—and much later for neighborhood health centers and emergency rooms. Having funded the construction of over 400,000 new beds and over 1000 outpatient facilities, the law was later taken up into the Health Planning and Resources Development Act but has gradually been phased out through declining appropriations.

In the early 1960s it had already become apparent in some areas that overabundance of hospital beds was more of a problem than scarcity. In 1964

New York State passed the first certificate of need (CoN) legislation, making use of its regional hospital planning councils (Hill-Burton agencies) to review the need for beds and reconstruction before granting permits. In 1968 the American Hospital Association, alarmed by the rising cost of hospital insurance, began a national drive to encourage enactment of CoN laws. The 1973 Health Planning and Resources Development Amendments made CoN laws mandatory for all states, and by 1979, some kind of CoN legislation existed in 39 states. Primarily a regulatory strategy aimed at hospital bed/ population ratios, CoN has provided very limited leverage for planning, with little impact even on total capital investment (Salkever and Bice, 1978). Control of the regional hospital councils by interests representing major medical centers has usually resulted in preserving the existing uneven concentrations of facilities.

The "Great Society" legislative initiatives of the mid-1960s produced two additional programs with parallel and sometimes conflicting health planning mandates. The President's Commission on Hearth Disease, Cancer, and Stroke, chaired by Dr. Michael DeBakey, recommended a network of Regional Medical Programs (RMPs). These organizations based in major academic medical institutions were to assist in making the latest scientific advances available to the medical profession at the grass-roots level. The Commission's report stressed the need for application of the research knowledge developed by medical schools as a result of the large-scale Federal health research funding in the 1950s and early 1960s. The regional centers would plan, oversee, and subsidize the dissemination of this knowledge. As a compromise to avoid confrontation with the AMA, the planning mandate of the original Administration proposal was restricted by stipulating that RMPs should seek "to preserve existing delivery facilities and arrangements" (Glaser, ca. 1972). They provided technical assistance and could award developmental grants to local health care institutions (Russell, 1966). Controlled by health care providers and heavily oriented toward academic, high-technology medicine, the RMP advisory groups concentrated on such installations as cardiac intensive care units and renal disease hemodialysis and transplant centers. They gave little emphasis to ambulatory, rehabilitative, or supportive care—even though the law was amended in 1970 to include these areas specifically in their mandate (Komaroff, 1969). In end effect, RMPs acted primarily as channels for funding and technical assistance to hasten dissemination of high-technology care and did little to improve overall planning of the health system (Bodenheimer, 1969).

As another outgrowth of the DeBakey Commission recommendations, Congress passed the Comprehensive Health Planning Act (CHP) later in the same session. The local and state CHP agencies created by the Act were given, at least as an abstract goal, a sweeping mandate to bring order into the chaos of the pluralistic health system. They were charged to "promote the highest level of health attainable for every person . . ." (by developing a regional master plan and reviewing all new proposals and existing programs for conformity) "but without interfering with existing patterns of private professional practice of medicine" (PL 89-749). Again, concessions had been necessary to prevent a head-on clash with the AMA and the AHA. Thus, from the beginning sentence of their authorizing legislation, CHPs were caught in the dilemma of being charged to rationalize a system without basically changing it. This inconsistent mandate only mirrored the political morass of conflicting pressures within which they had to function (Brown, 1972; Bruhn, 1973).

The "partnership for health" concept, the major innovation of CHP, grew out of the consumer and poverty group orientation of the Eighty-ninth Congress. The same concept characterized the Office of Economic Opportunity (OEO) strategies of the same period: "maximum feasible participation" of the affected community groups (Moynihan, 1969). Dissatisfaction with the responsiveness of hospitals to community needs, the Neighborhood Health Center movement with community dominated boards, and the OEO community-action principle of social advancement through participation in the power structure, all set the stage for the clause in the CHP Act requiring the local and state planning boards to have a majority of consumers. Unfortunately, the ensuing power struggles to determine who would speak for "the consumers" in each community absorbed the efforts of CHP agencies for many years and almost doomed them to impotence (Jonas, 1971; Levine, 1969). Nonetheless, the principle of consumer authority in health planning has survived in the new more viable generation of planning agencies. This was probably more important in the long run than the greater efficiency under the old pattern of provider domination (Gottlieb, 1974).

From 1966 to 1974 health planning also frequently devolved into internecine fights *between* the various planning agencies in an area—CHP, RMP, Hill-Burton agency, and later in some areas Experimental Health Services Planning and Development Systems (EHSPDS, later EHSDS) or public benefit corporations operating areawide health services like the New York City Health and Hospitals Corporation (Levin, 1972; Herman, 1972). All these agencies claimed the mandate to plan health services and facilities for the region (Lewis, 1969; Kaufman, 1969). The futility of this multiplicity of competing agencies gradually became obvious to the Administration and the Congress. The National Health Planning and Resources Development Act of 1973 superseded all of them with a new generation of planning agencies, called Health Systems Agencies (HSAs), State Health Planning and Development Agencies (SHPDAs), and State Health Coordinating Councils (SHCCs), closely resembling the old CHPs. Besides establishing the principle of consumer participation, the CHPs had served as training grounds for a cadre of health planners and for the development of techniques, data bases, and community experience in health planning politics. The new agencies seem to have profited from the CHP experiences and are off and running more quickly than the old ones (Ardell, 1973, 1974).

CHP "reviews and comments" on health proposals by influential provider groups were seldom more than pious recommendations. The new HSAs were given stronger "review and approval" authority over all Federal grant monies coming into their areas. The new agencies were also granted a major say in certification-of-need for all major capital investments under the state laws mandated by the Act (Cohen, 1973; Bicknell and Walsh, 1975). This was a logical extension of the more limited authority to approve capital projects first given to the CHPs under the 1972 Social Security Amendments. The new Act also provides for the development of National Health Planning guidelines by HEW. This responsibility moves the Federal government more centrally into the business of setting standards for appropriate levels of service throughout the country (Ingraham, 1972).

Proponents of comprehensive health planning have believed that inappropriate resource allocation and unresponsiveness to consumer needs were consequences of the decentralized nature of decision making, lack of communciation between consumers and providers, and absence of coordination between the various providers. Planning advocates assumed that if all the parties were brought together, a consensus could be reached about the "true" health care needs of the community. Priorities for meeting them could be agreed to, and the responsibility for achieving them could be assigned. This strategy attacks a *symptom*, lack of coordination, as if it were the primary cause of difficulty but fails to do anything about the deeper structure of the problem. The historical development of the health professions, hospitals, and other organizations has produced self-perpetuating social structures with vested interests in their technology and the social organizations built around it. These interests nurture goals and objectives that are no longer separable from the technological, organizational, and profes sional means for achieving them. Simply bringing provider groups together with consumers does not in itself overcome the problems that arise out of the pluralism of the present planning process. It may convert the implicit conflict between vested interests into an openly political struggle over competing goals and objectives, easily leading to deadlocks that divert attention and preserve the status quo. On occasion, an open political conflict can be an important step toward resolution. However, in the politics of health planning there is no executive branch (as in governmental politics) for implementing decisions. The parties at interest in the disputes also hold the power of implementation, making it unlikely that effective change will come about if it is contrary to their interests or objectives (Binstock, 1969).

As cost escalation has become an overriding issue in health policy matters in recent years, still another complication has been added to the planning process. Planning agencies (HSAs) have been assigned the role of holding down costs by certifying that facility expansion is really needed. Yet both consumers and providers often believe they have an interest in expanding services in their area (at the expense of other areas or at the cost of higher taxes spread over a much wider area). This can lead to a tenuous alliance between consumers and providers against government attempts to hold down costs. Thus, ironically, planning agencies often become platforms for providers to muster consumer support against government regulatory agencies in their struggle to gain approval of expansion plans. The National Health Planning Guidelines will help correct this situation by forcing agencies to make choices between alternative proposals—and not just serve as advocates for more and better programs and facilities. Regional capital budget limits of the kind proposed in Title II of the Hospital Cost Containment legislation of 1977 (Chapter 13) would provide an even more effective framework to make planning work. Even with regional capital budgets, however, there would still be no control over operating budgets, which constitute the bulk of health care expenditures and provide the major leverage over services and structure of the system. Given the present diffuse insurance reimbursement route for financing, there is no way that planning agencies can influence operating budgets. This severely limits any major potential for them to effect either cost containment or system reform.

HEALTH MAINTENANCE ORGANIZATIONS

Our analysis of the health care delivery system's mismatch with today's health care needs has disclosed problems of access to care, negotiability and continuity of service, responsiveness to patient needs, utilization patterns, and costs—all products of the way the delivery system is organized. In Chapter 8 it is argued that the primary organizational problem is the fragmented nature of the delivery system. This both results from and helps perpetuate a professional system that is much more responsive to technological prestige than to patient needs—or efficiency and cost consciousness. Because of the system of payment and the professional control of utilization, there is no financial counterpressure on physicians to organize services in a way that is more responsive to the needs of patients or more efficient in the use of costly resources.

Prepaid group practice (PGP) is an alternative form of organization for health care delivery and financing that allows more rational planning, integration, and efficient utilization of medical resources. The concept is not new; the first such group was organized in Elk City, Oklahoma in 1929 by Dr. Michael Shadid. This was the model studied by the Committee on the Costs of Medical Care leading to the recommendation in 1932 that such a scheme of organization be the basis for future development of the health care system (Chapter 11).

The first large-scale model was Group Health Association (GHA), established in 1937 as a co-op primarily for government employees in Washington, D.C. In 1942 the Kaiser Industries health system, which had been set up to provide medical care for construction workers at the remote Boulder and Grand Coulee dam sites, was established as the independent Kaiser-Permanente Health Plan (KPHP). It has since expanded throughout California, Oregon, Hawaii, and Ohio with a membership of over 4 million. Following World War II local PGPs under various auspices were established in many parts of the country (MacColl, 1966). The idea gradually spread, and the original plans grew, but slowly. By the time of the enactment of the Health Maintenance Organization (HMO) Act of 1973, only 5 million persons were enrolled in PGPs. The various plans have many differences in sponsorship and specifics of organization, but the basic philosophy and fundamental structure is nearly the same in each case. Kaiser is the largest and best known, and is taken here as the model in describing and analyzing the idea.

Subscribers are enrolled for a fixed anual premium, either individually or through an employee-group contract. Members receive comprehensive medical services from a contracting medical group with which they register as their base point for all services. Within the medical group, each enrollee chooses a primary-care physician and has access to its specialists by referral as needed. If hospitalization is required, the patient is sent to one of the Kaiser Foundation hospitals in the area. There he is treated by the full-time, Kaiser hospital staff physicians and followed by his own primary-care physician and/or the referring specialists from his physician group. All medical services are paid out of the single premium as long as the patient stays within the system to obtain them.* This feature, referred to as "closed panel" care, has been one of the principal objections by the rest of the medical profession. It is, however, a fundamental and necessary basis for organizing the plan to work as it should.

The medical groups in the plan, which are semi-independent corporate entities, contract to provide services for enrollees, and are paid by the central Kaiser Health Plan on a capitation basis for the number of patients who elect their group. The medical group in turn hires the necessary number of physicians on a salaried basis. Once the physicians become full partners, salaries are supplemented by incentive bonuses, which depend on hospital utilization and operating costs. Hospital, laboratory, office operating costs, *and* the physicians' incomes (including bonuses) all come out of the single basic premium. Therefore, the fewer hospital charges occur against patients from their medical group, the more money is left at the end of the year for bonuses. This creates a powerful incentive for PGP physicians to treat as many problems on an ambulatory basis as possible and not to order unnecessary procedures. Hospital physicians, also salaried, have no incentive to perform unnecessary surgery or to prolong hospitalization any longer than essential. As a consequence, members of PGPs use only about half as much hospital care as those cared for on a fee-for-service basis (Luft, 1978). This is the major source of cost saving for the system. It is sometimes argued that

---

* Certain highly specialized services such as unusual kinds of open-heart surgery, or very sophisticated radiation therapy may be provided by contract outside the plan, for example, with a university hospital, since they would be used too seldom to provide them efficiently within the system.

this represents undertreatment of PGP patients, but careful studies of the quality of care and output measures of the health of PGP members (such as mortality rates for various illnesses) confirm the fact that their care is at least as good as—and in many regards better than—fee-for-service patients.

Because of the group practice arrangement, it is possible to organize ambulatory care on an efficient basis, making it easy for physicians to provide many patient services in the office that would otherwise require hospitalization. Most groups have well-equipped laboratories on the premises, making it possible to do most of the necessary testing on-site. Tests too complex to be done in the local group setting can be arranged at a Foundation hospital on an outpatient basis. Specialist consultation is quick and easy, often on an informal basis by simply walking down the hall, much as in a hospital-based setting, but without added expenses to the patient. Since effective prevention tends to reduce the cost of medical services needed by the group's patients, PGP physicians have a vested interest in keeping their patients healthy through careful attention to preventive services (Roemer, 1962; Roemer & Schonick, 1973). Additional individual incentives payments are given to physicians to see that this occurs. Many plans pay bonuses to primary-care physicians whose patients maintain certain rates for preventive measures such as Pap smears. Studies have shown that PGP members generally receive better than average preventive care (Denson et al., 1960; Luft, 1978; Donabedian, 1969). This basic tenant of PGP philosophy—that they are paid to keep members healthy as much as to treat them when they are sick—is the reason that the term "health maintenance organization" (HMO) was coined (Ellwood, 1971; McNeil & Schlenker, 1974).

Besides the marked reduction in cost through decreased hospitalization, PGP has a number of advantages for patients (Saward, 1970). In view of the frequent difficulty in obtaining primary care (resulting from the geographic and specialty maldistribution of physicians), one of the most important features is the assured access to primary and referral care with no further arrangement required on the part of the patient. Negotiating the system is much simpler than in the fragmented fee-for-service system because nearly all services can be obtained under one roof. Unlike the situation in fee-for-service practice, PGP medical groups can hire the right number of physicians in each specialty to meet the needs of their patients. This creates a built-in planning mechanism to improve the efficiency of the operation as well as to assure patients access to needed services (Baehr, 1966; Feldstein, 1971).

Increasingly physicians are also coming to see the advantages of PGP for themselves. Because of the group arrangements for practice, they are able to lead more regular lives (McElrath, 1961). They are assured of an appropriate income from the moment of starting practice. Vacations and educational leave are no problem. Their patients are taken care of by other physicians of the group with no loss in continuity of care and no danger of their being lost to other physicians during their absence. Physicians do not have to be concerned with the mechanics and administrative problems of prac-

tice; this is all arranged for them. They can concentrate their efforts on patient care. Because of the corporate structure of the group, retirement plans
and other fringe benefits are automatic. Working in a group provides a
stimulating professional atmosphere. It creates built-in continuing education through frequent consultation and the incentives of professional pride,
constant looking over each other's shoulders, and seeing each other's patient
records. A feeling of mutual responsibility is fostered for the good reputation of the group. Essentially all the same incentives and sanctions that lead
to high technical quality of care in hospital-based practice also operate in
the group practice setting—except the highly selected case load of complex
problems. Ancillary services such as nutritional counseling and social workers, are available in many groups, making it possible to provide quality care
that goes beyond the direct medical or technical elements. Such potential
could be important for expediting the social support services so essential for
today's chronic diseases.*

Despite the strong advocacy of certain individuals and repeated studies
that showed their advantages, little public attention was given to PGPs until the escalating cost of medical care itself became a public issue. In the late
1960s, when the staggering costs of the Medicare and Medicaid programs
came to public notice, policy makers began to search for alternative more
economical methods of providing health care. The President's Commission
on Health Manpower (1967) carried out a study of the Kaiser-Permanente
plan and pointed out the magnitude of savings realized. Until then the primary arguments used by advocates of the concept had been the philosophical ones of more emphasis on preventive care and greater convenience or
continuity of care as a result of the one-stop arrangement. With the growing cost consciousness of the inflationary early 1970s, the Nixon Administration seized the idea under the rubric "health maintenance organization"
(HMO)† as a major initiative for economizing on health care expenditures.

* Unfortunately medical groups, whose policy is largely dominated by physicians, have
not yet made widespread use of ancillary and paramedical personnel in innovative ways.
Doing so could markedly improve the effectiveness and efficiency of their operation and
broaden the scope of care to deal with the increasing problems of chronic disabilities. The
organizational setting would lend itself to such practice if adequate incentives were provided through the insurance plans for moving in this direction.

† The HMO concept is broader than the original PGP idea and also allows so-called
"foundations for medical care" (FMC) or "independent practice associations" (IPAs) and
other looser forms of practice organization. FMCs create some of the same financial incentives to reduce hospitalization and other excessive utilization while leaving the organization of practice essentially in the old individual, fee-for-service format. As with PGP,
the patient pays a single premium that covers all health services. Individual physicians
contract with the foundation to provide these services and bill the foundation on a fee-
for-service basis, but fees are reduced proportionately if utilization goes up beyond the
total amount agreed to at the beginning of the contract year. Thus, the cost of care is
reduced, but the problem of fragmentation of services and difficulty in planning the
right mix of services and manpower remains. Although the organizational advantages of
group practice are lost in this scheme, physicians have been more amenable because it
represents less of a change from their traditional mode of practice.

The Department of HEW established an office to promote HMO development, and legislation was introduced eventuating in the HMO Act of 1973.
The Act authorized start-up grants, overcame some of the legal and professional barriers against PGP, and mandated that HMOs be made one option
for employee health benefits wherever such an organization (certified under
the Act) was available in the area.

Despite the considerable advantages of PGP, there are also drawbacks
and difficulties in convincing both patients and physicians to join in the
large numbers that were hoped for in the optimistic fervor of enacting the
HMO Act of 1973. The growth of existing groups has been slow. In 1979
only 4% of the population were receiving their medical care from such
plans, and only 20% of the country had such an option for their medical
care available in the geographic area (OHMO, 1980). As new PGPs have
opened in response to the funding made available by the HMO Act, it has
become obvious that there are also major problems in establishing such new
organizations and in recruiting enough enrollees to make them viable. A
major difficulty is simply that most middle-class consumers already have a
personal physician and are loathe to break the tie in order to enroll with
an HMO—even if they might choose it for the sake of saving if they were
just moving into the area. Over the years HMOs can compete favorably with
other modes of practice, but long start-up periods are usually necessary,
which requires large-scale financial backing to survive the lean years.

Patients often experience certain difficulties in obtaining their health care
through PGPs. The group practice setting easily fosters an impersonal clinic
atmosphere in which physicians tend to be preoccupied with the technical
aspects of care and less attentive to patients' personal problems and needs.
Physicians practicing in groups in general are more dependent on the approval of their colleagues in regard to professional standards of care and
less dependent on the pressures from patients for compliance with personal
desires (Freidson, 1970). These tendencies are intensified in PGP settings,
where the financial incentives toward responsiveness to patients' personal
needs are less than in a fee-for-service practice. PGP physicians tend to be
less tolerant of so-called "demanding patients" and more apt to perceive
nontechnical services to patients as a waste of their time (Mechanic, 1975).

The physician-patient relationship fostered by the group setting is also a
problem for many physicians. Because of the prepaid enrollment basis, there
tends to be more demand on the physicians by patients with problems that
physicians consider "trivial" (Freidson, 1973). Yet, no additional income is
gained for catering to such patients. Thus physicians are often impatient
and dissatisfied by these demands and feel trapped by such patients (Mechanic, 1975). There is no way they can easily unload them by referral to
another physician since the closed-panel arrangement will simply bring the
patient back on the next visit. Use of this referral tactic is also limited by
the possibility of incurring colleague resentment. In the attempt to operate
groups efficiently and with the difficulty that is sometimes encountered in

recruiting enough physicians, understaffing can be a problem. Since there is no financial rationing of health services, either an unlimited amount of services must be available or else nonfinancial means of rationing must emerge. Increased waiting time is the most likely and is perhaps almost inevitable in such an organization of care. On the other hand, careful comparative studies of satisfaction with care in fee-for-service and PGP settings show that most patients are generally quite happy with the care in both settings (Mechanic, 1975). As PGP is becoming more widely known and as medical costs have grown, the financial saving of PGP has increasingly become a factor in selection.

Even financially, there is a potential drawback with PGP. Although the total cost to families receiving care from HMOs is considerably less than from fee-for-service practice, the cost that is faced in advance (premiums taken out of the monthly pay check) is often somewhat higher than for other plans because the premium is comprehensive. Other plans tend to have co-payments and deductibles or do not cover many physician services. Thus, at the time that the choice is made, the potential enrollee is often faced with agreeing to a larger monthly payment, even though his total costs in the long run are apt to be lower. This can be hard to accept when one is healthy. Attempts to make the plans more competitive with fee-for-service by offering cheaper, more limited options or ones with co-payments have ironically been discouraged by the 1973 HMO Act itself, which requires that all approved plans provide very comprehensive coverage.

PGPs have met vehement resistance from other physicians, beginning with the AMA rejection of the Committee on the Cost of Medical Care's recommendations in 1932. In part this is a philosophical bias in favor of solo practice stemming from the guild tradition of the profession. In part this results from the fear of encroachment and limitation on the market created by the closed-panel structure of PGP. In part it is the very different style, incentives, and conditions of practice for physicians working in such settings. Local medical societies have resisted the development of PGPs in their areas from the beginning. In many instances they have made it difficult for physicians working for such organizations to get hospital privileges and have excluded them from membership in the county medical societies. Many states have been induced by state medical societies to pass laws against the so-called corporate practice of medicine. For large plans, such as Kaiser, it is an advantage for the plan to own separate hospitals, where costs and utilization can be more carefully controlled. But, new plans starting up are dependent on the use of community hospitals. Ostracism of group physicians from the local professional organizations is a serious drawback under any circumstances. In 1938 Group Health Association of Washington D.C. (GHA) brought suit against the District of Columbia Medical Society. The suit was finally settled in the Supreme Court in 1941 in favor of GHA. A similar suit against the King County Medical Society by Group Health Cooperative of Puget Sound forced its acceptance in Seattle. After these court battles were won, resistance of medical societies became much less overt, but many state laws continued to place severe restrictions on the development of PGPs (particularly those sponsored by consumer groups), for example, requiring the kind of capital reserves that would be necessary for true insurance companies (MacColl, 1970).

Besides the resistance of organized medicine, there are several factors that have made recruiting of physicians for PGP difficult and can create dissatisfaction of their staffs. The opportunity for the very high incomes that physicians sometimes make in certain specialties are not possible in PGP—although the average lifetime earnings (including fringe benefits) are quite comparable to fee-for-service practice. It is difficult, for example, to recruit radiologists, ophthalmologists, pathologists, and some kinds of surgeons, who are able to reach incomes of $150,000 to $200,000 per year in private practice. Young physicians coming out of medical school and residency training with considerable indebtedness may find it difficult to forego the hope of such incomes—even if most of them would never achieve such earnings in fee-for-service practice either.

Certain professional conditions in PGP also can create resistance from physicians. Most of PGP (like medical practice in general) consists of primary care. In the group setting, this is usually shared equally by the internists and pediatricians, who can therefore only concentrate on their more specialized training to a limited degree. In fact, this also happens to most internists and pediatricians in fee-for-services practice, but by default rather than by intent. In solo practice the hope remains that one will secure sufficient amounts of referral practice to be able to cut down on the portion of primary care. In PGP this is largely foreclosed except for those who get to practice full-time in a hospital owned by the health plan.

Many physicians dislike the bureaucratic setting of PGP—although it is considerably less hierarchical than the hospital-based setting in which most of them received their training. There tends to be a self-selecting process, however, by which physicians who are more inclined to work as part of a team come to practice in PGPs. Physicians who choose PGP are generally more ready to let their practice style and arrangements be governed by joint rules. However, the type of attitude that is self-selected also intensifies the tendency fostered in the group practice setting of being less responsive to patients' personal desires and needs than in the solo practice setting.

Despite the excellence of technical care in most HMOs, the crash program to encourage this form of practice as a means of economizing on health care costs (particularly government-paid costs), has not been without its dangers for abuse in the quality of services. Because of the difficulty involved in recruiting subscribers in order to get plans started or to get Medicaid patients to move into such plans for the sake of saving public funds, very questionable marketing practices have sometimes been employed. More emphasis has sometimes been given to rapid development or expansion than to the organization and assurance of quality care. The effort of the California

Medicaid system (Medi-Cal) to move rapidly into PGP for its beneficiaries was a particularly flagrant example of the abuse that can occur. In 1973 Medi-Cal divided the state into geographic areas and designated groups to recruit as many of the Medicaid beneficiaries as possible. Using "hard-sell" techniques, they often misrepresented the actual conditions of the service. Medical groups were quickly put together using large numbers of foreign medical graduates and were not adequately staffed to accomodate to the massive new load of patients. Patients often had to travel for miles to obtain care in second-rate clinics. Although the situation has since been rectified, the experience gave HMOs a bad image, which has made Congress and health advocacy groups more hesitant about major emphasis on PGP as a means of system reform (U.S. Compt. Gen., 1974; Roemer, 1976).

In summary, PGPs clearly make some significant contributions to resolving many of the basic problems of the health care system. PGP overcomes the fragmentation and misallocation of manpower and resources that is endemic in the fee-for-service system. It has a major impact on the part of the cost problem that is due to overutilization of hospitalization and unnecessary surgery. The enrolled population and group organization of practice could potentially serve as an appropriate structure for providing care that is better fitted to the needs of chronic illnesses. However, the dominant physician orientation favoring curative rather than supportive and rehabilitative services and the technological momentum toward acute, high-intensity, episodic care have continued to determine policy and planning in PGPs so that this potential has not been adequately realized. To make them a major lever for overcoming the mismatch of the medical care system, much stronger incentives will have to be provided in the desired direction. Most importantly, the slow rate of growth means that it cannot be a major vehicle of health system reform unless more radical measures are taken to give it a competitive edge.

TECHNOLOGY MANAGEMENT

There is growing awareness that unchecked implementation of new medical technologies is a major cause of cost escalation in the health care system. Frequently this concern is accompanied by a sense of bewilderment that there should be so little relationship between the expenditures or speed of dissemination of technologies and their efficacy. The real problem goes beyond the failure to test adequately for efficacy before dissemination. To be sure, careful testing for efficacy is an important step in technology management, which should actually go without saying, but this represents only a first step. The more difficult problem is to influence the utilization of technoloiges—discouraging the use of ineffective or inordinately costly ones and supporting the implementation of alternative technologies and strategies that are more appropriate for the health problems of the nation. Simply trying to reach consensus among providers about the best or most appropriate technologies to use in certain situations and to expect the profession to respond to the information is not apt to be an adequate solution. Questionably effective, high-cost technologies, oriented almost exclusively toward short-term intensive care are overly implemented and utilized because of professional incentives and a reimbursement system that reward their use disproportionately. Technologies and organizational structures needed for care of chronic illnesses do not get developed. Even where the tools are potentially available, such as computerized record systems and auxilliary health personnel, they neither are implemented for chronic care nor is use made of their potential for redirecting the system. The new technologies are only taken up by the system where they fit into the predominant specific-defect model, episodic, high-technology approach to disease—and there the dissemination occurs rapidly and without adequate controls.

The concern over medical technology began to be widely voiced in the early 1970s and was closely related to the growing concern about hospital costs. Wagner and Zubkoff (1978) note that the sudden suspicion expressed in regard to medical technology after decades of public enamourment was the result of three converging insights:

1. Studies of hospital cost increases began to demonstrate that growth in "intensity" of care was responsible for a major portion of hospital cost escalation (Chapter 12).

2. Disappointment with the ineffectiveness of Comprehensive Health Planning programs and certificate of need laws in stemming the rate of capital investment in health care led to studies of the process. It became clear that limiting increases in the number of beds did not decrease the overall rate of capital investment in hospitals—suggesting that it was going mainly into new technological intensity (Salkever & Bice, 1978; Salkever, 1976).

3. Increasingly, epidemiological studies and health policy analysts drew attention to the minimal effect that high-technology medical care was producing for the health of the population (Lalonde, 1974; McKeown, 1976, 1976a; Cochrane, 1971). They also linked overabundant technology and specialists using it to the serious incidence of unnecessary surgery and other unneeded procedures, which not only added to the cost of care but actually increased the risk to patients.

The sudden and dramatic appearance of several individual programs and procedures responsible for tremendous cost increases in the last few years created a final awakening shock in regard to the cost impact of health technologies—particularly on government health policy makers who had to deal with paying for them.

The development of hemodialysis for end-stage renal disease confronted policy makers with the ethical dilemma of having to deny life-sustaining technology to a group of persons who could not pay the bill necessary for their own survival. This led to the inclusion of a section in the 1972 Social Security Amendments authorizing payment for dialysis and kidney transplants under Medicare regardless of age. The cost of the program has increased far beyond the original estimates and has forced rethinking of such open-ended financing for new high-technology programs. The Administration is presently trying to encourage more treatment in the home dialysis mode, which is much less costly.

Coronary artery bypass surgery was developed early in the 1970s for the treatment of angina pectoris. Given the availability of large numbers of newly trained cardiac surgeons anxious to find new uses for their skills and the presence of third-party payment to cover the cost, use of the procedure spread rapidly. By 1977 the annual bill to the nation was over $1 billion—with no clear evidence of its efficacy. The one, well-controlled study of the procedure's effectiveness showed no increase in longevity at all (except for one small subgroup), and the supposed degree of symptomatic improvement was seriously questioned as "placebo effect" (Murphy et al., 1978).

In 1973 the Computerized Axial Tomographic X-ray scanner (CAT scanner) was developed in England as a method of improving the diagnosis of certain brain lesions. It had the advantage of frequently obviating the need to use potentially dangerous injection of air into the cerebrospinal space or X-ray contrast dyes into the carotid arteries. Quick to see its commercial potential, American companies rapidly developed whole body scanners and began a large-scale marketing program—before any careful evaluation was carried out of whether body CAT scanning made any significant contribution to diagnosis. Shocked by the costs being incurred, the Administration tried to limit the propagation by requiring certificate-of-need approval before placing any new orders. But the events had occurred too rapidly. By mid-1978 over 1000 CAT scanners were already in place—five times the number estimated necessary for the needs of the country even if they should turn out to have considerable value in certain diagnostic situations (OTA, 1978; Institute of Medicine, 1977). This has required an estimated investment of about $600 million and continuing annual operating cost to payors of $0.5 to $1 billion.

Reeling from this series of shocks and increasingly aware of the role that questionable technologies play in shaping our lives and contributing to costs, Congress established its Office of Technology Assessment (OTA) in 1972 to begin investigating such problems and to give advice about potential developments on the horizon. An early survey by OTA's medical division documented how extremely limited our knowledge is concerning the efficacy of most medical procedures. Of the 16 technologies surveyed (all in widespread use), they concluded that only six are probably effective enough to justify the extent to which they are being used. Of these, only three had been demonstrated effective in carefully controlled formal clinical trials of the kind that medicine takes for itself as the standard for proof of efficacy.

The OTA report called for a major program of medical technology assessment and regulation by the DHEW (OTA, 1978a). In early 1978 Senator Kennedy introduced legislation to implement this recommendation, and the Ninety-fifth Congress enacted a somewhat scaled-down version establishing a National Center for Health Care Technology to coordinate HEW departmental activities on technology assessment already underway and to make recommendations for encouraging behavior in the health system appropriate for the findings. The National Institutes of Health (NIH) have developed a framework for reviewing new and existing medical technologies and attempting to reach consensus among leaders of the professional community concerning their appropriate application. These so-called "consensus exercises" are followed by widespread dissemination of the findings and recommendations in the hope of influencing physicians to conform (Richmond, 1978).

This emerging interest in more careful testing of medical technologies for efficacy is encouraging—as is the attempt to create organizational arrangements for controlling their dissemination and use. Even if an adequate system of technology assessment can be established, however, moving the next step to a system of technology *management* promises to be much more difficult. In the first place, the highly visible new technologies such as CAT scanners and coronary artery bypass surgery, which are likely to be the focus of these assessments, represent only the tip of the iceberg. As much of the problem arises from unnecessary or inappropriate use of existing and/or basically effective technologies as from those that are new or clearly ineffective. For example, blood chemistries and similar clinical laboratory procedures are undoubtedly effective and important diagnostic procedures that must be available for the practice of high-quality medicine. Yet the expenditures for clinical laboratories have been growing at the rate of 14% per year since 1970, totaling $11 billion in 1976 (Fineberg, 1978). This increase in total costs has taken place despite decreasing cost per test as a result of the automated multichannel analyzers now widely available, indicating an even faster rate of increase in the number of tests being ordered. There is no evidence that so much additional testing contributes anything to the quality of care. The availability and ease of obtaining large numbers of tests from a single small blood sample (together with the financial incentives to physicians in many cases) seems to be a major reason for the rapid growth of such testing.

The problem for technology assessment in this case would not be to determine whether the tests are effective, but to establish guidelines for their appropriate use. This is a much more difficult task, which in the final analysis would require setting guidelines or standards for virtually the entire practice of medicine. A similar problem exists in relation to many surgical procedures. Appendectomies, hysterectomies, and cholecystectomies (removing the gall bladder) are effective procedures that have a legitimate place in the practice of medicine. Yet it is equally clear that they are tremenüously overused. "Assessment" of these procedures would primarily require establishing guidelines for their appropriate use—something that is not only very difficult but would also meet great resistance from physicians as encroachment on their professional judgement.

To reach a consensus about efficacy of a procedure is often no easy matter. Coronary artery bypass surgery is a case in point. The best controlled studies show no significant increase in longevity and very questionable validity for the apparent symptomatic improvement. The tremendous cost to society (and to patients) with a very poor cost/benefit ratio (even if the symptomatic relief is taken at face value) makes continued use of the procedure hard to justify. Yet, proponents of the operation continue to advocate vehemently for its use, condemning the studies that failed to demonstrate its effectiveness. However, the same proponents are usually not willing to limit its performance to series that are part of a controlled clinical trial where the results might allow eventual determination of its value under precisely specifiable conditions. A serious difficulty arises inevitably in evaluation studies of such procedures—in contrast to drugs and devices—from the fact that the technique must first be disseminated fairly widely in order to make the clinical trials possible. At this point, many physicians already have a strong vested interest in the procedure. Consequently, unless it is unequivocally demonstrated to be detrimental, a group of advocates will almost invariably continue to push it.

Even if consensus can be reached among professional leaders concerning a particular technology, this is a long way from guaranteeing that it will lead to rational management of the dissemination (or nondissemination) of the technology. Managing so-called "technology transfer" would require much greater leverage over the practice of medicine than is presently envisaged. There are several ways in which such leverage could be pursued. One possibility would be to extend the Food and Drug Administration's (FDA) regulatory strategy presently employed for drugs and devices. The FDA approach has worked very well in this country and has achieved a record of credibility matched by few other regulatory agencies. It is impossible, however, to control how the drug is used or what it is used for once it has been approved for marketing. Since the problem is frequently the appropriateness of usage, simply certifying a new technology for use would not solve the problem. Controlling the utilization of procedures is more difficult. For example, the agency would not only have to certify that a new model multichannel blood analyzer is effective; it would also have to determine, for example, that its use to obtain serum bilirubin is appropriate in suspected cases of appendicitis (to help rule out possible confounding liver or gall bladder problems), but is perhaps not appropriate (as the most cost-effective routine screening procedure) for all hospital admissions. There is no way that a regulatory agency of the FDA type could enforce such guidelines for the use of approved technologies short of complete regimentation of medical practice. This is neither possible nor poltically acceptable.

A second more commonly suggested strategy is denial of reimbursement as a lever to enforce compliance with guidelines for use of technologies. This could obviously be employed in cases where a procedure had been declared totally without benefit. For example, Medicare could refuse to reimburse surgeons for internal mammary artery ligation to relieve angina (a procedure which was shown to be quite ineffective in clinical trials). In most cases, however, it is a matter of judgment based on the special features of a particular case as to whether a procedure or technology is appropriate or not. It is only possible to say statistically that a surgeon is doing too many appendectomies or hysterectomies inappropriately and should have his reimbursement questioned. Only careful review of all the details of a case by a group of peers can justify the decision that therapy is inappropriate in a given individual case. This would be prohibitively expensive and time-consuming and could never be used as a routine method of determining appropriateness for granting or denying reimbursement. Professional Standards Review Organizations (PSRO) use some individual case reviews and utilization profile strategies selectively as means of utilization and quality review but are far from anything like management of technology transfer or control of its implementation.

For already disseminated technologies such as CAT scanners or coronary artery bypass surgery, where there is no definitive evidence that they are detrimental but serious question about cost effectiveness, one means of technology management might be to limit their use to organizational settings with incentives that discourage unnecessary utilization. Physicians should have nothing to gain financially by employing the procedure, and preferably both the physician and the patient should incur part of the cost (to offset the potential prestige rewards and the patient's unrealistic expectations). For example, certain procedures might be paid for only in settings such as HMOs or salaried physician organizations where the physician stands to decrease his share of the comprehensive premium or at least cannot profit by ordering or performing expensive procedures, and patients might be required to incur a significant co-payment. Congress is presently considering badly needed Social Security amendments that would prohibit "percentage-of-the-take" arrangements for radiologists and pathologists based in hospitals. These contracts not only lead to unconscionable incomes (quite unrelated to the amount of professional input entailed) but also create incentives to increase unnecessary utilization. Negotiated fee schedules or salaried arrangements for all physicians would be needed, designed to stop inordinant compensation from high-technology procedures (which may require much less of their time) and to reward them instead for hands-on care in proportion to the contribution of their own time (Chapter 12).

Clearly none of the strategies will make it possible to deal with technology management generically. This can be accomplished only within a much more general program of health care system reform. Nevertheless, technology assessment and management strategies can make important contributions to improve efficacy and cost effectiveness and represent important advances in thinking about the health system.

Because technology assessment is essentially a negative or limiting strategy in its present form, it leaves some important aspects of the technology problem untouched. Parallel to the problem of too rapid dissemination of any technology related to clinical intervention is the failure to implement (even existing) technologies for improvement of effectiveness and efficiency of the health care system. For example, computerized patient record systems, improved management systems for supportive services in chronic illnesses, and telecommunication systems for improving the effectiveness of paramedical personnel working in remote areas have all been shown to be effective. Yet, they have not been widely implemented. Such technologies do not create vested interests for physicians or other providers of care. They do not enhance prestige as do the pure medical technologies, which fit into the tradition of intervention against specific causes of diseases and on which the success of the profession was based. Computerized patient monitoring for intensive care units and clinical decision-assisting methods (which use technologies very similar to the management and record systems), on the contrary, were widely marketed as soon as they were developed. Effective technology management, therefore, would not only have to provide assessment and leverage to slow the dissemination and implementation of unproven or ineffective technologies. But it is also equally important to provide adequate incentives to speed the adoption and implementation of efficiency producing managerial technologies.

The technology assessment strategy *per se* likewise does nothing about the fundamental inappropriateness of the high-technology, episodic-care approach of the health professions, which is the root of the mismatch of the health care system to the chronic disease needs of today. Medical technology is carried by the momentum of its success in the direction of more intensive, specific intervention although it is increasingly less appropriate for many disease problems of today. The usual response to an unfavorable assessment is to start looking for another technology to do the same thing more effectively. This headlong search for new complex technological solutions to individual medical problems, "moon-shot" initiatives such as the "war on cancer," and the momentum and prestige of the clinical intervention approach to health problems stands to widen and intensify the mismatch of the health system to today's disease problems.

Technology assessment does nothing to change this basic problem of orientation within the health care system. In a sense, it even supports that orientation by focusing primarily on the individual technologies and specific disease problems. An adequate program of health technology assessment and management would have to go beyond assessing individual technologies, and move toward cost-benefit or social impact evaluation of entire approaches to health problems in juxtaposition to alternative strategies for dealing with them. A fundamental examination of the health goals of the nation is required within which the role of various types of technologies can be evaluated and potential tradeoffs assessed.

The high-technology, clinical approach is running up against the wall of ultimate human mortality and the inevitability of illnesses (or accidents) of some kind leading to that mortality. Improving the health status of a population in post-industrial society, if this is measured only by longevity, is a little like trying to reduce the temperature of some substance to absolute zero. After the major part of the reduction has been accomplished by simple means, each new tiny increment of improvement requires a new order-of-magnitude increase in cost and sophistication. Most of health technology investment today goes into so-called "halfway technologies" (Thomas, 1972), methods like hemodialysis for renal failure, which sustain failing organ systems without doing anything to cure or prevent the underlying disease process. They therefore contribute only an incremental postponement of the inevitable end at a higher and higher cost. Given the tradeoffs required in making many of these incremental advances, it is doubtful whether the general welfare and "health" (in the broadest sense) of the population will really be improved by most such attempts. In many cases it may well be that the best interest of the many is being sacrificed for the supposed benefit of a very few.

We certainly need to continue basic research that might someday produce the capability of fundamentally modifying, preventing, or arresting certain basic pathological processes like arteriosclerosis and some types of carcinogenesis. Until that lucky day comes, however, we must assess our medical technology investments in relation to potential tradeoffs. One of the serious dilemmas of post-clinical medicine is the setting of priorities. (1) Are the resources better spent in making last-ditch losing battles against fatal illnesses or in trying to provide supportive services that better match the immediate needs of patients as substitutes for such intensive intervention? (2) Would resources be better used to promote behavioral and environmental modification programs to decrease the incidence of some chronic illnesses like cancer, heart disease, and strokes? Can we justify the social and economic tradeoffs required to do this?

The necessary tradeoffs in social goals must be faced if any long-term improvement in health is to be realized. Because of the glamour and seemingly miraculous nature of medical cures, clinical medicine has gained an emphasis out of proportion to the real benefit that can be expected. This occurs at the cost of not providing resources vital to the improvement of preventive medicine and programs that improve health much more indirectly, such as providing better jobs, education, and even recreation. In order to make the difficult choices in the political arena, much better information will be needed concerning the relative effect on health and welfare produced by different options. For example, the costs in disruption to the economy, social structure, or personal freedom that would be required in some strategies to achieve decreased morbidity and social loss from accidents, homicide, coronary heart disease, or alcoholism might be too great to accept. On the other hand, it is quite conceivable that investment in mass transit or housing or schools or even subsidization of healthful personal life styles would do more for health (even in the narrower sense) than the same investment made directly in improved medical care. To make such choices wisely, we must learn to use not only technology assessments but also "health impact statements" for social investments and new programs in general—just as we try to evaluate the tradeoffs of other policy decisions in regard to their environmental or economic impact. The difficulties in making such evaluations are immense because we still know so little about the social factors determining the health status or diseases of a population, but a major effort in this direction would be necessary if health policy is to be rationalized.

REFERENCES

Ardell, Donald B., "Limitations and Priorities in CHP," *Inquiry*, 10(September):49–56, 1973.

Ardell, Donald B., "Communication, The Demise of CHP and the Future of Planning," *Inquiry*, 11(September):233–234, 1974.

Auger, R. C., and Goldberg, V. P., "Prepaid Health Plans and Moral Hazard," *Public Policy*, 22:353, 1974.

Baehr, George, "Pre-paid Group Practice: Its Strength and Weaknesses, and Its Future," *American Journal of Public Health*, 56:1898, 1966.

Banta, David H., and Bauman, Patricia, "Health Services Research and Health Policy," *Journal of Community Health*, 2, 1976.

Bicknell, William, and Walsh, Diana, "Certification-of-Need: The Massachusetts Experience," *New England Journal of Medicine*, 292:1054–1061, 1975.

Binstock, Robert H., "Effective Planning Through Political Influence," *American Journal of Public Health*, 59:808–813, 1969.

Bloom, Bernard, and Peterson, Osler, "End Results, Cost and Productivity of Coronary-Care Units," *New England Journal of Medicine*, 288:72–78, 1973.

Blum, Henrik L., *Planning for Health: Development and Application of Social Change Theory*, New York: Human Sciences Press, 1974.

Bodenheimer, Thomas S., "Regional Medical Programs: No Road to Regionalization," *Medical Care Review*, 26:1125, 1969.

Brian, E., "Foundation for Medical Care Control of Hospital Utilization: CHAP—A PSRO Prototype," *New England Journal of Medicine*, 288:878, 1973.

Brown, Douglas R., "Community Health Planning or Who Will Control the Health Care System," *American Journal of Public Health*, 62:1336, 1972.

Bruhn, John G., "Planning for Social Change: Dilemmas for Health Planning," *American Journal of Public Health*, 63:602–606, 1973.

Cochrane, A., *Effectiveness and Efficiency*, London: The Nuffield Provincial Hospitals Trust, 1971.

Cohen, H. S., "Regulating Health Care Facilities: the Certificate-of Need Process Re-examined," *Inquiry*, 10:3, 1973.

Comroe, J., and Dripps, R., "Scientific Basis for the Support of Biomedical Science," *Science*, **192**:105, 1976.

Conant, R. W., *The Politics of Community Health*, Washington, D.C.: Public Affairs Press, 1968.

Crystal, Royal A., and Brewster, Agnes W., "Cost Benefit and Cost Effectiveness Analyses in the Health Field: an Introduction," *Inquiry*, **3**(December):3–12, 1966.

Curran, William J., "A National Survey and Analysis of State Certificate of Need Laws for Health Facilities," in Havighurst, C. C., *Regulating Health Facilities Construction*, Washington, D.C.: American Institute for Public Policy Research, 1974.

Densen, Paul M., et al., "Prepaid Medical Care and Hospital Utilization in a Dual Choice Situation," *American Journal of Public Health*, **50**:1710–1726, 1960.

Donabedian, Avedis, "An Evaluation of Prepaid Group Practice," *Inquiry*, **6**(September): 3–27, 1969.

Egdahl, R. H., "Foundations for Medical Care," *New England Journal of Medicine*, **288**: 491, 1973.

Ellwood, Paul M., Jr., "Health Maintenance Strategy," *Medical Care*, **9**:291, 1971.

Feldstein, Paul J., *Prepaid Group Practice: an Analysis and Review*, the University of Michigan: Bureau of Hospital Administration, School of Public Health, **50**, June 1971.

Freidson, Eliot, *Profession of Medicine*, New York: Dodd, Mead, 1970.

Freidson, Eliot, "Prepaid Group Practice and the New 'Demanding Patient'," *Milbank Memorial Fund Quarterly, Health and Society*, **51**(Fall):473–488, 1973.

Gaus, Clifton R., et al., "Contrasts in HMO and Fee-for-Service Performance," *Social Security Bulletin*, May 3, 1976.

Glaser, William A., "Experiences in Health Planning in the United States," prepared for conference on "Health Planning in the United States: Past Experience and Future Imperatives," New York: Columbia University, School of Public Health, mimeo, undated, ca. 1972.

Glasgow, John M., "Prepaid Group as a National Health Policy: Problems and Perspectives," *Inquiry*, **9**:3–15, 1972.

Gottlieb, Symond, "A Brief History of Health Planning in the United States," in Havighurst, Clark, Ed., *Regulating Health Facilities Construction*, Washington, D.C.: American Institute for Public Policy Research, 1974.

Grosse, Robert N., "Cost Benefit Analysis of Health Services," *Annals of the American Academy of Political and Social Science*, **399**(January):89–99, 1972.

Harrington, D. C., "San Joaquin Foundation for Medical Care," *Hospitals, Journal of the American Hospital Association*, **45**(6):67, 1971.

Harvard Law Review Editors, "The Role of Prepaid Group Practice in Relieving the Medical Care Crisis," *Harvard Law Review*, **84**:887, 1971.

Havighurst, Clark C., "Regulation of Health Facilities and Services by Certificate of Need," *Virginia Law Review*, **59**:1143–1242, 1973.

Havighurst, Clark C., and Bovbjerg, Randall, "Professional Standards Review Organizations and Health Maintenance Organizations: Are They Compatible?" *Utah Law Review* (Summer): 41, 1975.

Herman, Harold, "Factors Affecting Comprehensive Health Planning in Large Urban Areas," Report/Comprehensive Health Planning Service, DHEW, Washington, D.C.: Linton, Mields, and Coston, mimeo, 1972.

Ingraham, Hollis, "National Health Planning: Structure and Goals," *Bulletin of the New York Academy of Medicine*, **48**(January):39–44, 1972.

Institute of Medicine, *Computer Tomography*, Washington, D.C.: National Academy of Sciences, 1977.

Jonas, Steven, "Theoretical Approach to the Question of 'Community Control' of Health Services," *American Journal of Public Health,* 61:916–920, 1934, 1937, 1971.

Kaufman, Herbert, "The Politics of Health Planning," *American Journal of Public Health,* 59:795–797, 1969.

Klarman, Herbert E., Francis, John, and Rosenthal, Gerald, "Cost Effectiveness Analysis Applied to the Treatment of Chronic Renal Disease," *Medical Care,* 6:48–54, 1968.

Komaroff, Anthony L., "Regional Medical Programs in Search of a Mission," *New England Journal of Medicine,* 284:750, 1971.

Lalonde, Marc, *A New Perspective on the Health of Canadians: A Working Document,* Ottawa: Government of Canada, 1974.

Lentz, Edward A. "Health Care Planning," *Annual Administrative Reviews,* 44:93–127, 1970.

Levin, Arthur L., "Health Planning and U.S. Federal Government," *International Journal of Health Services,* 2:367–376, 1972.

Levine, Naomi, "Community Participation and Some Hard Lessons," *Congress Bi-Weekly,* December 19, 1969.

Lewis, Charles E., "The Thermodynamics of Regional Planning," *American Journal of Public Health,* 59:773–808, 1969.

Lindaman, Francis C., and Costa, Marjorie A., "The Voice of the Community," *American Journal of Public Health,* September, 1972.

Luft, Harold S., "How do Health Maintenance Organizations Achieve Their 'Savings'?" *New England Journal of Medicine,* 298:1336–1343, 1978.

MacColl, William A., *Group Practice and Prepayment of Medical Care,* Washington, D.C.: Public Affairs Press, 1966.

Martin, Samuel P., Donaldson, Magruder C., London, C. David, Peterson, Osler L., and Colton, Theodore, "Inputs into Coronary Care during Thirty Years: A Cost Effectiveness Study," *Annals of Internal Medicine,* 81:289–293, 1974.

Mather, H. G., et al., "Acute Myocardial Infarction: Home and Hospital Treatment," *British Medical Journal,* 3(August 7):334–338, 1971.

McElrath, Dennis, "Perspective and Participation of Physicians in Prepaid Group Practices," *American Sociological Review,* 26:596–607, 1961.

McKeon, Thomas, *The Modern Rise of Population,* London: Edward Arnold, 1976.

McKeown, Thomas, *The Role of Medicine: Dream, Mirage or Nemesis,* London: Nuffield Provincial Hospitals Trust, 1976a.

McNeil, Richard, and Schlenker, Robert, "HMOs, Competition, and Government," Minneapolis: Interstudy, 20:December 1974.

Mechanic, David, *Public Expectations and Health Care: Essays on the Changing Organization of Health Services,* New York: Wiley-Interscience, 1972.

Mechanic, David, *Politics, Medicine, and Social Science,* New York: Wiley-Interscience, 1974.

Mechanic, David, "The Organization of Medical Practice and Practice Orientations among Physicians in Prepaid and Non-prepaid Primary Care Settings," *Medical Care,* 13:189–204, 1975.

Mechanic, David, *The Growth of Bureaucratic Medicine: An Inquiry into the Dynamics of Patient Behavior and the Organization of Medical Care,* New York: Wiley-Interscience, 1976.

Moynihan, David P., *Maximum Feasible Misunderstanding,* New York: Free Press, 1969. Foundations and Other Delivery Models," *Inquiry,* 12:10, 1975.

Newport, J., and Roemer, M. I., "Comparative Perinatal Mortality under Medical Care

Office of Health Maintenance Organizations (OHMO), USPHS, *Projections for HMO Development, 1980–1990,* Washington, D.C.: USDHEW (PHS), 1980.

Office of Technology Assessment, *Assessing the Efficacy and Safety of Medical Technologies,* Washington, D.C.: Congress of the United States, 1978.

Office of Technology Assessment, *Policy Implications of the Computed Tomography (CT) Scanner,* Washington, D.C.: Congress of the United States, 1978a.

Perrott, George S., "The Federal Employees Health Benefits Program," USDHEW, May 1971.

Platt, Roger, "Utilization of Facilities for Heart Surgery," *New England Journal of Medicine,* **284**:1386–1387, 1971.

Public Law 93–641, Health Planning Resources and Development Act of 1974, 1974.

President's Commission on Health Manpower, *Report of the National Advisory Commission on Health Manpower, The Kaiser Foundation Medical Care Program,* Vol. 2, 1–68, May 1967.

Richmond, Julius, Assistant Secretary for Health, DHEW, Testimony before the Subcommittee on Domestic and International Scientific Planning, Analysis and Cooperation, Committee on Science and Technology, U.S. House of Representatives, October 6, 1978.

Rienke, W. A., "An Overview of the Planning Process," in Rienke, W. A., Ed., *Health Planning: Qualitative Aspects and Quantitative Techniques,* Baltimore: John Hopkins University Press, 1972.

Roemer, Milton I., "On Paying the Doctor and the Implications of Different Methods," *Journal of Health and Human Behavior,* **3**(Spring):4–14, 1962.

Roemer, Milton I., and Schonick, W., "HMO Performance: The Recent Evidence," *Milbank Memorial Fund Quarterly, Health and Society,* **51**:271, 1973.

Roemer, Milton I., "Better Weather Ahead for California's Prepaid Health Plans?" *American Medical News,* October 25, 1976, 7–8.

Russell, John M., "New Federal Regional Medical Programs," *New England Journal of Medicine,* **275**:6, 1966.

Russell, Louise, "The Diffusion of New Hospital Technologies," *International Journal of Health Services,* **6**(4):557–580, 1976.

Salkever, David, "Health Planning and Cost Containment: a Selection of the Recent U.S. Experience," International Conference on Programs for the Containment of Health Care Costs and Expenditures, The Fogarty International Center, National Institutes of Health, Bethesda, Md., 1976.

Salkever, David, and Bice, Thomas, "Certificate-of-Need Legislation and Hospital Costs," in Zubkoff, M., Raskin, I., Hanft, R., Eds., *Hospital Cost Containment,* New York: Prodist, 1978.

Salmon, J. W., "The Maintenance Organization Strategy: A Corporate Takeover of Health Services Delivery," *International Journal of Health Services,* **5**:609, 1975.

Saward, Ernest W., "The Relevance of the Kaiser-Permanente Experience to the Health Services of the Eastern United States, *Bulletin of the New York Academy of Medicine,* **46**(September):1970.

Simmons, H. E., "PSRO Today: The Program's Viewpoint," *New England Journal of Medicine,* **292**:365, 1975.

Simmons, Roberta G., Klein, Susan D., and Simmons, Richard L., *Gift of Life: The Social and Psychological Impact of Organ Transplantation,* New York: Wiley-Interscience, 1977.

Spencer, F. C., and Eiseman, B., "The Occasional Open-Heart Surgeon," *Circulation,* February: 161–162, 1965.

Stebbins, E. L., and Williams, K. N., "History and Background of Health Planning in the United States," in Rienke, W. A., Ed., *Health Planning*, Baltimore: Johns Hopkins University Press, 1972.

Thomas, Lewis, "Guessing and Knowing: Reflections on the Science and Technology of Medicine," *Saturday Review of Science*, 55(December 23): 52–57, 1972.

U.S. Comptroller General, *Better Controls Needed for Health Maintenance Organizations Under Medicaid in California*, report to the Committee on Finance, U.S. Senate, September 10, 1974, Washington, D.C.: U.S. General Accounting Office, 1974.

Wagner, Judith L., and Zubkoff, Michael, "Medical Technology and Hospital Costs," in Zubkoff, M., Ruskin, I., and Hanft, R., Eds., *Hospital Cost Containment: Selected Notes for Future Policy*, New York: Prodist, 1978.

PART THREE

FINANCING AND COST
OF HEALTH CARE:

How the Economic
Superstructure Escalates Costs
and Perpetuates the Mismatch

Part 2 deals with the organizational momentum and professional incentives built around the new technology of medicine. These perpetuate and intensify the mismatch of the health system with the needs for care in post-clinical medicine. The objective of Part 3 is to explain how economic and financing mechanisms reinforce and intensify the organizational mismatch and are responsible for the uncontrolled cost increases.

Chapter 11 traces the evolution of health care financing in this country. This not only serves as a background for analyzing the problems of the financing system today but also illuminates the political and organizational forces and vested interests that have shaped it and must be countered in any attempt to reform it. At each step the new developments seemed a sensible extension of the existing financing system, disturbing it as little as possible while solving the most urgent new problems as they arose. Yet the final financing system that emerged stepwise was an incongruent mixture of mechanisms with no coherent means of providing corrective control over the amount or allocation of expenditures and resources.

Chapter 12 provides a basic analysis of the cost and financing problems, illustrating where the money goes and the apparent reasons for the rising costs. In addition the argument is made that the impact of health insurance on costs works primarily through providers rather than consumers. Chapter 13 reanalyzes the economics of the health sector from a new, structural perspective. It is argued that the problem of uncontrolled costs arises from the incongruent mixture of free market, public service, and regulated utility elements. Although no economic analysis has heretofore explicitly examined the effects and implications of these structural incongruities in the health economy, current political and ideological debate has highlighted them. Each major proposal for a strategy of cost control has focused on furthering one of the three economic structural types and eliminating as far as possible the elements of the other types that interfere with its most effective function. The incongruities of economic structures have freed health financing from most of the usual economic constraints that bring spending into line with need or demand in other economic sectors. Instead the financing system has taken on a momentum of its own, acting as a superstructure to the delivery system, which reinforces the present organizational mismatch and inordinate allocation of resources for high-technology care.

Unlike previous efforts to enact national health insurance programs in this country, the present round of political activity in regard to this issue (discussed in Chapter 14) has become quite conscious of the need to reform both the financing and the delivery system. The necessity of controlling costs and making the system more responsive to needs of patients and communities has become paramount. As a result, proposals for national health insurance, like those for cost containment, divide into those favoring free market, those favoring public service, and those favoring regulated utility approaches. The deep-seated ideological differences embodied in these approaches make it extremely difficult to work out compromises. The nature of the legislative process makes it unlikely that any sweeping reform of the system can be enacted—yet inaction or minimal action is a decision with equally significant consequences of continued escalating costs and failure to meet the needs of the population for appropriate care.

CHAPTER ELEVEN

The Development of
American Health Care Financing

Underlying the failure of the health care system to contain cost escalations and to meet the needs for service is a fundamental mismatch between the financing system and the problems of post-clinical medicine similar to the mismatch between the structure of the delivery system and the needs created by today's predominant diseases. Financing methods have a profound impact on the demand, supply, utilization, and allocation of health care resources and services. Any attempt to control the cost of care or improve the cost-effective allocation of services must also restructure the payment system. To understand the problems of achieving a workable solution for financing health care, it is useful to examine how our present health insurance system and health care financing policy arose step by step. Two questions will be foremost:

1. How did the cost-engendering features evolve as characteristics of the system; how were they institutionalized; and what organizational forces are apt to be encountered in any attempts to change them?
2. With an eye to proprosals for national health insurance and for health care organizational reforms, what political forces and philosophical perspectives were instrumental in shaping the evolution of the present system of financing?

This historical review illuminates the vested interests influencing today's philosophical and political positions in regard to health financing. It clarifies the problems awaiting any strategy for controlling the growth of health expenditures, for establishing more rational mechanisms of financing, and for governing the health system in an effective way.

THE BEGINNINGS OF HEALTH INSURANCE—
FAILURE TO CREATE A NATIONAL SYSTEM

The historic way of paying for medical care was the direct reciprocal relationship between doctor and patient, where the physician charged a fee for each service performed, so called "fee-for-service." Similar payment methods existed for hospitals, drugs, and so on. This arrangement derived from the independent guild tradition of the medical profession, and remains an important plank in its ideology. With this financing method, only those who could afford to pay directly could be assured of services. Therefore the professional service tradition enjoined physicians and hospitals to provide free medical care to those who could not afford to pay, or to adjust fees (sliding scales) in accord with the patient's ability to pay. Those needing free care or reduced fees had to ask for charity or document their poverty in some kind of "means test." The alternative of defaulting on payment of debts was equally humiliating and potentially entailed the danger of making medical care unavailable at some future date when it might be needed. For the truly indigent, at least in cities, free dispensaries or almshouses were available (Chapter 7).

After 1900, as the potential utility of medical care began to improve rapidly, assured access to medical services became more important. The trade unions, developing in the late nineteenth and early twentieth centuries, saw health care and other welfare benefits for their members as a natural rallying point for recruiting members, and established sickness benefit programs financed from the membership dues. In fact, many of the early craft organizations were first formed as mutual benefit societies to insure their members and families against various disabilities (Munts, 1967). They provided not only sickness benefits, but also the equivalent of unemployment insurance, disability benefits, death benefits to widows, and so on. Only later did the unions develop into collective bargaining representatives to negotiate with management over wages and conditions of employment. As the unions moved into confrontation with the powerful, growing industries in the post-Civil War period marked by alternating cycles of boom and depression, their sickness and welfare funds helped to retain membership and bargaining strength during the lean years. Samuel Gompers, a strong advocate of sickness benefit funds, used them to build his union base first with the cigar makers and later the American Federation of Labor (AFL). Not surprisingly, he later took a strong stand against government health insurance, which he feared might destroy the workers' solidarity with the unions. Some unions, such as the International Ladies' Garment Workers Union and later the United Mine Workers, operated clinics with physicians hired on a contract basis. This practice of contract medicine was threatening to many other physicians because it excluded them from part of the patient market.

Fear of its extension led medical societies to argue against all forms of health insurance (Burrow, 1963).

Management also saw the advantages of attracting employees and holding their loyalty by providing welfare and health care benefits. Company sponsored medical services were essential where employment took place in remote areas in such industries as railroad construction, mining, and lumbering where it was necessary to guarantee physician salaries in order to make them available. However, with the rapid growth of unionism during World War I many businesses, even in urban areas, began sponsoring employee benefit programs (including health care) as a countermeasure to the union plans. The improved employee and public relationships fostered by such plans were looked on as "good business" and referred to as "welfare capitalism" (Munts, 1967). In the 1930s this led to open conflicts between unions and management over who should control the welfare plans. These precedents set by the labor-management disputes over the control of health benefits were important in establishing the tradition of health insurance as an employment related prerogative rather than a government guaranteed service.

A second parallel but independent movement that influenced the health insurance question arose in the early decades of the twentieth century. During the so-called "progressive era" (Hofstadter, 1955) from 1900 to 1920, there was much state and Federal legislative activity aimed at ameliorating the lot of workers and protecting consumers from the excesses of business. The muckraking of publicists and the lobbying of social reformers (spearheaded by the support of the AMA Committee on Food and Drugs) led to the Federal enactment of the Pure Food and Drug Act of 1906. Urged on by active lobbying from the reform coalition called the American Association for Labor Legislation (AALL) between 1910 and 1920, 42 states passed worker's compensation and industrial accident insurance laws (Anderson, 1950). These made employers responsible for disability payment and medical costs of job related accidents or illness, whether or not negligence on the part of management was demonstrable. This responsibility came to be looked upon as a legitimate cost of production to be passed along in higher prices, thus distributing the financial risk of certain injuries and occupationally related illnesses over the population at large—a tradition also adopted later by fringe benefit financing of voluntary health insurance (Somers & Somers, 1954, 1961).

Passage of this important social legislation came about partly as a result of the general climate of public opinion in the period which favored humanitarian reform and stronger governmental control over corporate abuses. Pressure for social reform legislation also stemmed from labor unrest, effective organization by the AFL, Populism, American socialism, and from the example of European social reform legislation, especially in Germany and England (Hofstadter, 1955). Leadership of the agitation and lobbying for workers' compensation centered in the AALL, organized in 1906. The group was a coalition of prestigious academic and nonacademic social reformers. They commissioned studies of the consequences of industrial accidents and job related diseases, "placing great stress on the economic losses due to illness and premature death" (Anderson, 1968). The Association was by no means revolutionary—believing in the basic soundness of the free enterprise system—but saw that to increase productivity and protect individuals from the excesses of the industrial system, certain governmental regulation was necessary. This approach followed the prevailing philosophy of the progressive movement of the time. As a result, the organization was extremely effective in lobbying for state worker's compensation legislation in one state after another.

Heady with their first successes, the AALL saw enactment of government-mandated, general health insurance plans as the logical next step, following the examples instituted in Germany in 1883 and in England in 1911. The Committee on Social Insurance was established by the AALL in 1912 to study the problem of health insurance and press for legislation. Initially the AMA's top leadership cooperated, and three members of its executive council served jointly on the AALL committee and on a corresponding AMA committee to study the question. In 1914 the committee advocated preliminary standards for a potential health insurance system reflecting the dominant political attitudes of the time (Anderson, 1968):

1. The system should be compulsory with contributions from employer, employee, and the public.
2. Those who were not in covered groups should be able to join the system voluntarily.
3. There should be a system of disability insurance supplementary to health insurance.
4. The system should be administered by employers and employees under public supervision. Private insurance carriers properly supervised might be utilized.
5. There should be emphasis on prevention of illness wherever possible.*

* Anderson (1968) notes the following in regard to these points: (1) The compulsory nature of contribution was radical for its day, but the tripartite source of contribution was conservative. It was not thought advisable to rely completely on general tax funds, although some believed they would provide the most equitable means of sharing an economic burden: (2) Although payroll deductions would make it difficult to enroll those who were self-employed, it was still thought desirable not to rely solely on general taxation; voluntary insurance was thus a necessary additional component to complete the system. (3) It was recognized that medical bills were only one of the costs of illness for the wage earner. The broader social-insurance philosophy behind the movement required dealing with the problem of lost income and abnormally high expenses during periods of sickness. (4) This is a neat example of government negotiating and arranging with the private sector to carry out obligations government has been given a mandate to assume. (5) This principle reflects the early strength of the public health philosophy of immunization, early diagnosis, and routine physical examinations.

Thus the problem of devising an ideological compromise was recognized from the beginning—between compulsory and voluntary approaches, between public and private financing and control, between centralized (public) and decentralized (private) administration. Similar compromise elements have continued to dominate most serious national health insurance (NHI) proposals down to the present. It has come to be axiomatic that only such a mixed compromise strategy for NHI stands a chance of enactment because of the competing political philosophies. Yet, in the intervening 65 years, despite almost continuous efforts, it has not been possible to attain enactment of such a compromise. The conflicting vested interests, which were the reason for the compromise in the first place, have been strong enough to prevent enactment of the total package. Many pieces of the scheme have been implemented as solutions to pressing parts of the health financing problem. The piecemeal nature of arriving at the system, however, has left serious gaps, overlaps, and no overall plan or fiduciary responsibility. This incoherent financing system accounts for much of the exorbitant cost and unsatisfactory, inefficient organization of our health services (Chapters 12, 13, and 14).

In 1916 proposed legislation was introduced in several state legislatures. The positions of the various interest groups emerged very quickly in response to these legislative initiatives and have continued to dominate the debate since. The first and most surprising opposition came from within the ranks of the AALL itself, from none other than Samuel Gompers, labor's chief spokesman. Appearing in 1916 before the Committee on Labor of the U.S. House of Representatives, Gompers testified vehemently against a commission "to recommend a plan for the establishment of a national insurance fund" for fear that it would be prejudiced in favor of a compulsory national health insurance program. Because unions had attracted membership through their health and welfare funds, Gompers feared that their hard-won position could be undermined by government insurance plans or even by state regulation of the union operated funds. Ironically, he urged the course of stimulating voluntary health insurance plans, which the AMA was later to use as the keystone of its opposition to government sponsored health benefits. Gompers remained adamantly opposed to compulsory social insurance until his death in 1924. Although many top labor leaders disagreed with Gompers, his position held sway for almost two decades. Thus, organized labor, representing the workers who seemed to have the most to gain from compulsory subsidized health insurance, became the first major roadblock to its early enactment (Anderson, 1968).

The second source of opposition was the private insurance industry, which established the Insurance Economic Society in 1916 to fight government sponsored compulsory insurance. They argued that the state and Federal governments should limit themselves to providing medical care for the indigent because compulsory health insurance would be the entering wedge of socialism. Private insurance companies already had 37 million industrial group insurance policies in force as a result of workers' compensation laws. Little of this industrial group insurance represented health coverage, yet companies were moving in this direction and did not want the government as a possible competitor or regulator (Anderson, 1968).

The third major source of opposition, and in the long run the most powerful, came from the AMA. This was a surprise to many at the time in view of the strong initial support the AMA had given to the AALL and the liberal reform position of the AMA during the first decade of the century when the medical societies had fought hard for the Pure Food and Drug Act, legislation for a national department of health, workers' compensation laws, and reforms in medical education. As discussed in Chapter 7, however, a profound change had taken place within the AMA itself between 1900 and 1920 because of the massive expansion of its membership through organizing activity. This converted it from an elite, academically controlled, liberal, reform organization into a broadly based self-interest guild (Burrow, 1963).

. . . Compulsory health insurance was the first issue where the clash came between the residual old liberal leadership and the new conservative protectionist group that now held the majority of delegates. After their initial warm support of the AALL recommendations on health insurance, Dr. Isaac Rubinow and other reform members of the AMA's committee on social insurance had to quickly retrench in 1916 and to recommend that more study be undertaken before any decision could be reached on health insurance. Opposition continued to grow at the state medical society level, and in 1920 the House of Delegates passed a resolution that unequivocally rejected the idea of any plan for compulsory health insurance. (Anderson, 1968, p. 74)

Other interested groups also solidified their ideological positions on health insurance during this first active period of debate on the subject. Hospitals had benefited from the payments for otherwise indigent patients under the workers' compensation laws and generally supported the idea of health insurance. However, the American Hospital Association (AHA) was not yet a well-established spokesman for the hospital interests, so that no formal position was taken. The American Nursing Association and the National Association of Public Health Nurses favored national health insurance, as did the U.S. Public Health Service (USPHS) and the American Public Health Association (APHA). But the first major drive to secure enactment of national health insurance legislation in this country met serious resistance and quickly died. The AALL's fight continued at the state level, for example, in New York and California, for a number of years, but without the support of either labor or the medical societies no legislation was successfully enacted. In the abortive attempt, however, the ideological positions of most parties at interest in health care questions were established and remained essentially unchanged until the present (Anderson, 1950). The one important exception was organized labor, which changed its perspective radically as a result of the Great Depression and the new labor legislation that grew out of it.

One precedent setting piece of health financing legislation was nevertheless enacted in the 1920s. The Sheppard-Towner Act passed in 1921 provided Federal matching grants-in-aid to state health departments for implementing and improving maternal and child health programs. The legislation grew out of pressure from the social work movement in the first decades of the century and the activity of the Federal Children's Bureau (created in 1912). Its objective was to establish prenatal and child health clinics for low-income families. Such clinics had been pioneered in New York City with the goal of reducing maternal and infant mortality and preventing childhood diseases through better nutrition and immunization (Mustard, 1945). This legislation established the precedent of Federal support for specific (categorical) health programs through state matching fund grants-in-aid. Allowed to expire in 1929, it was reinstituted as the Maternal and Child Health Program in Title V of the 1935 Social Security Act. The strategy has been used repeatedly for Federal financing of health care since then; Medicaid is the largest such program. The AMA unsuccessfully opposed the Sheppard-Towner bill in 1921 claiming, as with national health insurance, that it constituted "Federal interference in state affairs and regimentation of medical practice." Better organized AMA opposition was instrumental in defeating renewal of the legislation in 1929 (Stevens, 1971).

The 1920s also provided important preparation for later health care financing strategies through the collection of information and studies of the health care system. From 1921 to 1924 the U.S. Public Health Service (USPHS) conducted the first large-scale American study on the incidence of disease in a population (Hagerstown, Maryland) by age, sex, and family income. This was the prototype for the National Health Survey begun by the PHS in 1935, repeated intermittently, and now conducted continuously. It supplies much of our information on incidence and social background of disease in this country (Anderson, 1968). From 1927 to 1932 the Committee on the Costs of Medical Care (CCMC) carried out studies on the utilization of health services, costs, and the organization of medical care that first provided baseline information necessary for planning and action. A milestone in American medicine, the CCMC demonstrated the tremendous unevenness of health problems within the population (less than 4% of the families incurring 80% of the costs and the disastrous effects of large medical expenses on those families that were struck; CCMC, 1932). It received the support and cooperation of virtually every major group involved in the health sector, but its recommendations widened the ideological split about health care policy and hardened these positions for many years to come (Stevens, 1971).

The majority report included two strong recommendations: (1) spreading the risk of medical expenses through the *insurance* or tax mechanism and (2) providing of care through *organized groups* of health professionals. The report was pessimistic about the potential for private health insurance plans because of the poor experience in Europe. The majority argued against the prevailing fee-for-service method of payment, asserting that prepaid group medical practice would provide more protection for both patients and practitioners. The minority (dissenting) report, which was supported by the AMA and private insurance companies, bitterly renounced both recommendations and called for restoring the solo general practitioner to his central role in American medicine. They demanded guarantees of free choice of physicians (i.e. no closed-panel practice) and only voluntary (private) health insurance (Anderson, 1968).

THE GROWTH OF VOLUNTARY HEALTH INSURANCE

Despite workers' compensation laws which led many industries to purchase health and disability insurance for their employees, only 2% of the labor force was covered by 1930. The Great Depression and the activity of the American Hospital Association (AHA) played key roles in the establishment and growth of voluntary health insurance, particularly Blue Cross. During the Depression, hospital occupancy and receipts fell precipitously and deficits rose, threatening many with bankruptcy. The hospitals had a pressing interest in developing a stable source of payment for services (Somers & Somers, 1961). Several plans were founded for insuring payment of hospital expenses. The one generally considered the progenitor of Blue Cross, was started in 1929 in Dallas, Texas, by Dr. Kimball, the vice president of Baylor University. Finding many upaid bills from local schoolteachers among the accounts of the university's hospital, he enrolled 1250 teachers in a program to prepay fifty cents a month to assure payment for 21 days of semiprivate hospitalization at the Baylor University Hospital (Law, 1974).

Other hospital groups took up the idea and the American Hospital Association soon endorsed what became the Blue Cross concept, hospital insurance on a nonprofit basis as a public benefit corporation. With the backing of the AHA, Blue Cross organizations spread quickly during the late Depression. Of 39 Blue Cross plans established in the mid-1930s, 22 obtained all of their initial funds from hospitals, and 5 were partially financed by hospitals. In the 1940s membership grew rapidly, reaching 39 million by 1950 and 78 million by 1971. This expansion, which initially was much faster than for commercial health insurance carriers, resulted largely from the favored position of Blue Cross as a nonprofit, tax-exempt organization and from its unique relationship to hospitals. Between 1934 and 1945 laws were enacted in most states that legitimized Blue Cross' special position in the community as a nonprofit, semipublic agency. Blue Cross plans are exempt from many of the stringent incorporation and reserve requirements imposed by state insurance departments on other insurance companies (commercials) and from taxes on earned income. Consequently, public hearings are usually required prior to approval of rate increases (Law, 1974).

Most Blue Cross plans also differ from commercial carriers in their special financial arrangements with participating hospitals. Coverage to subscribers is specified in terms of gross hospital benefits (e.g., number of days, type of accommodation, etc.). Hospitals are reimbursed directly by Blue Cross for their full costs of providing the services ascribed to Blue Cross beneficiaries—so-called retrospective cost reimbursement (Hedinger, 1968). Allowable costs include operating and capital expenditures, as well as depreciation of plant and equipment. The reimbursement procedure of most commercial insurers, on the contrary, pays the charges set in advance by hospitals for specific services obtained by subscribers. A smaller group of commercial insurers pays some fixed dollar portion of the charge for a service leaving the patient with the rest of the bill (indemnity payment). Neither the charge-paying nor cost-paying mechanism provides much incentive to hold down costs since hospitals are virtually guaranteed full recapture of any expenditures no matter what their costs (or charges necessary to cover them).

Originally Blue Cross used the so-called community rating method to establish the premium for coverage. Under this system, all subscribers were actuarialized together, with uniform premiums set for the entire community service area regardless of age, sex, employer, past history, and so on. This has the advantage that the financing of the poorer risks is spread over the entire group in a uniform manner. Over the last two decades community rating has given way to so-called experience rating (Chapter 12). Introduced by commercial insurance companies, experience rating depends on group purchase of insurance (e.g., employees of a single company) and sets premiums on the basis of actual costs of services and utilization patterns of the specific group. Such a system holds down premiums for those in the prime of life, but it is a severe hardship for segments of the population in less perfect health. Elderly people (prior to Medicare), or the disabled and unemployed, have to purchase their insurance individually at a residual community rate. This results in much higher premiums because they are not members of a group that balances out their higher health costs. Blue Cross plans eventually also had to adopt experience rating for group policies to remain competitive with the commercials (Anderson, 1975). This development soon pushed residual individual policy premiums for the aged and the unemployed out of reach—making Medicare and Medicaid legislation more urgent. Co-insurance payments and deductibles, two other characteristics of private insurance, have also increasingly been incorporated into Blue Cross plans to reduce premiums through cost sharing and as a financial disincentive to hold down utilization.

COLLECTIVE BARGAINING FOR HEALTH INSURANCE

The Great Depression, the New Deal, and World War II brought a marked change in organized labor's position regarding health insurance. During the Depression many company sponsored health and welfare benefit plans collapsed. The Federal government took over the largest of these, the Railway Retirement System. In the early years of the Depression labor was not strong enough nor interested enough in health benefits to make this a major issue in collective bargaining (or to push for including health insurance in the Social Security Act of 1935). Strengthened by the Wagner Act (National Labor Relations Act of 1935), however, and under the powerful leadership of John L. Lewis of the United Mine Workers (UMW), the major heavy industries (steel and automobile manufacturing) were finally organized in the late 1930s. As the labor movement grew, so did the conviction that health and welfare benefits should not be at the discretion of paternalistic employers, but rather should be considered part of workers' compensation for their labor, to be negotiated at the bargaining table (Munts, 1967).

During World War II the wage stabilization policies stimulated nonwage forms of remuneration including health insurance because of a wage freeze and the special tax exemptions for such contributions. Unilaterally granted, however, the benefits remained under the control of management. In 1946 the new heavy-industry unions—inspired by the example of the UMW control over the health and welfare fund paid for by the employers—made such fringe benefits the chief target of collective bargaining (Becker, 1963). The employers resisted, claiming that the legal mandate to bargain in good faith over "wages and other conditions of employment" (included in the Wagner Act) did not mean such fringe benefits. The result was a series of court battles between management and unions. The most significant was the 1948 Inland Steel case and Supreme Court decision that ruled that management was required to negotiate over health benefits as "other conditions of employment" (Munts, 1967). By 1948 ten major unions had succeeded in negotiating health and welfare plans as fringe benefits. Thus a tremendous market for underwriting group health benefits emerged as a result of collectively bargained agreements.

Commercial life insurance companies moved quickly into this market. These companies became especially successful in negotiating with unions or employers to provide benefits agreed upon in collective bargaining for a group of employees. Group policy coverage is carefully tailored to the specific needs and finances of the union or company soliciting bids for their insurance plan and priced at the cost of their own utilization plus administration. Such experience-rated premiums on group policies are considerably lower than for the same coverage offered to the individual consumer by the same insurance company because the members tend to be healthier and because of lower marketing and administrative costs. Carriers return up to

95% of the group premiums in claims, but only about 50% on individual policies, making the latter very expensive. At the end of the year the carriers adjust group policy rates in accord with the benefits paid. Thus the carrier may make a refund to the employer, trust fund, or mutual company. This procedure is not applied to individual policy holders where a lower payout than the premium is simply profit, while an increase in payout is reflected in premium rate increases the following year (Marcus, 1980).

Over the last 30 years the share of the health insurance market controlled by the commercials has grown tremendously. This growth was largely a result of collective bargaining for health insurance as a fringe benefit of employment (Becker, 1963). Commercial policies accounted for only about 10% of all accident and health insurance in 1930. Even in 1940 only 25% of hospital insurance was commercial (covering 1.3 million Americans) because Blue Cross had expanded so rapidly. In the next decade, however, as fringe benefit contracts expanded the health insurance market, the large commercial carriers won a lion's share of the new group policy sales. By 1974 the commercials accounted for 115 million (56%) of the 208 million hospital policies, and approximately 78% of these were group policies (Health Insurance Institute, 1979).

Similar developments have since taken place in the underwriting of surgical expenses and, more recently, of major medical expenses. Nevertheless, in the 1950s it became apparent that voluntary health insurance alone could not solve the problems of paying for health care. Premium costs were rising at a rate that threatened to make insurance unmarketable, and still it had not been possible to expand benefits beyond the point of paying 25% of the total health expenditure bill. Certain groups were essentially excluded from coverage: the poor who were unemployed or employed at jobs with no health benefits, such as migratory workers and domestics; and the aged, retired, or disabled for whom nongroup health insurance could scarcely be brought because of the high utilization and premium rates (Falk, 1973).

ORIGIN OF MEDICARE AND MEDICAID

As part of the social reform legislation of the mid-1960s, Medicare and Medicaid were intended to provide from tax revenues the benefits for the aged and the indigent that employees enjoyed under insurance from fringe benefits. Between 1929 and 1965 many precedents were set that helped shape the final form of Medicare and Medicaid legislation. The Federal Emergency Relief Act of 1933 included a provision for medical care for those on relief. There was hope that the Social Security Act would include some form of national health insurance. However, the well-organized opposition from the AMA convinced many that such an attempt might jeopardize the chances for enactment of the more urgent unemployment and old age retirement benefits of the act. Title V of the Social Security Act reinstated the maternal and child health grants-in-aid to states of the Sheppard-Towner act. This reaffirmed the responsibility of the Federal government to support health care for certain special indigent or dependent groups. This principle of shared Federal and state responsibility for "welfare medicine" was never seriously challenged again (Anderson, 1968).

Studies on health, medical care, and health insurance of Americans conducted by the Social Security Board demonstrated conclusively that available services fell far short of needs. This study set in motion a series of legislative initiatives that eventually culminated in Medicare. President Roosevelt appointed the Technical Committee on Medical Care in 1937, which recommended major expansion of Federal assistance to local public health services, hospital construction, and a "general program of medical care." This was interpreted by many as a new call for national health insurance and led to a series of such bills in Congress beginning with the Wagner Bill of 1939 and continued in almost every session of Congress until 1965. Although these bills were supported by President Roosevelt and then even more strongly by President Truman, none succeeded in getting beyond committee hearings. However, the Hill-Burton legislation enacted in 1946 provided Federal financial assistance for the construction of hospitals and health centers enabling widespread expansion of facilities in underserved areas during the ensuing 25 years. During World War II Emergency Maternal and Infant Care (EMIC) established the Federal precedent of paying providers in accord with stated costs for services to beneficiaries. This method became the norm for later Federal health care financing programs (Sinai & Anderson, 1948; Anderson, 1968).

Congress repeatedly rejected national health insurance legislation in spite of the clear evidence of need and the growing majority of sentiment among the electorate in favor of it. The well-organized, well-financed, lobbying effort of the AMA against national health insurance was undoubtedly one important factor—though not the only one. Several liberal senators who had supported the Truman proposals were defeated in the 1948 election with the help of large-scale AMA campaign contributions to their opponents. The AMA conducted an intensive advertising campaign against "government interference in the privacy of the doctor-patient relationship" (financed by a special "war chest" assessment from each member). This campaign brought hundreds of letters pouring into Congressmen's offices and helped defeat the 1951 bill (Burrow, 1963). There was no equally well-organized or financed lobbying effort from proponents of the national health insurance bills during this period. In the 1950s organized labor, though favoring the bills, was preoccupied with establishing its strength and prerogatives in collective bargaining as a means of obtaining health insurance benefits for its members. The rapid growth of voluntary health insurance in the early 1950s convinced many that government sponsored health insurance programs would not be necessary except for those "outside the mainstream" such as the poor or those with disabilities like tuberculosis, blindness, or mental illness—who had always depended on charity or public assistance.

Underlying this hope that private insurance could solve the health care financing problem was a long-standing ideological dichotomy in American attitudes toward the welfare system. Nearly all public welfare programs in this country include a division between the "social insurance" and the "residual welfare" concepts of assistance (Wilensky & Lebeaux, 1965). The social insurance concept, which is embodied in the Social Security system and private health insurance, is built on the "promote the general welfare" (collective action) tradition of government. In these programs government or private institutions assist individuals to attain "satisfying standards of life and health" by providing certain services in times of need as "entitlement" because of previous participation or contribution to the system. The concept is one of sharing the risk by collective action, prepayment, or mitigation of chance misfortune through the insurance principle. Government may act as the organizing and fiscal agent in such programs but does not directly provide services or pay for them out of general tax revenues. Such assistance is not looked upon as charity but rather as "one's just due" resulting from prudence on the part of the participant. Whether such planning was actually intended or simply occurred as a result of employment, there is no stigma attached to assistance gained through such entitlement (Marmor, 1970).

The "residual" concept of public welfare, which is embodied in such programs as Aid to the Blind (AB) and Aid to Families of Dependent Children (AFDC), is an outgrowth of the charity tradition. Historically this has been combined with the mandate for the social control of undesirable or fear-evoking members of society. Hospitals prior to the medical technological revolution exhibited both features of the charity tradition. They provided asylums of last resort for the indigent sick and prisonlike regulation of such persons. Direct government support of services through general tax revenues has been considered proper only for such residual welfare programs, based on its responsibility to guarantee at least certain minimal standards of subsistence for all citizens (Chapter 7). Because of the charity aspect of residual welfare programs, they always carry some degree of social stigma. The person accepting such help is looked upon as "undesirable"— at the very least unfortunate, but more likely as a failure, lazy, or even immoral. Because welfare recipients are a drain on the public purse, so-called "means tests" are required to prove that candidates are both in need of assistance and deserving of it. Demonstration of "need" entails examination of the person's finances and personal life circumstances. Demonstration that one is "deserving" usually requires showing the proper attitude and readiness to submit to the life-style regulation imposed by the welfare agencies. Administration of such programs is often paternalistic, punitive, and imposes control in accord with the values and norms of the agencies. Residual welfare programs tend to be piecemeal (categorical) for special groups, such as dependent children, and left to local authorities to administer. Residual welfare programs are usually noncontributory and supported by general tax revenues (or philanthropy), which are *progressive* taxes having an income redistribution effect. On the contrary, social insurance welfare programs like Social Security or voluntary health insurance are traditionally paid for by payroll taxes or equal contributions from all participants, which are *regressive* taxes having little or no income redistribution effect (Wilensky & Lebeaux, 1965).

The combination of different administrative, ideological, and taxation characteristics involved in the two approaches to welfare, often leads to peculiar political coalitions and legislative strategies in securing their enactment. Nongovernmental social insurance programs are the easiest. They require negotiation only between the few parties directly involved and have the ideological support of the prevailing free-market philosophy of this country. Government social insurance programs are very difficult to enact. They require broad middle-of-the-road coalitions, which in turn necessitate either a massive public mandate arising from dire need (such as the Depression leading to the Social Security Act) or a very delicate compromise to secure political agreement (combined with public pressure), as with Medicare. Despite the stigma attached and the general dissatisfaction with residual welfare programs, they can be easier to enact. It is often possible to put together a coalition of liberal Congressmen who favor the income redistribution or support a special disadvantaged group, moderates who recognize the need and accept government's responsibility for it, and some conservatives, who see the approach as a hedge against the danger of broader social insurance programs. A compromise is necessary between adequately meeting the needs of the recipients (to please the liberals) and sufficiently stringent limits on the size of the program (to satisfy the conservatives). As a result of the philosophical conflicts in each welfare approach, it is difficult to get a solid alliance for any single legislative strategy. Subtle shifts in public opinion or minor changes in the composition of Congress can profoundly influence the chances of success (Marmor, 1970). Many of the same arguments, coalitions, and strategies that shaped the history of the Medicare-Medicaid legislation will undoubtedly arise again in the coming struggle over national health insurance (Chapter 14). It is, therefore, worth examining its final emergence in some detail.

After the failure of the Wagner-Murray-Dingell Bill in 1949 and 1950, the Truman Administration saw that a new strategy was necessary. The unsuccessful bill had called for universal entitlement through a compulsory 3% payroll tax (divided equally between employer and employee), with grants from general revenues for the unemployed and destitute not reached by the contributory plan. Thus, it was essentially a social insurance type program with appended residual welfare features for those who would otherwise be excluded. The prospect of a new regressive payroll tax, which would hit the working man hardest, made it unpopular with the moderates. Voluntary health insurance, which appeared capable of dealing with the problem at the time, was preferable to most of the middle-of-the-road members of Congress needed to pass the bill. Federal administration of the program (as well as universal entitlement) raised the fear of government interference with medical practice among physicians and challenged the vested interest of the insurance companies and Blue Cross, so that both the AMA and the AHA staunchly opposed it—as did the conservative members of Congress (Hyde & Wolff, 1954). Thus in spite of the popular support for national health insurance, which Truman had made a successful issue in the 1948 election, there was no chance for this approach even to get out of committee, especially the fiscally conservative Ways and Means Committee (Feingold, 1966).

Searching for a new legislative strategy, Oscar Ewing, Administrator of the Federal Security Agency (predecessor to the Department of Health, Education, and Welfare), decided to concentrate on Federal health insurance only for the *aged* using the Social Security System. This was to serve as an entering wedge, and then coverage could be expanded to other groups. Limiting the program to the aged and using the Social Security system as the fiscal mechanism was meant to bridge the two welfare strategies and attract members of both potential coalitions. Social Security had become the most respected of the social insurance approaches. Participatory entitlement freed it of stigma, and the efficient record of administration made it the most popular of government programs. The aged as a group were financially poorly off so that universal entitlement seemed justified while nevertheless convincing conservatives that the program was limited to the needy. Not only were the elderly generally living on low fixed incomes, but they were also subject to the highest medical expenses and had to pay exorbitant rates for health insurance because of the rapid move toward experience-rated premiums for employed groups—or were denied insurance entirely. In order to avert the fear of physicians about government regulation, only hospital services were included. To counter the concern about cost from high utilization, the plan was limited to 60 days of hospitalization per year, acknowledging but accepting the remaining danger of incurring catastrophic sickness costs (Marmor, 1970).

The legislation, soon dubbed "Medicare," was first introduced in 1952 and in every subsequent year until its passage in 1965. However, President Eisenhower's election and opposition to any form of national health insurance deferred hearings on the bill until 1958 when it was sponsored by Rep. Aime Forand (Dem., R.I.). Despite the careful attempt to draft a bill that would threaten the medical establishment as little as possible, it was violently opposed in Congressional hearings by both the AHA and the AMA. An extensive public advertising campaign against the bill was waged by the AMA. Organized labor for the first time carried on a similar but unsuccessful counterattack. The bill was overwhelmingly rejected in the Ways and

Means Committee. Conservatives believed that the measure would be too expensive for the Social Security system to absorb and that it needed to be limited to the truly indigent aged by using a means test. Liberals feared it would not be adequate to deal with catastrophic illness expenses (Feingold, 1966).

The following year Sen. Robert Kerr (Dem., Ok.) and Rep. Wilbur Mills (Dem., Ark.) introduced and Congress quickly enacted an opposing bill that dealt with both objections by reverting to the opposite (residual welfare) strategy. The Kerr-Mills bill limited coverage to the aged with insufficient financial resources to meet medical expenses, but provided them comprehensive benefits including physician services, hospitalization, drug, and nursing home care. It was financed from (progressive) general tax revenues, by matching grants to states, and was administered by the states. It was known that this method of financing would severely limit utilization and cost because most states would not set high enough eligibility levels to require very significant matching funds. This made it more acceptable to the fiscal conservatives of the Ways and Means Committee. After three years of operation, 90% of the Kerr-Mills funds were being used by five of the largest industrial states with good tax bases and a long history of liberal social welfare policies, but having only 32% of the population over 65 (Greenfield, 1966). Eighteen states had no programs at all. The AMA initially opposed the Kerr-Mills proposal but soon recognized it as a convenient hedge to prevent passage of the more extensive Forand Medicare legislation. The Kerr-Mills proposal was enacted in 1960, but the election of President Kennedy the same year, who was pledged to universal hospital insurance for the aged, foreshadowed a continuing fight over Medicare (Marmor, 1970).

A modified Forand bill was introduced in 1961 as the King-Anderson medicare proposal, but was repeatedly held up in the Ways and Means Committee by the fiscally conservative, powerful chairman, Wilbur Mills, and a coalition of conservative Democrats and Republicans. Unwilling to face a showdown with Mills, the new administration waited for the composition of the committee to be gradually changed by new appointments from the more friendly House leadership (Marmor, 1970). During this period the AMA stepped up its campaign against Medicare and acquired much of the onus for its delay, which was actually more a result of the fiscal concerns of the Ways and Means Committee. One other change in the political alignment occurred in 1962. An agreement was reached with the AHA to support Medicare in exchange for the concession that the Social Security Administration would use "fiscal intermediaries" to handle the payment of claims and protect hospitals from interference by government administrators.

The Johnson landslide of 1964 on a platform of the "Great Society" social reforms made the passage of Medicare almost a certainty in 1965. If the Mills coalition had chosen to resist, it would have been possible to override the Ways and Means Committee with the new Democratic majority in the House of Representatives. Seeing the inevitability, the Republicans and the AMA abandoned open opposition and attempted instead to influence the content of the final version of the law by proposing substitute measures. The AMA sponsored "Eldercare," a bill that would have extended the Kerr-Mills program by authorizing states to buy private health insurance for the needy aged, while retaining the means tests, state matching fund requirement, and state administration. The Republicans introduced the Byrnes bill, which would add insurance for physician services and drugs to the King-Anderson hospital benefits. It also required voluntary premium contributions from participants (matched by Federal general revenues) and imposed more extensive co-insurance and deductibles. Hearings began almost immediately and were completed quickly because of the accumulated testimony from past Congresses and the desire for rapid Congressional action (Feingold, 1966).

Instead of reporting out any one of the bills (presumably King-Anderson), however, Mills put together a new compromise bill containing elements of all three. King-Anderson became Medicare (Title XVIII) Part A, hospital care financed completely by the Social Security system with universal entitlement for Social Security beneficiaries, but with increased co-insurance and deductibles. The Byrnes Bill became Medicare part B, voluntary, contributory, physician-services insurance for Social Security beneficiaries, partially subsidized by the government, but without coverage for out-of-hospital drugs. Eldercare (the extension of Kerr-Mills) was incorporated as Medicaid (Title XIX) with a broad range of benefits for the indigent (no longer limited to the elderly poor) leaving the states discretion to set eligibility and precise benefits. It was financed out of general revenues as matching grants to states, which would administer their own programs. Medicare claims processing and payment was to be handled by the fiscal agent chosen by the hospitals in each area, which predictably was Blue Cross in most cases. Under Medicaid the choice of fiscal mechanism was left to the states. Thus the final legislation involved both welfare approaches, as well as compromises on cost control and administrative policies (Marmor, 1970; Radovsky, 1965).

Medicare did succeed in bringing the elderly back into the main stream of medical care by paying most of their health bill, but at a cost that has exceeded all expectations (U.S. Senate Finance Committee, 1970). Medicaid on the other hand, which is administered with different standards by each state, has tended to perpetuate a second-class system of health care for the poor (Stevens & Stevens, 1974). Parallel to the new government health financing programs, continuation of private health insurance (subsidized by tax write-offs and pass-alongs to consumer prices) has created a morass of indirect financing devoid of responsibility for budget control or resource allocation. Simply pouring more dollars into the present system of care through the existing mechanism of third-party reimbursement has not solved the problem of providing access to adequate health care to all (Davis, 1973, 1975, 1976). The effect has been the highest rate of health cost inflation in history without evidence of equivalent improvement in quality or availability of services (Chapter 12). Fundamental changes will be needed in the organization and distribution of services, as well as financing, to accomplish that. The health insurance system has become a mutually supportive superstructure to the present, intensive technology-oriented delivery system—both a product of it and a major mechanism for its perpetuation and expansion. The 1965 legislation intensified this situation by channeling a massive influx of tax dollars through the same financing system.

REFERENCES

Anderson, Odin W., "Health Insurance in the United States 1910–1920," *Journal of the History of Medicine & Allied Science,* 5:363–396, 1950.

Anderson, Odin W., *The Uneasy Equilibrium,* New Haven, Conn.: College and University Press, 1968.

Anderson, Odin W., "The Politics of Universal Health Insurance in the United States," *International Journal of Health Services,* 2:577–582, 1972.

Anderson, Odin W., *Blue Cross Since 1929: Accountability and the Public Trust,* Cambridge: Ballinger, 1975.

Becker, Harry, "Voluntary Health Insurance," *Current History,* 45:(August):92–97, 1963.

Burrow, James G., *AMA: Voice of American Medicine,* Baltimore: Johns Hopkins University Press, 1963.

Committee on the Costs of Medical Care, *Medical Care for the American People,* Chicago: University of Chicago Press, reprinted, USDHEW, 1970, 1932.

Davis, Karen, "Theories of Hospital Inflation: Some Empirical Evidence," *Journal of Human Resources,* 8(Spring):181–201, 1973.

Davis, Karen, "Equal Treatment and Unequal Benefits: The Medicare Program," *Health and Society,* 53:449, 1975.

Davis, Karen, "Achievements and Problems of Medicaid," *Public Health Reports,* 91(4): 316, 1976.

Falk, Isador S., "Medical Care in the USA—1932–1972. Problems, Proposals and Programs from the Committee for National Health Insurance," *Health and Society,* 51:1, 1973.

Feingold, Eugene, *Medicare: Policy and Politics: A Case Study and Policy Analysis,* San Francisco: Chandler, 1966.

Feldstein, Paul J., *Health Associations and the Demand for Legislation: The Political Economy of Health,* Lexington, Mass.: Ballinger, 1977.

Fennor, R., "The Internal Distribution of Influence: The House," in Truman, D., Ed., *The Congress and the America's Future,* Englewood Cliffs, N.J.: Prentice-Hall, 1965.

Fennor, R., *Congressmen in Committees,* Boston: Little, Brown, 1973.

Fried, Charles, "Equality and Rights in Medical Care," *Hastings Center Report,* 6(February):29–34, 1976.

Greenfield, Margaret, *Health Insurance for the Age: The 1965 Program for Medicare,* Berkeley: Institute of Government Studies, University of California, 1966.

Health Insurance Institute, *Health Insurance Fact Book, 1979,* Chicago: Health Insurance Association of America, 1979.

Hedinger, Frederick R., "The Social Role of Blue Cross: Progress and Problems," *Inquiry,* 5:12, 1968.

Hofstadter, Richard, *The Age of Reform,* New York: Random House, 1955.

Huitt, R., "The Internal Distribution of Influence: The Senate," in Truman, D., Ed., *The Congress and America's Future,* Englewood Cliffs, N.J.: Prentice-Hall, 1965.

Hyde, David R., and Wolff, Payson, "The American Medical Association: Power, Purpose, and Politics in Organized Medicine," *Yale Law Journal* 63:938–1022, 1954.

Law, Sylvia A., *Blue Cross: What Went Wrong?,* New Haven: Yale University Press, 1974.

Marcus, Glenn, "Group Health Insurance Premium Setting," Washington, D.C.: Congressional Research Service, 1980.

Marmor, Theodore, *The Politics of Medicare,* Chicago: Aldine, 1970.

Munts, Raymond, *Bargaining for Health: Labor Unions, Health Insurance, and Medical Care,* Madison: University of Wisconsin Press, 1967.

Mustard, Harry S., *Government in Public Health,* New York: Commonwealth Fund, 1945.

Radovsky, Saul S., "The Advent of Medicare," *New England Journal of Medicine,* **278**: 249–252, 1965.

Sinai, Nathan, and Anderson, Odin W., *Emergency Maternity and Infant Care,* Ann Arbor, 1948.

Somers, Herman M., and Somers, Anne R., *Doctors, Patients and Health Insurance,* Washington, D.C.: Brookings Institution, 1961.

Somers, Herman M., and Somers, Anne R., *Workman's Compensation,* New York: Wiley, 1954.

Stevens, Robert, and Stevens, Rosemary, *Welfare Medicine in America: A Case Study of Medicaid,* New York: Free Press, 1974.

Stevens, Rosemary, *American Medicine and the Public Interest,* New Haven: Yale University Press, 1971.

U.S. Senate, Finance Committee, *Medicare and Medicaid: Problems, Issues, and Alternatives, Report of the Staff,* Washington, D.C.: Government Printing Office, 1970.

Wilensky, Harold L., and Lebeaux, Charles N., *Industrial Society and Social Welfare,* New York: Free Press, 1965.

CHAPTER TWELVE

Cost and Financing of Health Care

Much of the controversy about the American health care system in recent years has centered around the problem of rising costs. Over the last decades expenditures for health care have been increasing more rapidly than most other major items in the consumer market basket. In 1950 a total of $12.7 billion ($82 per capita) was spent in the United States for health services, including both private and public expenditures.* In 1978, $192.4 billion ($863 per capita) was spent for health services (Figure 12-1; Table 12-1†). Thus expenditures increased fifteenfold in the 28-year period. During the same time the Gross National Product (GNP), the usual index of overall economic activity and growth, increased only sevenfold. As a result health expenditures accounted for 9.1% of the GNP in 1978, as compared with 4.5% in 1950. The present national expenditure for health care is three-fourths of the total national outlay for food, or more than half again as large as the budget for national defense. If the rate of growth in health expenditures were to continue at the same rate in relation to the GNP as between 1966 and 1978, in 30 years 25% of national production would go into health care. This would be more than the portion of the GNP that now goes into the entire Federal budget for all public goods, services, and transfer payments.

How is the nation to decide what fraction of GNP is "too much" or the "right amount" to spend for health care? And who is to make the decision or implement it? Swedish health planners, for instance, anticipate health care expenditures amounting to 12 to 15% of their GNP within the next few years (Anderson, 1980). It is sometimes argued that no amount is too much to pay for health care, because without one's health nothing else matters. Few challenged this argument as long as health care represented a small

---

* Unless otherwise stated, all statistical and cost data used in this chapter are taken from the *Statistical Abstract of the United States* (U.S. Bureau of the Census, 1979); *Health, United States, 1979* (USDHEW, 1980); or "National Health Expenditures, 1978" (Gibson, 1979).

† All tables referenced in this chapter appear in the Statistical Appendix at the end of the chapter and are intended as more detailed information to supplement the figures.

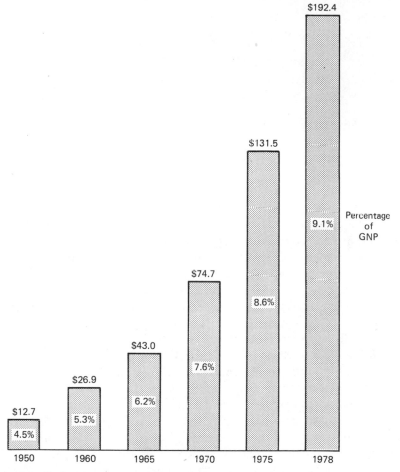

Figure 12.1. National health expenditures (in billions) and percent of gross national product for selected calendar years from 1950–1978 (compare Table 12.1). Source: Gibson, R. M., "National Health Expenditures 1978," *Health Care Finance Review*, 1(1), 1979.

part of national production and the economy was expanding rapidly. Additional health costs could be absorbed with little burden. Under today's economic conditions, however, we are forced to come to grips with the fact that medical care is but one of many basic needs essential to sustain health. Since a society's productive resources and financing are limited, national (and individual) consumption must be budgeted among competing goods and services. If the growth of health costs continues so out of proportion to the general economic growth, corresponding reductions will be necessary in the country's nutrition, housing, education, defense, or other vital budget items. Faced with these tradeoffs, many are questioning whether the present rate of escalation in health care spending makes sense (Kisch, 1974; Fuchs, 1974; Cochrane, 1971; McKinlay & McKinlay, 1977).

The proper question regarding health expenditures is not whether, considered in isolation, it is good to spend so much on medical care. The question is whether the general welfare is better served by allocating a larger portion of the total available resources for medical care and less for other goods and services or vice versa. According to economic theory, to maximize utility from a limited budget, we should apportion it among competing demands in such a way that the marginal benefit from each additional dollar spent for any item just balances the benefits lost by taking it away from other items (P. Feldstein, 1979). Unfortunately we do not have precise methods of estimating the health benefits to be expected from additional expenditures for health care—or agreement about the relative value (utility) of health benefits versus benefits from other budget items.

This is, of course, true for most other commodities as well. Yet it usually presents no problem in appropriately allocating budgets. Each consumer can make the choice for himself on the basis of his subjective evaluation of how much he wants to use of one commodity as opposed to another at their relative prices. Collectively through the market these individual decisions lead to an allocation of the national consumer budget that maximizes perceived utility. This occurs without explicitly evaluating the relative marginal utilities of the various commodities competing for the limited budget. However, the indirect (tax and insurance) method of paying for health care makes it both unnecessary and impossible for each consumer to decide individually how much he prefers to spend for health care rather than other commodities. As a result, the market cannot provide a collective evaluation of the relative utility of health care as it does for most commodities. We are forced to rely on expert judgments and the political process representing public opinion to decide whether the expenditure level for health care is too high or too low. Using these guides, we must attempt to weigh the benefits of additional health care against the personal and societal tradeoffs necessary to pay for it.

THE BURDEN OF HEALTH CARE COSTS

Medical costs have become a heavy burden on all Americans. This is most dramatic when hospitalization or other expensive care leads to a financial catastrophe if insurance benefits are exceeded. In 1977 some 7 million Americans had uninsured *out-of-pocket* medical expenses exceeding 15% of their income (USDHEW, 1979). But these cases of catastrophic out-of-pocket expenditures represent only a tiny fraction of the total impact of medical costs. The average citizen—who might not even have an episode of illness in a given year—bears a heavy burden of health costs. Most of this is paid so indirectly that it is seldom perceived as outlays for health care at all. Nonetheless, the financial drain on personal resources is just as real. National health care expenditures per family were over $2800 in 1978, 12.6%

of the median family income. If this had to be paid directly the average household would find it onerous indeed. Because it is diffused and disguised for most, the impact is felt instead through the effect on their general economic situation—by way of higher taxes, higher prices, and lower wages. Regardless of how indirectly the cost is imposed, the average family had $2800 less to spend on food, housing, or other goods and services because of its hidden contributions to health expenditures.

Almost 40% of total health care payment takes place directly through the tax system. Thirteen cents of every Federal tax dollar, personal and corporate, is used for health expenditures. This includes the portion (one-sixth) of the Social Security tax that goes for Medicare hospital coverage which is supplemented for medical services by general revenues in addition to premiums. Additional state and local tax funds are paid for Medicaid, public hospitals, and preventive care. Another 12% of health care expenditures is financed indirectly through the tax-reduction subsidies to private health insurance premiums, which must be made up in other tax payments (Sunley, 1980). Thus an appreciable portion of the family's tax burden, which subtracts from its disposable income, actually represents payment for health care.

Another way that health costs strike the average family indirectly is through their contribution to inflation, "the cruelest tax." From 1965 to 1978 hospital and physician prices outpaced the overall Consumer Price Index (CPI) by a wide margin (Figure 12.2; Table 12.2 and 12.3). However, the medical care component is given only a small weight in the CPI corresponding to the small portion of health costs and health insurance paid *directly* by consumers—*not* the portion of the GNP accounted for by health spending (Dyckman, 1978). Therefore the *direct* impact of health care inflation on the CPI appears quite small. But the largest portion of health payments do not appear in the CPI under the label of "health costs" at all. Private health insurance, which pays 27% of the health bill, is mostly obtained as a fringe benefit of employment. Employers pay 85% of the premiums on the average, and these costs are largely passed on to consumers as inflation of the prices for the goods and services produced. Yet, this impact on inflation is not accounted to health costs in the CPI. Employer payroll and corporate income taxes used to support government health programs are similarly passed on in higher prices but also do not appear under the health label in the CPI. This *indirect* impact on inflation of these indirect payments for health care is many times larger than its direct contribution to the cost of living. The Congressional Budget Office, for example, estimates that the total inflationary impact of hospital costs is three to four times their direct effect on the CPI (C.B.O., 1979). Some analysts estimate that through all its direct, indirect, and ripple effects, health care inflation accounted for as much as 14% of all inflation in the economy from 1974 to 1978 (USDHEW, 1979a). Other experts estimate the inflation impact of health costs is somewhat less by assuming that a larger part of the employer costs are passed back to employees as lower wage settlements rather than forward as higher

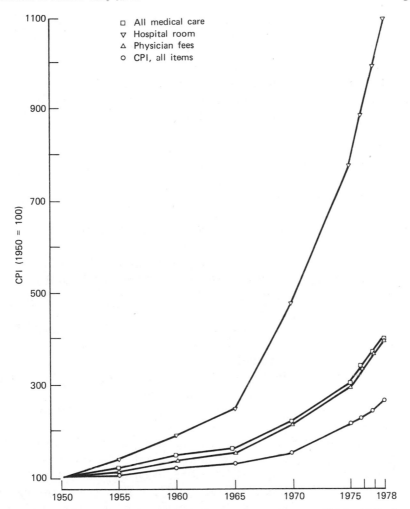

Figure 12.2. Consumer Price Index for selected items (compare Table 12.2). Source: USDHEW, 1979.

prices.* But the net impact on real consumer purchasing power is just as great either way.

Inflation is widely perceived as the number one domestic problem be-

---

* A more precise appraisal of hospitals' contribution to the total economy's inflation rate would require a macroeconomic model in which one could test the sensitivity of overall inflation to changes in the rate of hospital cost increases. Such a detailed model is not currently available. Even if all other components were in place, there are no good data for estimating the extent to which cost increases of hospital fringe benefits are passed forward as higher product prices, backward in lower wage settlements, or absorbed by the employer as lower profits (Schultze, 1978). Since 45% of hospital costs are paid in this way, such an estimate would be critical to the accuracy of the model. If the fringe benefit costs were entirely passed forward in higher prices, as recent collective bargaining settlements suggest, the estimate of 14% contribution to the total inflation rate would be correct.

cause it drains consumer purchasing power, destroys investor confidence, and ultimately cripples the economy. Since health expenditures contribute such a major portion to that inflation, the burden must be seen as serious in weighing it against potential benefits. Until recently, however, most individuals have not been aware of the major inflationary impact from health costs because so little comes directly out of their own pockets. Even employees' own contributions to health insurance premiums are usually deducted from the pay check, so they seem like diminished wages rather than higher costs. Thus despite the growing concern about inflation and taxes, few consumers have perceived the connection to health costs.

Business outlays for employee health benefits and tax contributions to health programs are a major element in production costs and therefore a significant obstacle in hiring considerations and business productivity (Schultze, 1978). Rising health costs have become a stumbling block to labor in collective bargaining. Premium payments by employers drain off funds that might otherwise go to workers in the form of higher wages, pensions, or other benefits. Health fringe benefit payments take an ever larger piece out of wage settlements because of the open-ended costs. Union health and welfare trust funds are being depleted by high health care outlays. For instance, one of the major issues delaying settlement of the prolonged 1977 coal strike was the cutback in health benefits as a result of insolvency in the United Mine Workers' trust funds.

The impact on government budgets and taxes is another source of the growing discontent about health costs. Many states have had to cut back on Medicaid eligibility and benefit levels and other health programs because of the drain on their budgets (Stevens & Stevens, 1974; Dukakis, 1978). The Federal budget for Medicare and Medicaid in fiscal year 1980 increased by $5.9 billion over fiscal year 1979 with no significant increase in services. This *increment* alone is more than HEW's entire social services budget or all its discretionary health services programs including manpower training, prevention, maternal and child health, community health services, and so on. Such an escalation in costs for entitlement (nonappropriated) programs severely limits any new social programs and jeopardizes attempts to balance the Federal budget. Without effective health cost containment, government either has to raise taxes, increase deficits, or cut back on health benefits, throwing the burden back onto the aged and others who are most vulnerable to rising health costs.

While we all value health care and want to ensure its availability when needed, the severe impact of health care costs on consumers, businesses, governments, and the general economy raises doubts whether the money is well spent in this way. A consensus is emerging that the growth in expenditures for medical care is out of proportion to the improved benefits it provides (Benham & Benham, 1975; Auster et al., 1969). Even if the single goal of maximizing health is considered (without taking into account the necessary tradeoffs with other societal goals), it is still questionable whether increased spending for medical care is the best way to improve the health of the population. There is considerable evidence that much medical care produces little demonstrable marginal benefit for the patient. Allocating more resources for housing, education, environmental protection, mass transit, new jobs, or even recreation might improve the population's health more than spending the same amount for medical care (Fuchs, 1974). The chronic disease problems of post-clinical medicine (Chapter 5) are even less likely to be helped by growth in spending for clinical care. They could probably be impacted more by greater investment to improve the social and physical environments. Similarly, social and economic support to improve the quality of life of the aged and those who suffer from chronic disabilities would probably contribute more to their well-being than increased spending for medical care in the narrower sense.

THE CAUSES OF RISING HEALTH CARE COSTS: WHERE DOES THE MONEY GO AND WHY?

Why, then, do we increase our spending for medical care so rapidly if it is already such an economic burden and there is so little evidence that it contributes commensurately to improving the nation's health? To track down the causes of rising health care costs, two questions must be answered: (1) Where do the growing expenditures go? (2) What factors account for their going there?

Expenditures for hospital services make up the largest item in the health budget, accounting for 40% of the spending for health services in 1978 (Figure 12.3; Table 12.4). They also account for the largest part of the increase, taking a bigger slice of the health budget each year. From 1967 (the first year with a full impact of Medicare) until 1978, the average rate of increase in expenditures for hospitals was 14% per year—nearly doubling total outlays every five years (Table 12.5).* Even from 1950 to 1965, prior to the stimulus of Medicare and Medicaid payments, the growth rate of hospital costs was half again as fast as the GNP growth (Davis, 1972, 1973a). This massive budget share and rate of growth is the major reason for so much emphasis on the problem of hospital costs. Strategies for controlling health expenditures are forced to deal foremost with hospital outlays. Nursing homes, which were little used in 1950, now provide a great deal of long-term care (much of which might otherwise be given in general hospitals). Nursing

---

* The growth rate was even faster if only short-term general hospitals are considered. Expenditures for long-term psychiatric and tuberculosis hospital care which made up 25% of total hospital expenditures in 1950 declined to 3% by 1960. The decrease was due to a declining number of psychiatric and TB patient days per capita, and to lower rate, of cost increase in these hospitals than in general hospitals.

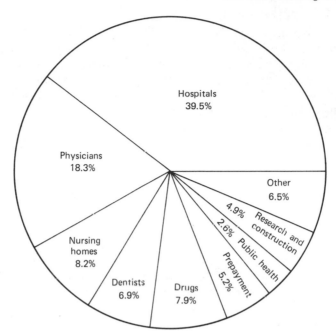

Figure 12.3. National health expenditures by category of service, 1978 (compare Table 12.4). Source: Gibson, R. M., "National Health Expenditures 1978," *Health Care Finance Review*, 1(1), 1979.

homes account for another 8% of the growth in the health services budget. Together hospitals and nursing homes absorbed almost half of the funds spent for health services in 1978.

Expenditures for physician services make up the second largest item of the health care budget. In 1978 physician services comprised almost 20% of the total spent for medical care. Like hospital costs, total physician expenditures have grown rapidly in recent years, at an average annual rate of 9.5% from 1950 to 1978—compared to 7.3% for the GNP—and even more rapidly (11.9% per year) since 1966 (Table 12.5). Although physician expenditures make up a smaller part of the total annual increment in health care costs than do hospital costs, 34% of physician expenditures are uninsured and paid directly out of pocket compared to only 10% of hospital costs (Figure 12.4; Table 12.7). As a result patients feel the increases in physician costs more directly. The elderly are particularly hard hit. The combination of their Medicare physician insurance premiums, deductibles, 20% co-insurance, and the large portion of physician billings beyond the maximum allowable Medicare fees results in their paying almost 60% of their health costs out of their often very limited incomes (Gibson & Fisher, 1979).

Besides these direct costs, in the process of rendering their own services physicians also make the decisions leading to 80% of all medical costs—generating $3.40 in other health costs for every $1 paid directly for their own

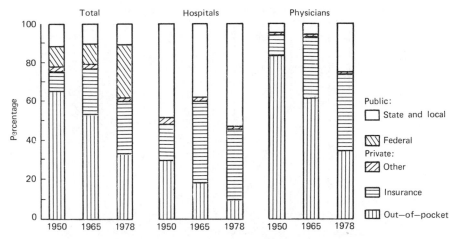

Figure 12.4. Percentage distribution of personal health care expenditures by type of service and source of financing (selected years). Other includes philanthropy, employee health services, and so forth. (Compare Table 12.7.) Source: Gibson, 1979.

services (Blumberg, 1978). These decisions are influenced by the same factors responsible for the rapid expansion of direct physician costs. Consequently physician expenditures and reimbursement mechanisms have an economic importance far greater than the actual amount spent on this item.

A second way of characterizing where the problem of health care inflation lies is to ascertain what portions of cost growth are attributable to more illnesses, more services per illness, or just higher prices. Both the pattern of diseases (incidence and prevalence) and the kinds of health care provided for many illnesses have changed radically in the last 25 years. Thus the changes in the cost of health care are also a result of several factors: (1) higher fees and costs for the same services ("pure inflation"); (2) use of more and higher-cost modes and inputs for the diagnosis and treatment for the same illnesses (growth in the so-called "intensity" of care); (3) more illness per capita (and/or more of the illness appearing for treatment); and (4) growth and aging of the population. The total cost of health care is a product of these factors.*

$$\text{total cost} = (\text{price per service}) \times (\text{services per illness}) \times$$
$$(\text{treated illness per capita}) \times (\text{population})$$

The DHEW has recently developed an input price index for the various components of health care that makes it possible to calculate the portion that each factor contributes to the total cost growth (Waldo, 1979; Gibson, 1979). Between 1969 and 1978, 63% of the increase could be attributed to

* For discussion of the theory and method of attributing cost increases to the component factors see Klarman, 1965.

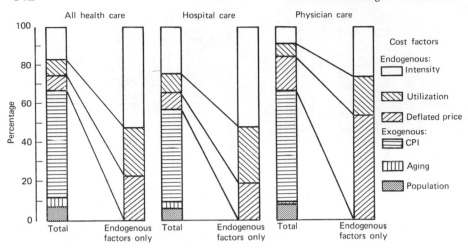

Figure 12.5. Contribution of specific medical care cost-factors to expenditure growth 1969–1978 (compare Table 12.8). Sources: Gibson, 1979; USDHEW, 1979; Dyckman, 1978.

price increase (Figure 12.5; Table 12.8). But of this amount 54% is due to loss of purchasing power of the dollar from general inflation, leaving 9% as inflation in the medical care sector beyond the general economic inflation rate.

Of the expenditure increase 7% was due to *population* growth. A meaningful comparison of the per capita expenditures for health care from one period to another, however, must take into account the important effect of *age distribution* on health care utilization. The total population of the United States grew by 8.1% between 1969 and 1978, but the number of persons over 65 increased by 22.7% in the same period. Older patients not only tend to have more illnesses, but also more chronic ones, which leads to frequent physician visits and more hospitalization (Shanas, 1968; Berg et al., 1970). Persons over 65 average 50% more physician visits per year than those under age 65 and spend over three times as many days in the hospital. The aged account for almost all of the increase in nursing home utilization since 1950. As a result 27% of the total health care budget goes to pay for services used by persons 65 and over, although they make up only 11% of the total population (Gibson, 1979). Thus the shifting age distribution contributes additional demand for health services beyond the simple growth of population. Nevertheless, only 4% of the increase in health expenditures between 1969 and 1978 can be attributed to this factor.

This leaves 27% attributable to increased outlays per capita (age-adjusted) in constant (deflated) medical care dollars. Part of this is a result of increased utilization of services due to a higher *rate of illness* in the population appearing for treatment. Part is due to utilization of more services for the same kinds of illnesses, the so-called *"intensity* of medical care." In order to factor out increased utilization due to more illnesses being treated as opposed to use of more intensive care for the same illnesses, approximations must be made of the major factors influencing age-adjusted utilization rates—trends in the incidence and prevalence of illnesses.

For hospital care, admission rates can serve as a proxy for illness dependent utilization rates; and for physician services, "visits" can serve as such a measure. But no composite index like the one for prices exists for illness incidence and prevalence. We would need such a measure of health status to assess the extent to which growth in utilization occurs on the basis of increased "need" for services per capita. It is also uncertain how constant the relation is between (1) actual incidence of illness, (2) reported indicators of need for care, and (3) incidence of illness appearing for care. Nevertheless, a spectrum of indicators consistently suggests that the age-adjusted increase in illness (and illness appearing for treatment) is somewhat less than 1% per year. The days of restricted activity per person (adjusted for age) increased by 0.5% per year from 1969 to 1977. The incidence of acute conditions (reported to the Health Interview Survey) increased 0.7% annually in the same period. The age-adjusted rate of hospital admissions per capita increased 1.4% per year from 1969 to 1978 in one estimate and not at all in another (USDHEW, 1979). The number of days of hospital care did not increase at all, and the number of (office plus outpatient) physician visits per capita actually declined. Together these indicators suggest that 1% annual growth of utilization on the basis of increased illness in the population is a reasonable approximation. This would account for 8% of the escalation in health care expenditures during this period. Factoring out these estimates of need for more care due to greater incidence of illness leaves 17% for increased intensity of care in the narrower sense of more services for the same illness (Table 12.8).

Aging and growth of the population and general economic inflation are factors outside the health sector (exogenous) that influence its costs but cannot be even potentially controlled by anything done within the sector. A better indication of the relative importance of causes for health cost inflation is the apportionment of the increases among the factors endogenous to the health sector. Looking only at endogenous factors, intensity accounts for 52.5% of the age-adjusted, per capita increase in constant (consumer-buying-power) dollar outlays (Figure 12.5; Table 12.8). Increased utilization due to more illness accounts for 25%, and growth in medical care specific prices accounts for 22.5%. Similar calculations can be carried out for hospital and physician services separately showing the somewhat different nature of the problem for these sectors of care. The preponderance of hospital costs in the overall health care budget and the predominant role of intensity in accounting for the growth of health expenditures represent an economic description of the trend toward high-intensity care discussed in Chapters 5, 6, 7, and 8.

A detailed study of the actual services provided (and their individual costs) for a number of common diseases in 1951, 1964, and 1971 yields a very similar picture (Scitovsky and McCall, 1975). A steady increase in the price of individual services was found, generally at a higher rate than the CPI. For nearly all diseases there was a significant increase in the amount of X-ray and laboratory testing. For those diseases whose treatment involved hospitalization, there was a marked rise in the percentage of cost going to hospital services. For diseases where antibiotics made a major breakthrough in treatment during those years, there was a net reduction in inputs; for those diseases with a shift in mode of treatment to a new high-technology approach (coronary care units for heart attacks), there was a major increase in the service inputs and by far the largest overall growth in the cost of treatment. Diseases with no major change in mode of treatment had cost and service trends between these extremes. Scitovsky concludes that, in the net, changes in modes of treatment were cost-raising and seriously questions whether this increased intensity and cost of treatment provides any significant improvement in outcomes.

THE PROBLEM OF RISING HOSPITAL COSTS

Physician and hospital services differ somewhat in the way cost increases have occurred. For hospitals, a much larger portion of the cost increase has taken place in the intensity of services *within* the day of care, the unit that was traditionally taken as the measure of "price." In fact, the day of care is an aggregate basket of many diverse services that has changed markedly over the years, mostly as a result of the more sophisticated and intensive care for the same illness. Thus the components of the input cost of providing care are better indicators of the causes of rising expenditures than the output prices—per diem or per admission costs. DHEW in cooperation with the AHA has recently developed indices of input prices and service intensity that make this analysis possible (Freeland et al., 1979). The input price index is a weighted average of the wages and prices hospitals pay for the goods and services that they must procure to produce their care, the so-called hospital market basket, analogous to the consumer market basket used in determining the CPI. Using this index it can be calculated that 57% of the constant-dollar, age-adjusted, per capita growth in hospital costs was due to greater intensity of services per admission, 20% to hospital specific price inflation, and 23% to increased admissions per capita (Figure 12.5; Table 12.8).* For the last decade the input price index has been increasing about 1.3 percentage points per year faster than the CPI. There are two reasons for this.

* Using admission rates as the measure of utilization corresponding to the amount of illness needing such treatment assumes, as a first approximation, that the case mix of illnesses and the admitting criteria of physicians have not changed appreciably over the period in question.

1. Hospital care is very labor intensive, 50% of the hospital input costs are wages, and wages generally go up faster than nonwage prices.* Hospital wages have gone up even faster than general manufacturing or service sector wages in recent years. Traditionally, wages and fringe benefits for unskilled hospital workers were lower than prevailing community wages for equivalent jobs in industry. In the last 15 years (although only about 10% of hosiptal workers have been unionized), this gap has closed as hospital wages caught up for most work categories. Catching up has meant a higher rate of increase. Hospital personnel standards have also been rising (M. Feldstein, 1971). The rapid investment in sophisticated technology for diagnosis and treatment has required more highly quali- fied personnel to operate the new equipment. Wages and salaries for skilled hospital workers with no counterparts outside the health industry have risen even faster than those of the unskilled workers. This trend toward more highly skilled and expensive hospital personnel will un- doubtedly continue.

2. Another large part of hospital procurement is specialized equipment and supplies with limited competition among producers and little buyer re- sistance from the (cost-reimbursed) hospitals to hold down prices.

Nevertheless, the rate of increase of the hospital market basket beyond the CPI only accounts for 22% of the rise in per diem costs. By far the largest component of increase beyond the general inflation rate is the growth in in- tensity of care—increased utilization of new inputs and new services per day of care. Using an independent method, Feldstein and Taylor (1977) also found that, from 1955 to 1975, 75% of the cost increases in excess of the gen- eral economy's inflation rate (prices and wages) could be attributed to in- creased labor and nonlabor inputs per patient day.† Thus most of the in- crease in hospital service expenditures is actually utilization of more inten-

---

* Ironically, as inflation has climbed into the double digit range since mid-1979, the large portion of wages in hospital input costs has actually had the reverse effect of slowing the rise of the hospital market basket relative to the CPI. During this period consumer price inflation has outpaced the rise in wages, which are only periodically due for renegotiation unless there is an inflation indexing clause in the contract. As a result, 50% of the hos- pital market basket is now rising more slowly than consumer prices.

† The actual growth of service intensity is even greater than the method of either Feld- stein or HCFA indicates. The AHA has also developed a direct survey method for mea- suring service intensity that shows an even greater growth of new inputs per patient day—averaging about 6% per year since 1974 (Phillip et al., 1976). This total (gross) growth of services per day has been partially offset by improved productivity and efficiency, for example, use of labor-saving equipment, such as computerized billing and disposable syringes, more efficient scheduling of personnel, and so on. These improvements make it possible to produce more services from the same inputs. Therefore the net dollar increase in inputs is less than the gross increase in the intensity of services actually supplied to patients per diem because part of that growth comes from increase in service for the same dollars due to productivity improvements.

sive care in the form of more and higher priced man-hours per patient day and more expensive technology, equipment, and facilities.

FACTORS INFLUENCING THE GROWTH OF INTENSITY OF CARE AND COSTS

What is the nature of this growth in service intensity, and can it be slowed without jeopardizing improvement in the quality of hospital care? No definitive studies are available to give a final answer, and experts disagree. Some insight can be gained by examining the components of the new inputs to see what parts of hospital services are growing most rapidly. From 1955 to 1975 nonlabor inputs grew almost three times as rapidly as increases in personnel-hours per patient day, and since 1966 the differential has been even higher (Feldstein & Taylor, 1977). This is interpreted by many analysts as indicating that a major factor in rising hospital costs is the proliferation of new technology used by hospitals in patient care (Wagner & Zubkoff, 1978). Other authorities dispute this interpretation, pointing out that there is no direct measure of "technological input" as distinct from other inputs into hospital care (Klarman, 1977). There is further evidence, however, that tends to support the technology interpretation. Hospitals also classify their expenditures into "routine care" and "ancillary care" categories. Routine care includes the so-called hotel functions of a hospital plus general duty nursing, overall maintenance, and the like. Ancillary care includes operating rooms, laboratories, special services like intensive care units, X-ray departments, and so forth. Ancillary costs have been growing twice as rapidly as routine costs and now comprise 60% of hospital expenditures.

An example of a technology-based increase in ancillary costs is the growth in use of clinical laboratory tests, which rose at an average rate of 16% per year from 1970 to 1975. Total expenditures for clinical labs increased sharply despite a steady decline in the unit cost of such tests as a result of automated blood chemistry analyzers and similar innovations. Increased utilization due to easier availability has more than balanced the greater productivity from these machines (Fineberg, 1978). Both patients and physicians tend to equate "quality of care" with technological sophistication. Hospitals, under virtually no economic constraint in regard to new inputs, therefore attempt to maximize revenue by attracting more physicians and patients with additional investment in prestigious, high-technology services and showpieces like CAT scanners and cobalt radiation units (Lee, 1971; Pauly & Redisch, 1973). Consequently, they invest in new equipment far beyond the point where marginal utility gains for service output would outweigh marginal cost—the point where a price competitive industry would stop investment.

The pertinent question for strategies of reform is not whether technology or "other" new inputs are responsible for rising costs but how much of the intensity growth is cost-effective in improving the outcomes of care. In attempting to reduce hospital expenditures, it is important to know how much constitutes inefficiency or unnecessary services resulting from the lack of budget constraint that would force hospitals to decide which investments really improve outcomes. A number of studies do indicate an excessive amount of waste, inefficiency, unneeded capacity, and unnecessary utilization of services in the hospital industry (U.S. Comptroller General, 1980). Another indication that a large portion of expenditures for added service intensity is unnecessary is the experience of nine states that have instituted mandatory hospital budget review and rate setting. These states have managed to reduce the rate of increase in net service intensity below 1% per year compared to almost 4% per year for the rest of the country (USDHEW, 1979a). There is no evidence that the reduced rate of growth of intensity in these states has reduced the quality of care or rate of technical improvement (McMahon, 1978).

Thus a large factor in the growing intensity of health care seems to be the use of increasingly sophisticated and more expensive technologies developed by medical science for diagnosing and treating illnesses (Gaus, 1975). In most economic sectors consumers must be convinced of the desirability of new technologies to create demand for their use. Health care is different in that the decision to utilize particular technologies in any situation is largely controlled by physicians (Wagner & Zubkoff, 1978). Since payment for most technological procedures is usually covered under health insurance plans, there is little financial impediment to deter physicians from ordering them. Because of the great stress on the scientific approach to medicine throughout their careers, physicians come to believe that using technology that is more sophisticated is apt to hold greater promise for helping their patients. For any particular technology this attitude is encouraged by the developers, promoters, and manufacturers, all of whom have vested interests in its wider use.

Professional standards, prestige incentives, practice habits, and financial rewards, all reinforce physicians' inclination toward use of any technology available. Whatever *can* be done *will* be done for more intensive treatment or in the search for more precise diagnoses (the so-called "technological imperative"; see Chapters 5 and 6). Because of this unique situation of the health care market, any new technology almost immediately and automatically creates its own demand, often even before the full risks, benefits, and costs are well enough understood to allow intelligent judgment about its efficacy. Because of the indirect way we pay for medical care, physicians seldom have to take cost into account in weighing their decision to use a technology. They only have to decide whether *any potential benefits* alleged by promoters outweigh the risks—*not* whether the *marginal benefits (utility) outweighs the marginal cost,* as in most sectors of the economy.

On the cost side, too, health care technology presents an unusual and perplexing situation. Unlike technological innovation in most industries, very little new medical technology substitutes for labor inputs to reduce net cost. Certain administrative and backup service investments, like automated bookkeeping and billing or disposable syringes and dishes, may save on labor costs. Most medical innovations, however, represent an additional service or more sophisticated versions of old technologies, adding to the total intensity of care for a given illness (Fineberg, 1977). More, rather than less, personnel is usually required, further increasing the cost of care. In fact, on the average, for each new dollar of capital investment in hospitals, operating expenses go up by about $0.50 per year (USDHEW, 1977a) increasing the cost of care still further. In some instances innovations have clearly improved the outcomes for certain illnesses, shortened the episodes, and resulted in an overall saving in cost. Antibiotics are a prime example. In other cases new technologies improve outcomes, providing further useful and happy life for the patient but at the same time creating additional demand for care of the chronic illness that must be sustained by the life-supporting technology. Diabetes and end-stage kidney failure are two examples (Rettig, 1978). On the other hand, sophisticated technology also often leads to prolonging of life in cases where little is gained for the patient. The additional few days or months of miserable or unconscious existence often come at a tremendous cost to society and to the patient's family.

The development of medical technology exerts a second, *indirect* effect on the utilization and cost of services. The much publicized successes of medicine during the last 50 years and the dramatic nature of some medical technologies have led to unrealistic expectations about the efficacy of medical care. As noted in Chapter 5, the impact of these expectations on the demand for medical services has been so striking that it is referred to as the "revolution of rising expectations" (Somers & Somers, 1961). The Consumer Movement, the Civil Rights Movement, and the War on Poverty with its program of community organization all included health care as a rallying point, further raising expectations among groups that were previously resigned to lack of service. Rising consumer expectation is part of a general trend in American society, but the phenomenon is particularly strong in health care because of the dramatic nature of the developments in this field and the personal urgency felt in regard to health problems.

The resulting consumer demand for access to health care has fed the cost escalation in two ways. Through the political process, public opinion has helped channel funds into medical research, manpower training, and facility construction, all of which tend to increase the intensity and utilization of care (Strickland, 1972a). Through the collective bargaining process consumer demand fueled the growth of health insurance. Insurance financing of medical services, in turn, has stimulated greater intensity of care and also radically modified the market for the production and utilization of medical care (see Insurance section, this chapter and Chapter 13).

Excess capacity is also a problem in the hospital industry contributing to unnecessary costs. The number of general care beds in the United States expanded from 3.3 per 1000 population in 1950 to 4.5 beds per 1000 in 1978, and the number of patient days per 1000 population increased by almost the same ratio. In such a monopoly and provider-dominated market, the prices of medical services are not held down through competition by increasing the supply (Chapter 13). In fact, it has become axiomatic among health policy makers in recent years that a major means of controlling health care costs is to *reduce* the supply of hospital beds and other expensive facilities. The availability of hospital beds, for instance, seems to create its own demand. The higher the ratio of beds to population in a community, the greater the utilization of hospital services. This fact concerning hospital utilization was first observed by Roemer (1961; Roemer & Shain, 1959), and has been well enough confirmed that it is referred to among health planners and administrators as "Roemer's law."

Some have argued that the causation might be in the other direction, that hospitals are built or expanded where demand exists. Yet, the differences in bed ratios from one community to another are too great to be accounted for on the basis of differential need. Careful studies have shown that a major factor explaining the variation in hospital utilization rates in different areas (after standardizing for other factors) is the difference in availability of beds (May, 1975). There are at least two reasons that might explain this phenomenon. First, physicians (particularly specialists) tend to establish their practices in areas where there are more hospital facilities. Physicians in turn generate more utilization not only of their own services but also of the technology they command, including hospital services. Second, the availability of beds seems to influence (both directly and by way of pressure from administrators) physician norms as to how long a stay is appropriate, or how urgently in-hospital care is needed in a given type of case (Derzon, 1978).

Excess capacity, even without increased utilization, creates additional costs that ultimately accrue to the various payers because of the (cost determined) method of reimbursement (see Insurance section, this chapter). The capital costs (interest and depreciation) continue to accrue even if the unit is totally unused. Unless a whole unit is completely closed, partial staffing of facilities to keep them in readiness creates considerable costs. It is estimated that an empty bed on an active unit incurs routine operating costs equal to 80% of an occupied one (USDHEW, 1978b). Similar "maintenance" costs probably occur for all unused hospital services or those not used to capacity. Despite tighter restrictions on further hospital investment, the cost reimbursement financing and lack of effective enough community health planning still allow hospitals to invest in unnecessary self-sufficient units for all services. Several hospitals in a local area often duplicate services that have limited need. They compete for prestige and patients, rather than coordinating and distributing services in the best interests of the community.

THE PROBLEM OF RISING PHYSICIAN COSTS

The nature of the problem and the causes of growth in physician costs are somewhat different than for hospitals, and therefore require different strategies of control. As with hospital costs, the increases in expenditures for physician services are a product of growth in utilization, greater intensity of care for the same illness, and inflation of prices for the same services. We can calculate the percentage of the total increase attributable to each factor. For physician services the growth rate of personnel and other inputs into office visits has been much slower than for hospitals. Additional laboratory services are commonly billed separately so that escalation of fees, unlike hospital daily room charges, does not include a large factor of intensity growth. Therefore the physician-fee component of the CPI is usually taken directly as the input price index (Waldo, 1979). Since 1950, by this measure, physician fees have generally risen about 40% more rapidly than the overall cost of living. During most of this period, however, the real rate of growth in fees was even faster. The CPI component underestimates the actual rate of increase in physician fees because it is based on "customary" (list) fees rather than average fees actually charged, which were traditionally adjusted to the patient's ability to pay. The rapid growth in physician payment by way of insurance, with Medicare for the aged and Medicaid for the poor, reduced the need for physicians to engage in this practice. As a consequence of this decrease in fee discounting, average fees actually rose about 1 percentage point per year more rapidly than the CPI component has seemed to indicate, 60% faster than the overall cost of living and 30% faster than other services components or wages (Dyckman, 1978).

Taking these adjustments into account, fee inflation constitutes about 75% of the increase in physician expenditures since 1969—of which 18% is the medical care sector's endogenous inflation component beyond the CPI growth (Figure 12.5; Table 12.8). It is difficult, however, to say how much of this should be attributed to increased intensity of care during a visit and how much is "pure" inflation for the same service. Of the remaining 32% of the increase in physician expenditures, approximately 12% can be attributed to population growth and 10% to the growth of office visits per capita. Most of this must be due to aging since the *age-adjusted,* per capita visit rate to offices and outpatient clinics did not increase from 1970 to 1978. This leaves a residual 10%, which is most likely attributable to growth of services provided in hospital settings or other services not counted as "visits," such as fees collected for interpreting laboratory findings and the like, that is, hidden increased intensity (Dyckman, 1978). Considering only the factors endogenous to the health sector, of the per capita, constant (consumer-buying-power) outlay increases, physician fee (excess) inflation accounts for 54%; increased utilization (mostly due to aging) accounts for 20%; and greater intensity accounts for 26%.

Thus unlike the situation for hospitals, "pure inflation" of fees for essentially the same services accounts for a much larger portion of expenditures than does greater intensity of office care or more visits per capita. Sixty percent of physician revenues go into their net earnings, and over half of their operating expenses go to employees' wages. Consequently, physician fees comprise largely (80%) wages and "salaries" (their own income), which ordinarily rise faster than prices. Yet, although their office expenses have also grown somewhat more rapidly than consumer prices, net physician incomes have climbed much faster than other professional incomes and 10% more rapidly than average wages (Table 12.9). In 1978 the median income for physicians was almost $70,000—twice that of dentists or lawyers and five times that of full-time workers in general. Physician incomes vary widely by specialty and type of practice so that some groups have average incomes far in excess of this median. For example, hospital-based radiologists and pathologists who contract for a percentage of their departmental gross revenues had average earnings of $122,400 and $138,200 respectively in 1976 (compared to $52,600 and $49,200 respectively for salaried radiologists and pathologists), while GPs on the average earned only $46,000 (Dyckman, 1978).

The reasons for this high rate of fee and physician income inflation are complex, and the balance of contributing factors has shifted over time (Dyckman, 1978). Prior to 1965 the rapid growth of fees was primarily a consequence of limited competition due to restriction of physician supply in the face of rapidly growing consumer demand. From 1930 until 1960 the supply of new physicians was severely restricted by the limitation of medical school class sizes imposed by the AMA Council on Medical Education following the reforms of medical education in the early part of the century (Rayack, 1967; Chapter 6). During this period the physician-to-population ratio of the country was maintained at an almost constant level—despite the rising demand for services based on higher consumer expectations as the efficacy of medical treatment improved. This decreased competition between physicians probably was a major factor in allowing them to raise their fees at almost twice the rate of increase in the cost of living (Dyckman, 1978). Physician incomes rose almost twice as rapidly as the national average income from 1939 to 1955.

In the early 1960s two factors changed which began to increase the number of physicians rapidly. (1) The AMA reversed its opposition to the expansion of medical schools. The resulting Health Manpower Training Act of 1963 provided support for establishing new medical schools and incentives for enlarging the class size of existing ones. The training of more physicians picked up speed over the next decade and had doubled by 1976 (Rayack, 1967). (2) Faced with pressure from hospitals in need of more physicians to fill their enlarging residency programs and to provide services for their growing number of more complex cases, the U.S. Immigration Service lowered barriers to the influx of foreign medical graduates (FMGs) in the late 1950s. Large numbers of foreign trained physicians began to flow into the country (Stevens & Vermeulen, 1972). Between 1968 and 1976 (when immigration was again restricted) as many FMGs as new American graduates entered medical service. As a result the ratio of physicians to population increased from 139 per 100,000 in 1960 to 177 in 1975. To be sure, an increasing percentage of these physicians are practicing in hospital settings, so that the number of physicians competing in office practice has not increased as rapidly as the total supply (Chapter 8). However, the new physicians are also not locating their practices in areas of shortage, but primarily in the metropolitan areas, which are already oversupplied.

Nevertheless, the increasing density of physicians has not slowed the rate of increase in fees as might be expected from the converse effect of decreased competition in earlier years. Physicians continue to achieve high income growth almost independent of the apparent competitive density of physicians in an area. From 1965 to 1978 the CPI for physician services and the average physician income grew more rapidly (even compared to the total CPI and the average service wage increase) than from 1955 to 1965. Moreover, physicians in areas of higher density command even higher fees than in areas of lower supply—even after an adjustment is made for differences in cost of living (Blumberg, 1978; Dyckman, 1978). Analysts suggest that in effect physicians have a "target" income growth rate that they are able to meet either by increasing their fees or increasing the number of services (Blumberg, 1978; Evans, 1974). In areas of greater physician density, physicians tend to charge higher fees to make up for the fewer patients per doctor in order to achieve the same incomes.

Two factors underlie this loss of the sensitivity of physician fees to competition since 1965: increased physician control over utilization of their own services and expansion and modification of the insurance reimbursement system for physician services. First, the increase in physician control over demand for their own services stems in part from the accelerated development of high-technology procedures coming to fruition from the intensified medical research after World War II. Because of the power of physicians as gatekeepers to all medical care, the consumption of medical services today is more influenced by the supply side of the production-utilization equation than by "demand" in the usual consumer-dependent sense. Unlike the situation 30 years ago when a newly graduated physician might require many years to build up a practice, physicians today can fill their offices almost from the day they enter practice. Blumberg (1978) estimates that 80% of physician income derives from "self-generated" services, for example, return visits, referral visits (where the principle of reciprocity assures increasing one's own business by referring to another), hospital visits, and other technical procedures. As a result the utilization of physician and other medical services in a community is to a large extent a function of the number of physicians (May, 1975).

There is considerable evidence, for instance, that the amount of surgery done in a community is strongly influenced by the number of surgeons available (Lewis, 1969). Bunker (1970) first noted this in a comparison of the rates in England and in the United States of various surgical procedures. Almost twice as much surgery per capita is done here as in England, where the number of surgeons per capita is only half as great. Such a correlation has since been confirmed by comparing areas within the United States (May, 1975). Equally striking is the fact that the structure of practice and the incentive system within which the physician is working makes a major difference in the amount of surgery performed. In HMOs where the physician is paid on a comprehensive capitation basis (so much per patient per year, no matter what services are rendered), there is only half as much surgery per capita as there is among patients cared for on a fee-for-service basis (Luft, 1978; Gaus et al., 1976).* Insofar as excessive surgery is unneeded it not only leads to cost escalation but also places the patient in unnecessary jeopardy, since any anesthesia or surgical procedure carries some degree of risk in addition to the inconvenience and unpleasantness involved (U.S. House of Representatives, 1975).† With (nonsurgical) medical services, the extent of overutilization is more difficult to evaluate. Since the same motivations and organizational structure of practice are operating as in the case of surgery, it seems reasonable to assume that similar behavior occurs.

The second reason for decreased sensitivity of physician fees to increasing competition is the change in the amount and type of physician insurance coverage that has come about since 1960. Before looking at the specific nature of these changes, we must examine the general structure of the health insurance system and its effects on costs.

HEALTH INSURANCE, TAX SUBSIDY, AND PUBLIC FINANCING OF MEDICAL CARE

The insurance method of financing is a major reason why more funds flow into health care than seems appropriate for the marginal benefits—and are

---

* These differences in rates of surgery can, of course, be interpreted in two ways, that one group is getting too little surgery, or that the other group is getting too much. There is no evidence that the English or HMO enrollees suffer more deaths from diseases such as appendicitis or gall stones, where insufficient surgery might lead to life-threatening complications.

† This is not meant to imply that most unnecessary surgery takes place through purely pecuniary intent. That probably seldom occurs. The decision whether or not to operate is, in many instances, a very difficult one; many factors of risk and possible benefit, which are not always comparable or clearly definable, must be weighed. An empty operating schedule or, conversely, the prospect of squeezing still more work (without additional compensation) into a busy group practice, can influence a physician's perspective in subtle ways such as *how soon* to intervene. For example, delay may resolve a case favorably without the need to intervene, as seemed to be the case earlier. Although this shifts the balance on any particular case only very slightly, it can nevertheless have an important statistical effect on the total amount of surgery done.

allocated in a way that is inappropriate for present needs (M. Feldstein, 1973, COWPS, 1976). Health insurance developed as a means of protection against the high cost of medical care (Chapter 11). As new medical technologies raised the cost of care, families could be forced into bankruptcy by medical bills—or hospitals could be closed if they were unpaid. Unlike most items in the family budget, the incidence of serious illness leading to such "catastrophic" costs is very uneven and unpredictable in the population and not related to ability to pay. Thus it seemed appropriate to use the insurance mechanism to spread the risk and convert it into a predictable budget item. Paradoxically, however, the emergence of private and then publicly financed health insurance as the principal mechanism of paying for care has been a major cause for the uncontrolled increases in those costs. Once in place, health insurance, encouraged by tax laws, changed the entire structure of the health care market in a way that is responsible for a major portion of the excessive utilization and cost of care (M. Feldstein, 1977). The insurance mechanism of financing care has several economic effects on the health market: (1) It lowers the apparent (out-of-pocket) price to the patient; (2) it removes revenue constraints for providers; (3) it serves as a cost pass-through mechanism from health outlays to remote payers who are not involved in expenditure decisions. As a consequence, neither normal market constraints nor other budget limiting mechanisms can control costs. Each of these effects of insurance by itself could theoretically account for the disproportionate cost growth in the health sector. Yet quite different reforms in the financing system would be necessary to ameliorate the inflation impact of each factor. Therefore it is important to ascertain the degree to which each of the mechanisms contributes to the inflation problem—to determine where to place the major emphasis in attempting reform.

The Apparent Price-Lowering Effect of Insurance

The most obvious influence of the insurance system on the health care market (though probably not the most significant) is the apparent price-lowering effect. This occurs through the shift in the direct burden of payment away from the patient at the time of using services (Figure 12.4; Table 12.6). In 1950, 75% of all personal health services were paid for from private sources, with almost 66% coming directly out-of-pocket and only 9% from insurance benefits. The Federal, state and local governments' share was 22%—mostly in the form of direct services such as veterans hospitals, state mental hospitals, and county or city hospitals for the indigent. From 1950 to 1965 the major change was the growth in payments through private ("voluntary") health insurance. During this period insurance benefits increased tenfold and became the conduit for 23% of all health expenditures. Then from 1966 until 1978, mostly as a result of Medicare and Medicaid, the government share of the total health care budget increased to almost 40%. Private insurance benefits also continued to rise after 1966, although somewhat less rapidly, so that in 1978 insurance payments accounted for 27% of the total—while only 33% was paid by patients out-of-pocket.

What ordinarily influences decisions to procure most commodities is not the average price but the *marginal* (out-of-pocket) price—the additional money needed to obtain a unit of the commodity at the time of purchase— with little regard to the amount of payment up to that point. Once insurance has been paid for, the use of additional insured services adds little extra cost for the patient, unless there is appreciable co-insurance (sharing in the cost of each unit of service used). Thus the apparent "price" of insured health care is much less than either the average or marginal cost of producing it. Such an artificially lowered price, like a purchasing subsidy, ordinarily raises demand. If health care utilization were actually determined by the free-market choice of consumers, this price-lowering effect of insurance might account for much of the increase in consumption of services.

For health expenditures, however, this price-lowering effect does *not* account for much of the increase. This is demonstrated by econometric studies that estimate the influence of various factors on the utilization and cost of hospitals and physician services. Multiple studies of this kind have produced varying and rather confusing results, which seem to depend on the techniques used and the type of data employed. Thus they require cautious interpretation. The major divergences occur between studies using individual data based on surveys and studies using aggregate statistical data (P. Feldstein, 1979). With survey data each person's utilization of services can be correlated with the type of insurance he holds and with other individual characteristics such as income. Aggregate data studies are usually based on state or other geographic area expenditures, utilization rates, levels of insurance, average income, and so forth.

Individual data should reflect most strongly and accurately the influence of out-of-pocket price and other personal factors on utilization decisions that the patient controls. Such studies show that whether a person is admitted to a hospital or not (or has surgery) is quite sensitive to whether he has insurance coverage at all (Chart 12.1).* Once admitted, however, the hospital (or surgical) expenses per admission (or length of stay) vary little with the amount of co-insurance (out-of-pocket price) borne by the patient or with his income. The patient apparently has a veto or postponing power

---

* As with the similar decrease of hospital use in HMOs, it is an open question whether these rate differences represent too much hospitalization and surgery for the insured or too little for the uninsured. In HMOs, where there is less financial incentive to hospitalize patients, admissions and surgical rates are also lower by about the same degree, and studies show HMO members to be at least as healthy as beneficiaries of plans with high hospitalization rates (Chapter 10). HMOs, however, are organized to provide many of the same services on an ambulatory basis. A 40% lower hospitalization and surgical rate for uninsured patients, who do not have this other source, probably means that some needed services go unprovided. In any case, it would be unacceptable policy to hold down utilization by intentionally leaving some parts of the population totally without coverage while striving to increase the *completeness* of coverage for others.

Chart 12.1 Comparison of Sensitivities (Elasticities[a]) of Expenditure and Utilization Rates as Determined by Different Study Methods (and with Factor Contribution to Total Cost Growth)

	Hospital Care				Physician Services			All Medical Care
	Admission Rates	Cost per Admission	Patient Days	Total Expenditures	Visit Rates	Cost per Visit	Total Expenditures	Total Expenditures
Individual data studies:								
Insurance "elasticity"[h]	40%[g]							
Price elasticity		0.04[g]	0.2[f]		0.18[g] to 0.2[f]		0.19[g]	
Income elasticity		0.0[g]			0.03[g]		0.05[g]	
Aggregate data studies:								
Price elasticity	0.45[d]		0.67[c]	0.48[d]	1.0[b]		0.15[e] to 0.35[e] 0.56[d] to 0.85[d]	0.35[i] to 1.5[i] 0.6[d] to 1.2[j]
Income elasticity								
Contribution of factor to expenditure growth	22.9%[k]	77.1%[k]			20.5%[k]	79.5%[k]		

[a] Negative signs for price elasticities of coinsurance are omitted.
[b] Davis & Russell, 1972.
[c] Feldstein, M., 1971a.
[d] Feldstein, P., & Severson, 1964. (Price elasticity of insurance effect)
[e] Fuchs & Kramer, 1973.
[f] Newhouse & Phelps, 1976.
[g] Phelps, 1975.
[h] Reduction
[i] Rossett & Huang, 1973.
[j] Silver, 1970.
[k] Table 12.8.

over elective hospital admissions and surgery but no longer controls intensity of care (expenditures per admission) once he is admitted.

Yet the relative contribution of the admission rate versus intensity factors to increases in hospital expenditures is exactly opposite to the way insurance influences patients. The great majority of the real (constant-consumer-dollar) growth in hospital expenditures per capita from 1970 to 1978 is attributable to increased cost per admission (77%; including 57% for intensity and 20% for the relative hospital input price inflation rate). Only 23% of the expenditure growth is attributable to increased admission rates (Table 12.8). The influence of insurance coverage on admission rates has not contributed appreciably to expenditure escalation because there has been little change in the percentage of persons with hospital and surgical insurance in recent years. At the beginning of the 1970 to 1978 period both insurance markets were already nearly saturated (except for those below the poverty level but without Medicaid) so that little change in insurance coverage rates could occur (Health Insurance Institute, 1979).

Studies based on *aggregate* data appear at first sight to contradict those based on individual data. They generally show what seems to be a higher sensitivity of hospital expenditures per admission to the patient's share of payment and to income levels than do studies with individual data (P. Feldstein, 1979). This is surprising since aggregate data usually blur the sensitivity of consumption to factors like price and income that presumably influence demand through consumer choice. One possible explanation for the apparent paradox would seem to be as follows: The aggregate statistics are actually measuring different variables than are the individual data. The aggregate statistics measure *features of the area* that characterize in total how expensive facilities and provider services are—rather than measuring averages of the features that exert their supposed influence on individual patient choices. Thus the direction of causality is reversed for aggregate compared to individual data studies. In aggregate studies the "price" (i.e., the co-insurance rate, defined as the patient's share of total payments) appears low in areas where expenditures are high *because* the hospital costs per admission are high, rather than the other way around.

Per-admission hospital expenditures in an area are a function of the medical facilities and under the control of providers in the area. Thus they are similar for all patients regardless of co-insurance. In areas where facilities provide more intensive care or where there are more providers, expenditures for hospital care per admission tend to be higher. Since most hospital insurance pays whatever costs or charges are incurred (with only certain exclusions and deductibles), higher expenditures are simply reflected in higher insurance payments to hospitals in the area. Deductibles are more uniform (for each carrier) across the nation than hospital expenditure rates (e.g., the Medicare hospital deductible was $180 per episode of illness nationwide in 1980). Therefore the portion paid by patients (which is used as the measure of "price") is lower in comparison with total hospital expenditures in those states with higher hospital costs per admission. This makes it appear that *because* price to the patient is lower, total expenditures are higher. In fact, the opposite is the case. Where hospital expenditure rates are higher, the *apparent* "price" to the patient (the rather constant patient contribution divided by the total cost) is lower in relation to the total. Thus the characteristics of the medical facilities and providers in these geographic areas are the determiners of the higher rate of hospital expenditures—rather than a lower out-of-pocket price influencing patients to buy more services per admission. Otherwise, the sensitivity of expenditures to variation in out-of-pocket price would be even greater in individual data studies than with aggregate data where these variations are much more averaged out.

A similar relationship occurs with income levels. Areas with higher median incomes tend to attract more physicians and have more expensive health facilities. Funds for investment are usually more easily available and public expectations promote the availability of more sophisticated care facilities. The individual patient living in that area, however, has little choice as to how much he will pay for his hospital care no matter what his own income is relative to the mean in the area.

For physician services, too, similar relationships exist between individual and area influences, and between patient and provider control of utilization decisions. The effects are less marked and less obvious than for hospitals. The separation between what the physician controls and where the patient has a veto or delaying power is not as clearly divided in relation to office visits and fees as it is between hospital admissions and expenditures per admission. Presumably the first visit in an illness is determined by the patient, but other visits (indistinguishable in the statistics) may be at the instigation of the physician. Conversely, patients may neglect a return visit or extra tests and services suggested in the office setting, while this is more difficult in the hospital. Individual-data studies show that for physician visits co-payment rates do make a difference in utilization, but income has little influence. Co-insurance rates in turn have little relation to cost per visit, while income has a moderate influence. This suggests that persons with higher incomes tend to go to higher priced physicians regardless of their co-payment rates.

As with hospital insurance, in *individual-data* studies, the relative influence of co-insurance (price) on physician visit rates as opposed to expenditures per visit does *not* parallel the relative contribution of these factors to the growth of physician expenditures. The major portion of physician cost increases is attributable to rising cost per visit (primarily due to pure fee increases for the same services and much less due to greater intensity of care associated with physician services) while the rate of physician visits has actually declined. Thus what is most under the patient's control and is most influenced by the patient's co-insurance rate—visit utilization rates—accounts for little or none of the expenditure increases. What is most under physician control and least influenced by the patient's co-insurance rate—expenditures per visit—accounts for most of the escalation.

As with hospitals, studies using *aggregate* data show greater sensitivity of total physician expenditures to the patient's share of the payment and to income than do the individual data studies. The same difference is found, though less marked, in regard to sensitivity of physician visit rates. Again, the explanation is the same. Variables used in aggregate studies actually measure features of the geographic areas. These features are either characteristics of the providers, such as their fee schedules, or act through them to influence expenditures and utilization—rather than through the patient's sensitivity to out-of-pocket price. This suggests that the aggregate influence of insurance on physician expenditures is mediated primarily by the effect on providers, which allows them to raise their fees with ease (Dyckman, 1978).

Reimbursement Methods of Providers

The special methods of determining providers' reimbursements account for the large effect of insurance financing on the *supply* side of the equation. These modes of paying providers remove essentially all economic brakes on their revenues and costs. Because of the early dominance of Blue Cross plans closely linked to hospital associations (Anderson, 1975), a method of open-ended retrospective cost reimbursement emerged as the dominant mode of paying for hospital services (Chapter 11). Whatever costs a hospital incurs in supplying benefits are simply added up at the end of the year, and this becomes the bill owed by the insurance carriers (Berki, 1972).* All patient-care operating costs, interest and depreciation on capital investments, and most teaching costs (indirectly) are recaptured from all major payers. Many Blue Cross plans allow uncollectable debts as reimbursable costs. Each carrier pays the percentage of those costs attributable to the portion of services used by its beneficiaries. Most patients are not involved in the transaction at all and may never see a bill (except for noncovered services). Thus hospitals are guaranteed payment for almost any costs they incur for insured patients. This removes most constraints on their budgets unless they have a large number of charity cases or uninsured patients who default on their debts. As a result, there is little incentive to economize on the purchase of equipment, hiring and wage setting of personnel, or through improving efficiency and eliminating unnecessary services. When combined with the dominance of physicians in making decisions about equipment and services and with the prestige incentive governing the behavior of health providers (Chapters 6 and 7), this reimbursement mechanism provides a major im-

---

* Some insurance carriers pay on the basis of charges, but Medicare regulations, in effect, require that these charges be at least as high as the equivalent cost basis so that the end effect on reimbursement is no different.

petus for expansion of hospital costs (Altman & Eichenholz, 1976). It removes consumer reticence in using high-cost hospital care and does away with any concern the physician might have about financial impact on his patients. It also removes constraint on hospitals in supplying whatever services or inputs they or their physicians want to provide.

A similar phenomenon occurs in regard to physician reimbursement. The early dominance of Blue Shield plans, largely controlled by medical societies, established a system of paying physicians whatever they declared as their so-called usual, customary, and reasonable (UCR) fees for each service rendered (Somers & Somers, 1961). This allows physicians virtually open-ended, self-determined income for insured services, just as with hospitals, leading to the same problem of cost escalation. Between 1955 and 1978 the portion of physician payment by way of health insurance grew from 10 to 67%. Beginning immediately after World War II, surgical expenses began to be included in most health insurance benefit packages; by 1960, 60% of the population was covered, and by 1977, 80%. A similar development took place in medical (nonsurgical) physician reimbursement with a lag of about 5 to 10 years. By 1967, 60% of the population was covered for medical expenses, and by 1977, 80% (Figure 12.6; Health Insurance Institute, 1979). Thus there has been a major expansion in the number of persons covered for surgical and medical fees.

Since 1965 the comprehensiveness and portion of fees reimbursed have also increased sharply because of Medicare and Medicaid and a change in type of private policies being written. Beginning about 1960, a new development in the reimbursement policy of physician insurance took place that was accelerated by the policies of Medicare established in 1966. Prior to 1960 most physician insurance was written on an indemnity or fixed-fee basis, where the patient was left to pay any difference between the charges billed by the physician and the amount allowed by the insurance for each service. Since the payments allowed were usually considerably below the average customary physician fees, patients were responsible for a major portion of the fee, which increased directly in relation to the physician's charge. Since 1960 there has been a rapid increase in so-called major medical policies, which typically use the UCR fee reimbursement method. Within certain "reasonable" limits, generally established in relation to what other physicians in the area charge, these policies pay a fixed (usually fairly high) percentage of whatever customary fee the physician charges. The Medicare law also confirmed and added to this trend by mandating that physicians be reimbursed according to a UCR schedule or "customary, prevailing, and reasonable" (CPR) as it came to be called because of the provision that "reasonableness" be established on the basis of the 75% percentile of fees prevailing in the area (Institute of Medicine, 1976; Holahan et al., 1979).

This reimbursement system makes it possible for physicians to establish their fees with very little constraint from price competition since the pa-

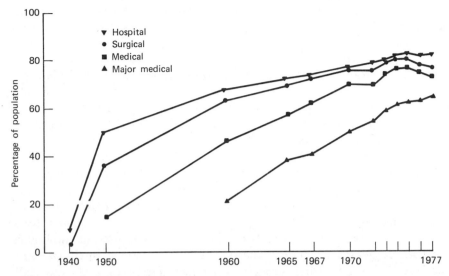

Figure 12.6. Private insurance coverage by category of benefits, 1940 to 1977. (Medicare and Medicaid coverages are not included.) Source: Health Insurance Institute, 1978–1979.

tient pays only a small percentage of the fee, no matter how much is charged (within reasonable limits). The higher the percentage of fees covered by insurance in this way, the faster the level and growth of physician incomes, as for example with surgeons, pathologists, anaesthesiologists, radiologists, obstetricians, and gynecologists. In those specialties where patients have traditionally paid a larger share of the fee directly, such as general practitioners, pediatricians, and psychiatrists, physician incomes have grown more slowly (Dyckman, 1978).

The reasons behind this major shift in the mode of physician reimbursement since 1960 are not entirely clear. With Blue Shield plans the high portion of physician membership on the boards of directors might explain their offering plans with payment formulas especially favorable to physicians. However, the commercial insurers sell UCR medical policies just as frequently as the Blue Shield plans—largely under group contracts. Consumers are apparently as desirous of such policies as physicians because they transfer a larger portion of medical expenses to "someone else" (i.e., to the common pool of payers). The higher premiums constitute little obstacle since they are largely borne by employers and highly subsidized by tax exemptions (Dyckman, 1978). The most likely explanation seems to be that, under the pressure of tax incentives and collective bargaining, this was simply the next logical area for expansion of benefits after hospital, surgical, and regular physician insurance markets were nearly saturated (Mellman, 1980). Hospital cost reimbursement and UCR fee schedules (with greater limitations in relation to so-called prevailing fees) were incorporated into Medicare and to a large extent into Medicaid. These reimbursement methods, combined with provider control of most utilization decisions, encourage the highest justifiable prescription of services and escalation of costs.

Insurance Bias Toward High-Technology Care

Health insurance has another indirect influence on the utilization and cost of care. The benefit structure and reimbursement methods reinforce the bias of American medical practice toward hospital, specialist, and high-technology care. They encourage greater use of services that drive up costs and further amplify the mismatch between the kind of care needed today and the system for providing it. Hospital care, surgical fees, and certain other high-technology procedures were the earliest to generate high unanticipated medical costs. Consequently, these services were the first to be covered by insurance benefits and continue to be reimbursed at the highest rate with the least patient cost sharing (Health Insurance Institute, 1979). The new Federal health insurance programs enacted in 1965 (especially Medicare), maintained essentially the same benefit structure as in the established private plans, greater coverage for hospital services, surgical and high-technology care.

The differences in patient cost sharing for various health services under many insurance benefit plans distorts the apparent relative price to the consumer (Table 12.7). Despite total expenditures for hospital care that were twice as great as for physician services in 1978, out-of-pocket payments for physicians were almost twice those for hospital care. Out-of-pocket payments for drugs, dental services, and other health care items were three times as great as for physicians and four times as much as for hospitals although the total expenditures for these items were only half as large as for hospital care. Since physicians largely decide which services are to be used, however, the reimbursement ratios probably have less effect than the differences suggest. Differential insurance coverage probably does make a difference in regard to hospital admissions for diagnostic workups and minor surgery, however. When expensive diagnostic tests or operating room facilities are called for, the patient often presses to have the procedures done in the more expensive hospital setting, where they are covered by the insurance, even when they could be done equally well on a less expensive outpatient basis.

The UCR reimbursement method is also a major factor encouraging physicians to increase the use of hospital care and other high-technology procedures. This reimbursement method has perpetuated previously existing customary fee schedules that reward in-hospital visits and high-technology procedures at a higher rate per unit of professional time than for simpler hands-on office services (Blumberg, 1978). Blumberg calculates that on the average a physician has a much higher *net* hourly income for hospital visits than for office visits. This reinforces the prestige-oriented professional tendency to overuse high-technology procedures and hospitalization. Reimbursement schedules also perpetuate the higher fees for specialists as opposed to primary-care physicians, for hospital-based as opposed to office-based practice, and in urban as opposed to rural areas (Burney et al., 1978). The resulting financial incentives reinforce the present geographic and specialty maldistribution of the profession. Because the kind of practice encouraged by these fee differentials also tends to generate proportionately more additional nonphysician health expenditures, this system is a major cause not only of higher physician costs but also other medical costs. These secondary medical expenditures contribute more to the rising cost of health care than do the direct physician expenditures.

Cost reimbursement for hospitals removes fiscal constraint on the adoption and utilization of new technology or other expansion of hospital services. The insurance mechanism of payment frees hospitals and physicians from having to compete in price for patients. Therefore competition is based largely on professional and organizational prestige, which is heavily dependent on the sophistication of the technology employed (Chapter 7). In sum, the health insurance system acts as a mutually supportive superstructure to the present, increasingly mismatched, technology-oriented delivery system—both a product of it and a major mechanism for its perpetuation and expansion.

Insurance Channeling of Funds and the Cost-Pass-Through Effect

Health insurance also stimulates demand, utilization, and cost of health care in another less obvious way. By earmarking resources as usable only for health care, this financing method injects large amounts of funding into the health care market creating new service demand. This is particularly true when it is channeled through tax-financed health insurance (Medicare, Medicaid) or employer-paid fringe benefits. But preferential earmarking of funds also occurs when prepayment by the consumer himself sets aside his own contribution ("precommitment"; Fuchs, 1979). Such predesignated authorization of funding for one commodity removes it from potential use to procure other competing commodities and thereby artificially increases preferential demand for the one. M. Feldstein (1977) argues similarly that health insurance (particularly as marketed through group arrangements) forces individuals to procure more inclusive coverage than they really want. The predetermined package requires families to buy more health care than they actually would if it were marketed with options for lesser coverage. Given the demonstrated consumer preference for extensive coverage (Davis, 1980), however, it seems unlikely that packaging is a major factor in excessive health expenditures—though insurance as a commitment of funds certainly is.

The feature of the health care financing system that makes the channeling effect so strong is the "cost-pass-through" nature of the third-party payment mechanisms. As already noted, the cost-reimbursement and UCR methods of payment enable hospitals and physicians to recover almost any costs (or revenue to achieve desired incomes) in the form of reimbursement from third-party payers, the public and private insurance carriers. As a result of methods of setting premiums, the carriers, in turn, can recover whatever they pay out in benefits from their sources of payment, the taxpayers or premium contributors (employers, employees, and individual policy holders). Thus, just as providers pass through their costs (and revenue requirements) to the carriers, the carriers pass through their pay-out costs to their subscribers. For public insurance programs this is obvious; Medicare, Medicaid, or other health laws set the benefits and method of determining payment to providers. Whatever those benefits cost must be paid out of taxes. For private insurance this pass-through is less obvious but equally the case, in end effect. Most private health insurance (90%) today is obtained on a group basis primarily as a fringe benefit of employment. Only 10% is sold on an individual policy basis. The premiums for virtually all such group insurance is set by experience rating* in one of three ways (the following discussion of premium setting is heavily indebted to seminars and materials from Marcus, 1980). With any of these methods whatever benefit costs are paid out to providers are automatically passed-through to whomever is responsible for bearing the premium costs.

About one-third of the dollar volume is self-insured, mostly by large firms that simply contract with an insurance carrier to handle their claims processing. In these cases premiums in the usual sense do not exist. This avoids state premium taxes averaging about 2% of total payments—which is the major attraction of this rapidly growing method of insuring health benefits. There is no underwriting in this method unless the employer reinsures himself to avoid catastrophic losses. All medical expenses incurred by employees for covered benefits are simply paid by the employers. The average cost per beneficiary is, in effect, the "premium" after the fact. This system acts as a complete pass-through of medical costs, a blank check at the insurance level quite analogous to the cost-reimbursement method of hospital financing.

---

* There are two basic methods of establishing premiums for health insurance: experience rating and community rating. The former is only used for setting premiums for insurance sold on a group basis. Premium rates are computed by actuaries on the basis of the actual pay-out experience for benefits to the particular group so that the premiums just cover the cost of benefits plus administration plus retention (for profit or capital growth). The underwriting role of carriers is minimized using this method. Experience rating is advantageous to younger, healthier groups with lower than average utilization of health care.

Community rating is used primarily for policies sold on an individual basis. The basic premium rates are set actuarially as if an experience rate were being calculated for the residual group (in the area) not covered under any of the experience-rated group plans. Since each carrier has little control over who from this residual community buys its policies, and premiums cannot be so easily adjusted, underwriting (risk insuring) plays a major role in the final premium determination, and higher underwriting margins are necessary. Because of the individual marketing and administration of claims, much higher administrative costs are also included in the premiums.

At least another third of group policies (dollar volume) is sold on a retrospective or negotiated premium basis. Although these policies technically involve underwriting, in fact, the carrier is again virtually acting as a fiscal intermediary for the employer. There is complete knowledge of actual payment rates by actuaries on both sides of the contract, and periodic adjustments are made to correspond to the group's actual pay-out experience. This may occur retrospectively or in negotiating premiums for the following period. (Retrospective premiums are increasingly the dominant mode in order to minimize state premium taxes.) But in either case, this method of premium setting also serves as cost-pass-through financing at the insurance level. Since premiums are determined actuarially by the actual pay-out experience of the one group, there is little to be gained through seeking competitive premium rates from one carrier or another. Because risk underwriting is virtually eliminated, the major competitive factor is limited to cost of administration, which also varies little from one carrier to another. Choice of carrier usually is made on other grounds. The same insurance companies also manage pension funds and serve as sources of capital financing for many of the employers. Competition in regard to these other functions is often a more important factor in selecting the carrier than the health insurance function per se (Marcus, 1980).

A smaller portion of the dollar volume of group policies is sold by the third method of experience rating, pooling of many smaller firms by a carrier to spread the underwriting risk. Premiums are set on the basis of actuarial calculation adjusted for the particular population characteristics of the group and the pay-out experience of the beneficiary population of the pool into which their carrier places them. There is true underwriting for these policies. If a carrier has a beneficiary population with higher utilization rates than other carriers for the same actuarial group, an employer may move to another carrier that offers a lower premium for his group. Conversely, if a group has a higher utilization compared to its actuarial characteristics than others in the pool, the carrier will pay out more than its premiums for that group. Losses will only be recaptured in future years when the increased payment experience of the pool leads to higher premiums for all. However, pooled experience rating *as a system* also acts in the aggregate as a cost-pass-through mechanism from the providers to premiums. Thus, although voluntary health insurance (together with publicly financed health insurance) has in fact become the major financing system for health care, it continues to function simply like *insurance*—it merely spreads over a larger population the risk of what is viewed as an *uncontrollable* cost. It does not function as a business seeking competitive ways to offer its customers more efficient forms of the health care prepayment system that it has become. Any underwriting losses or gains only redistribute premium costs among groups and pass profits and losses back and forth among carriers. There is no net market-restraining effect on providers as a result of underwriting competition.

Carriers (with a few limited exceptions, such as the SAFECO primary physician capitation plan) do not attempt to be premium competitive by bargaining with providers for lower rates for their beneficiaries or by other methods to reduce their pay-out experience. Even the largest employers are not in a position to negotiate with providers for better rates or to hold down costs through restricting utilization, no matter which method of experience rating they use. Some *are* promoting development of HMOs in their areas, but any appreciable impact of this strategy lies years in the future (Chapter 13). Thus the only restraint on costs lies in the cost sharing required of beneficiaries. As we have seen, this has little influence on utilization and no effective market restraint on provider charge schedules. Moreover, the tax advantage to both employee (exclusion from income tax) and employer (exclusion from payroll taxes) is a powerful incentive to encourage taking a larger portion of each new wage settlement in the form of such fringe benefits. This inevitably increases the percentage of medical expenditures covered and decreases the employee cost sharing.

Employers (and employees to the extent they share premium costs) must absorb in their premiums whatever costs are generated by the utilization of their beneficiary group. Approximately 40% is subsidized by the income and payroll tax exclusions and in this way passed through to the tax system. The remainder must be divided in some way between the employee and employer. Nationally, on the average, employers pay about 85% of the total premium burden for fringe benefit health insurance, employees pay about 15%. The employers' portion, in turn, is largely passed through to customers as a cost of production in the form of higher prices for goods and services marketed. Thus the experience-rating method of financing health care through employment related insurance has a pass-through effect that is virtually indistinguishable from financing it through taxes.

STATISTICAL APPENDIX

Table 12.1   Gross National Product and National Health Expenditures:
United States, Selected Years 1929 to 1978 (Data are compiled by the
Health Care Financing Administration)

Year	Gross National Product (in billions)	National Health Expenditures		
		Amount (in billions)	Percent of Gross National Product	Amount per Capita
1929	$ 103.1	$ 3.6	3.5	$ 29.49
1935	72.2	2.9	4.0	22.65
1940	99.7	4.0	4.0	29.62
1950	284.8	12.7	4.5	81.86
1955	398.0	17.7	4.4	105.38
1960	503.7	26.9	5.3	146.30
1965	688.1	43.0	6.2	217.42
1966	753.0	47.3	6.3	236.51
1967	796.3	52.7	6.6	260.35
1968	868.5	58.9	6.8	288.17
1969	935.5	66.2	7.1	320.70
1970	982.4	74.7	7.6	358.63
1971	1063.4	82.8	7.8	393.09
1972	1171.1	92.7	7.9	436.47
1973	1306.6	102.3	7.8	478.38
1974	1412.9	115.6	8.2	535.99
1975	1528.8	131.5	8.6	604.57
1976	1700.1	148.9	8.8	678.79
1977	1887.2	170.0	9.0	768.77
1978[a]	2107.6	192.4	9.1	863.01

SOURCE: USDHEW, 1979.

[a] Preliminary estimates.

Table 12.2 Consumer Price Index (1967 = 100) for All Items and Medical Care Components: United States, Selected Years 1950 to 1978 (Data are based on reporting by samples of providers and other retail outlets)

Item and Medical Care Component	Consumer Price Index (year)								
	1950	1955	1960	1965	1970	1975	1976	1977	1978[a]
CPI, all items	72.1	80.2	88.7	94.5	116.3	161.2	170.5	181.5	195.3
CPI, less medical care	—	—	89.4	94.9	116.1	160.9	169.7	180.3	193.9
CPI, all services	58.7	70.9	83.5	92.2	121.6	166.6	180.4	194.3	210.8
All medical care	53.7	64.8	79.1	89.5	120.6	168.6	184.7	202.4	219.4
Medical care services	49.2	60.4	74.9	87.3	124.2	179.1	197.1	216.7	235.3
Hospital service charges[b,c]	—	—	—	—	—	132.3	148.7	164.1	111.1[d]
Semiprivate room	30.3	42.3	57.3	75.9	145.4	236.1	268.6	299.5	331.6
Operating room charges	—	—	—	82.9	142.4	239.4	274.8	311.3	—
X-ray diagnostic series, upper GI	—	—	—	90.9	110.3	156.2	174.6	189.4	—
Professional services:									
Physician fees	55.2	65.4	77.0	88.3	121.4	169.4	188.5	206.0	223.3
Dentist fees	63.9	73.0	82.1	92.2	119.4	161.9	172.2	185.1	199.3
Other professional services:									
Examination, prescription, and dispensing eyeglasses	73.5	77.0	85.1	92.8	113.5	149.6	158.9	168.2	—
Eyeglasses[c]	—	—	—	—	—	—	—	—	104.4[d]
Routine laboratory tests	—	—	—	94.8	111.4	151.4	160.5	169.4	—
Drugs and prescriptions	88.5	94.7	104.5	100.2	103.6	118.8	126.0	134.1	143.9
Prescriptions	92.6	101.6	115.3	102.0	101.2	109.3	115.2	122.1	132.1
Over-the-counter items	—	—	—	98.0	106.2	130.1	138.9	148.5	159.1

SOURCE: USDHEW, 1979.

[a] Owing to the 1978 revision of the Consumer Price Index, hospital service charges include nursing and convalescent home care and hospital emergency room care. Semiprivate room includes all hospital rooms. Also, detail on physician fees is no longer collected. These data are available for the years 1950 to 1977 in *Health, United States, 1978*.
[b] January 1972 = 100 for 1975, 1976, 1977.
[c] December 1977 = 100 for 1978.
[d] Unadjusted Index for December 1978.

Table 12.3 Consumer Price Index, Average Annual Percent Change for All Items and Medical Care Components: United States, Selected Years 1950–1978 (Data are based on reporting by providers and other retail outlets)

Item and Medical Care Component	Average Annual Percent Change (year)							
	1950–1955	1955–1960	1960–1965	1965–1970	1970–1975	1975–1976	1976–1977	1977–1978a
CPI, all items	2.2	2.0	1.3	4.2	6.8	5.8	6.5	7.6
CPI, less medical care	—	—	1.2	4.1	6.7	5.5	6.2	7.5
CPI, all services	3.9	3.3	2.0	5.7	6.5	8.3	7.7	8.5
All medical care	3.8	4.1	2.5	6.1	7.0	9.5	9.6	8.4
Medical care services	4.2	4.4	3.1	7.3	7.6	10.1	9.9	8.6
Hospital service charges	—	—	—	—	—	12.4	10.4	11.1c
Semiprivate room	6.9	6.3	5.8	13.9	10.2	13.8	11.5	10.7
Operating room charges	—	—	—	11.4	10.9	14.8	13.3	—
X-ray diagnostic series, upper GI	—	—	—	5.1	7.2	11.8	8.5	—
Professional services:								
Physician fees	3.5	3.3	2.8	6.0	6.9	11.3	9.3	8.4
Dentist fees	2.7	2.4	2.4	5.3	6.3	6.4	7.5	7.7
Other professional services:								
Examination, prescription, and dispensing eyeglasses	1.0	2.0	1.7	4.1	5.7	6.2	5.9	—
Eyeglasses	—	—	—	—	—	—	—	4.4b
Routine laboratory tests	—	—	—	3.3	6.3	6.0	5.5	—
Drugs and prescriptions	1.4	2.0	0.8	0.7	2.8	6.1	6.4	7.3
Prescriptions	1.9	2.0	2.2	0.1	1.6	5.4	6.0	8.2
Over-the-counter items	—	—	—	1.6	4.1	6.8	6.9	7.1

SOURCE: USDHEW, 1979.

a Owing to the 1978 revision of the Consumer Price Index, hospital service charges include nursing and convalescent home care and hospital emergency room care. Semiprivate room includes all hospital rooms. Also, detail on physician fees is no longer collected. These data are available for the years 1950–1977 in Health, United States, 1978.
b January 1972 = 100 for 1975, 1976, 1977.
c Unadjusted percent change from December 1977 to December 1978.

Table 12.4   National Health Expenditures—Percent Distribution, According to
Type of Expenditure: United States, Selected Years 1950 to 1978 (Data are
compiled by the Health Care Financing Administration)

Expenditure	Amount (in Billions)						
	1950	1960	1965	1970	1975	1977	1978a
Total	$12.7	$26.9	$43.0	$74.7	$131.5	$170.0	$192.4
	Percent Distribution						
All expenditures	100.0	100.0	100.0	100.0	100.0	100.0	100.0
Health services and supplies	92.4	93.6	92.0	92.9	93.7	94.9	95.1
Hospital care	30.4	33.8	32.4	37.2	39.7	40.0	39.5
Physician services	21.7	21.1	19.7	19.2	19.0	18.4	18.3
Dentist services	7.6	7.4	6.5	6.4	6.3	6.9	6.9
Nursing home care	1.5	2.0	4.8	6.3	7.5	7.9	8.2
Other professional services	3.1	3.2	2.4	2.1	2.0	2.2	2.2
Drugs and drug sundries	13.6	13.6	13.4	11.3	9.0	8.1	7.9
Eyeglasses and appliances	3.9	2.9	4.3	2.8	2.3	2.0	2.0
Expenses for prepayment	3.6	4.1	3.4	3.1	2.8	4.6	5.2
Government public health activities	2.9	1.5	1.9	1.9	2.4	2.5	2.6
Other health services	4.2	4.1	3.0	2.8	2.8	2.4	2.3
Research and construction	7.6	6.4	8.1	7.1	6.3	5.2	4.9
Research	0.9	2.5	3.4	2.5	2.4	2.2	2.2
Construction	6.7	3.9	4.7	4.6	3.9	3.0	2.7

SOURCE: USDHEW, 1979.

a Preliminary estimate.

Table 12.5 National Health Expenditures—Average Annual Percent Change,
According to Type of Expenditure: United States, Selected Years 1950 to 1978
(Data are compiled by the Health Care Financing Administration)

	Average Annual Percent Change					
Expenditure	1950–1978	1950–1960	1960–1965	1965–1970	1970–1975	1975–1978
All expenditures	10.2	7.8	9.8	11.7	12.0	13.5
Health services and supplies	10.3	8.0	9.4	11.9	12.1	14.1
Hospital care	11.2	9.9	7.1	14.8	13.4	13.4
Physician services	9.5	7.5	8.3	11.1	11.7	12.2
Dentist services	9.8	7.5	7.3	11.1	11.6	17.3
Nursing home care	17.2	10.9	31.5	17.7	16.1	16.8
Other professional services	8.9	8.1	3.7	9.1	10.4	17.7
Drugs and drug sundries	8.1	7.8	9.6	7.8	7.0	8.5
Eyeglasses and appliances	7.7	4.7	19.2	2.4	7.3	9.2
Expenses for prepayment	11.7	9.1	5.9	9.5	10.2	39.2
Government public health activities	9.9	1.4	14.7	11.8	17.3	16.6
Other health services	7.8	7.7	3.4	9.5	12.4	5.5
Research and construction	8.5	5.9	15.2	8.8	9.3	4.6
Research	13.7	18.9	17.2	4.9	11.3	10.4
Construction	6.7	2.2	13.8	11.4	8.1	0.6

SOURCE: USDHEW, 1979

Table 12.6 Amount and Percentage Distribution of Personal Health Care Expenditures[a] by Source of Funds, Selected Calendar Years 1929 to 1978

		Source of Funds						
		Private				Public		
Calendar Year	Total	Total	Direct Payments	Insurance Benefits	Other	Total	Federal	State and Local
			Aggregate Amount (in Millions)					
1929	$ 3,202	$ 2,913	$ 2,829[b]	—	$ 84	$ 289	$ 87	$ 202
1935	2,663	2,269	2,195[b]	—	74	392	91	301
1940	3,548	2,980	2,886[b]	—	94	570	145	425
1950	10,885	8,445	7,133	$ 922	320	2,440	1,136	1,304
1955	15,708	12,100	9,132	2,536	432	3,608	1,646	1,962
1960	23,680	18,523	12,990	4,996	537	5,157	2,199	2,958
1965	37,267	29,387	19,900	8,729	758	7,880	3,784	4,095
1966	41,055	30,873	20,957	9,142	775	10,182	5,292	4,890
1967	45,923	30,752	20,426	9,545	781	15,172	9,572	5,600
1968	51,543	33,745	21,574	11,344	827	17,798	11,455	6,344
1969	57,888	37,721	23,786	13,069	866	20,167	13,211	6,956
1970	65,723	43,281	26,543	15,744	995	22,442	14,561	7,881
1971	72,115	46,395	27,548	17,714	1,134	25,721	16,804	8,917
1972	79,870	51,042	30,406	19,433	1,203	28,828	18,967	9,861
1973	88,471	56,408	33,647	21,513	1,248	32,063	21,126	10,937
1974	100,885	62,266	35,682	25,171	1,413	38,619	25,865	12,755
1975	116,297	70,164	37,803	30,902	1,459	46,133	31,532	14,601
1976	132,127	80,531	41,869	37,070	1,592	51,596	36,283	15,314
1977	149,139	91,048	48,596	40,492	1,960	58,091	41,096	16,996
1978[c]	167,911	102,870	55,317	45,363	2,189	65,042	46,503	18,539
			Percent Distribution					
1929	100.0	91.0	88.4	—	2.6	9.0	2.7	6.3
1935	100.0	85.2	82.4	—	2.8	14.7	3.4	11.3
1940	100.0	84.0	81.3	—	2.6	16.1	4.1	12.0
1950	100.0	77.6	65.5	9.1	2.9	22.4	10.4	12.0
1955	100.0	77.0	58.1	16.1	2.8	23.0	10.5	12.5
1960	100.0	78.2	54.9	21.1	2.3	21.8	9.3	12.5
1965	100.0	78.9	53.4	23.4	2.0	21.1	10.2	11.0
1966	100.0	75.2	51.0	22.3	1.9	24.8	12.9	11.9
1967	100.0	67.0	44.5	20.8	1.7	33.0	20.8	12.2
1968	100.0	65.5	41.9	22.0	1.6	34.5	22.2	12.3
1969	100.0	65.2	41.1	22.6	1.5	34.8	22.8	12.0
1970	100.0	65.9	40.4	24.0	1.5	34.1	22.2	12.0
1971	100.0	64.3	38.2	24.6	1.6	35.7	23.3	12.4
1972	100.0	63.9	38.1	24.3	1.5	36.1	23.7	12.3
1973	100.0	63.8	38.0	24.3	1.4	36.2	23.9	12.4
1974	100.0	61.7	35.4	25.0	1.4	38.3	25.6	12.6
1975	100.0	60.3	32.5	26.6	1.3	39.7	27.1	12.6
1976	100.0	60.9	31.7	28.1	1.2	39.1	27.5	11.6
1977	100.0	61.0	32.6	27.2	1.3	39.0	27.6	11.4
1978[c]	100.0	61.3	32.9	27.0	1.3	38.7	27.7	11.0

SOURCE: Gibson, 1979.

[a] Includes all expenditures for health services and supplies other than (1) expenses for prepayment and administration; (2) government public health activities.
[b] Includes any insurance benefits and expenses for prepayment (insurance premiums less insurance benefits).
[c] Preliminary estimates.

Table 12.7   Amount and Percentage Distribution of Personal Health Care Expenditures, by Type of Expenditure and Source of Funds, Selected Calendar Years 1950 to 1978

Expenditure and Calendar Year	Total	Source of Funds				
		Private				Public
		Total	Direct Payments	Insurance Benefits	Other	
Aggregate Amount (in Millions)						
Hospital care						
1950	$ 3,851	$ 1,967	$ 1,152	$ 680	$ 135	$ 1,884
1955	5,900	3,172	1,318	1,679	175	2,728
1960	9,092	5,338	1,804	3,304	230	3,754
1965	13,935	8,539	2,469	5,790	280	5,396
1966	15,640	8,706	2,445	5,993	268	6,934
1967	18,259	8,242	1,867	6,133	242	10,017
1968	21,016	9,544	1,964	7,322	258	11,472
1969	24,019	11,013	2,397	8,356	260	13,006
1970	27,799	13,227	2,879	10,008	340	14,572
1971	30,769	14,309	2,665	11,263	382	16,460
1972	34,974	16,370	3,749	12,199	421	18,604
1973	38,585	18,085	4,343	13,308	434	20,499
1974	44,857	20,298	4,493	15,274	530	24,560
1975	52,138	23,304	3,967	18,869	468	28,834
1976	59,806	27,037	4,085	22,469	482	32,769
1977	67,914	30,964	6,268	23,956	740	36,950
1978[a]	76,025	35,107	7,533	26,724	849	40,918
Percentage Distribution						
Hospital care						
1950	100.0	51.1	29.9	17.7	3.5	48.9
1955	100.0	53.8	22.3	28.5	3.0	46.2
1960	100.0	58.7	19.8	36.3	2.5	41.3
1965	100.0	61.3	17.7	41.5	2.0	38.7
1966	100.0	55.7	15.6	38.3	1.7	44.3
1967	100.0	45.1	10.2	33.6	1.3	54.9
1968	100.0	45.4	9.3	34.8	1.2	54.6
1969	100.0	45.9	10.0	34.8	1.1	54.1
1970	100.0	47.6	10.4	36.0	1.2	52.4
1971	100.0	46.5	8.7	36.6	1.2	53.5
1972	100.0	46.8	10.7	34.9	1.2	53.2
1973	100.0	46.9	11.3	34.5	1.1	53.1
1974	100.0	45.2	10.0	34.1	1.2	54.8
1975	100.0	44.7	7.6	36.2	0.9	55.3
1976	100.0	45.2	6.8	37.6	0.8	54.8
1977	100.0	45.6	9.2	35.3	1.1	54.4
1978[a]	100.0	1.1	53.8	46.2	9.9	35.2

Table 12.7   (cont.)

Expenditure and Calendar Year	Total	Source of Funds				
		Private				Public
		Total	Direct Payments	Insurance Benefits	Other	

		Aggregate Amount (in Millions)				
Physicians' services						
1950	$ 2,747	$ 2,604	$ 2,285	$ 312	$ 7	$ 143
1955	3,689	3,441	2,576	857	8	248
1960	5,684	5,318	3,716	1,593	9	366
1965	8,474	7,890	5,202	2,680	8	584
1966	9,175	8,324	5,484	2,831	9	851
1967	10,142	8,093	5,120	2,964	9	2,049
1968	11,104	8,619	5,119	3,489	10	2,485
1969	12,648	9,819	5,780	4,029	10	2,829
1970	14,340	11,253	6,335	4,908	10	3,087
1971	15,918	12,463	7,012	5,440	11	3,454
1972	17,162	13,223	7,154	6,056	12	3,939
1973	19,075	14,635	7,889	6,731	14	4,441
1974	21,245	15,913	7,979	7,922	13	5,332
1975	24,932	18,395	8,946	9,435	14	6,537
1976	27,658	20,592	9,654	10,922	15	7,066
1977	31,242	23,136	10,890	12,228	17	8,106
1978[a]	35,250	25,811	12,013	13,779	19	9,439

		Percentage Distribution				
Physicians' services						
1950	100.0	94.8	83.2	11.4	0.3	5.2
1955	100.0	93.3	69.8	23.2	0.2	6.7
1960	100.0	93.6	65.4	28.0	0.2	6.4
1965	100.0	93.1	61.4	31.6	0.1	6.9
1966	100.0	90.7	59.8	30.9	0.1	9.3
1967	100.0	79.8	50.5	29.2	0.1	20.2
1968	100.0	77.6	46.1	31.4	0.1	22.4
1969	100.0	77.6	45.7	31.9	0.1	22.4
1970	100.0	78.5	44.2	34.2	0.1	21.5
1971	100.0	78.3	44.1	34.2	0.1	21.7
1972	100.0	77.0	41.7	35.3	0.1	23.0
1973	100.0	76.7	41.4	35.3	0.1	23.3
1974	100.0	74.9	37.6	37.3	0.1	25.1
1975	100.0	73.8	35.9	37.8	0.1	26.2
1976	100.0	74.5	34.9	39.5	0.1	25.5
1977	100.0	74.1	34.9	39.1	0.1	25.9
1978[a]	100.0	73.2	34.1	39.1	0.1	26.8

Table 12.7 (cont.)

Expenditure and Calendar Year	Total	Source of Funds				Public
		Private				
		Total	Direct Payments	Insurance Benefits	Other	
		Aggregate Amount (in Millions)				

All other services[b]

Year	Total	Total	Direct Payments	Insurance Benefits	Other	Public
1950	$ 4,287	$ 3,874	$ 3,695	—[c]	$ 178	$ 413
1955	6,119	5,487	5,238	—[c]	249	623
1960	8,904	7,867	7,470	$ 99	298	1,037
1965	14,857	12,958	12,228	259	470	1,900
1966	16,240	13,844	13,028	318	498	2,396
1967	17,522	14,416	13,439	447	530	3,106
1968	19,423	15,582	14,490	533	558	3,842
1969	21,221	16,889	15,609	683	596	4,333
1970	23,584	18,802	17,329	828	645	4,783
1971	25,429	19,622	17,871	1,011	740	5,807
1972	27,734	21,449	19,503	1,177	769	6,285
1973	30,812	23,688	21,414	1,474	800	7,124
1974	34,783	26,055	23,210	1,975	869	8,728
1975	39,227	28,464	24,890	2,598	976	10,763
1976	44,663	32,902	28,129	3,679	1,094	11,761
1977	49,983	36,948	31,438	4,308	1,202	13,035
1978[a]	56,637	41,952	35,771	4,861	1,321	14,684
		Percentage Distribution				

All other services[b]

Year	Total	Total	Direct Payments	Insurance Benefits	Other	Public
1950	100.0	90.4	86.2	—	4.2	9.6
1955	100.0	89.7	85.6	—	4.1	10.3
1960	100.0	88.4	83.9	1.1	3.5	11.3
1965	100.0	87.2	82.3	1.7	3.2	12.8
1966	100.0	85.2	80.2	2.0	3.1	14.8
1967	100.0	82.3	76.7	2.6	3.0	17.7
1968	100.0	80.2	74.6	2.7	2.9	19.8
1969	100.0	79.6	73.6	3.2	2.8	20.4
1970	100.0	79.7	73.5	3.5	2.7	20.3
1971	100.0	77.2	70.3	4.0	2.9	22.8
1972	100.0	77.3	70.3	4.2	2.8	22.7
1973	100.0	76.9	69.5	4.8	2.6	23.1
1974	100.0	74.9	66.7	5.7	2.5	25.1
1975	100.0	72.6	63.5	6.6	2.5	27.4
1976	100.0	73.7	63.0	8.2	2.5	26.3
1977	100.0	73.9	62.9	8.6	2.4	26.1
1978[a]	100.0	74.1	63.2	8.6	2.3	25.9

SOURCE: Gibson, 1979.

[a] Preliminary estimates.
[b] Includes dentists' services, other professional services, drugs and drug sundries, eyeglasses and appliances, nursing-home care, and other health services.
[c] Included in direct payments; data not available separately.

Table 12.8 Annual Percentage Increase in Medical Care Cost Factors and Their Contribution to Expenditure Growth 1970 to 1978 (All values are percentages)

	Total Expenditures	Population	Aging	Price	CPI	Deflated Price	Utilization (per Capita, Age-Adjusted)	Intensity
All Personal Health Care:								
Rate of increase	12.6	0.9	2.3 (0.5)[b]	7.7	6.8	0.9	1.0	2.1
Contribution to expenditure growth	100.0	7.4	4.1	63.1	55.7	7.4	8.2	17.2
Contribution to endogenous growth						22.5	25.0	52.5
Hospital Care:								
Rate of increase	14.8	0.9	2.3 (0.5)[b]	8.0	6.8	1.2	1.4	3.5
Contribution to expenditure growth	100.0	6.3	3.5	55.9	47.3	8.4	9.8	24.5
Contribution to endogenous growth						19.7	22.9	57.4
Physician Care:								
Rate of increase	12.1	0.9	2.3 (0.2)[b]	8.9[a]	6.8	2.1	0.8	1.0
Contribution to expenditure growth	100.0	7.6	1.7	75.4	57.6	17.8	6.8	8.5
Contribution to endogenous growth						53.8	20.5	25.6

SOURCE: Gibson, 1979; DHEW, 1979; Dyckman, 1978.
a As adjusted by Dyckman (1978) for decreasing rate of physician fee discounting.
b Equivalent additional population growth due to aging.

Table 12.9   Income of Physicians, Dentists, and All Professional, Technical and Kindred Workers, 1939 to 1976

| Year | Median Net Income | | | Average Wages and Salaries for Full-Time Employees |
	Office-Based Nonsalaried Physicians	Office-Based Nonsalaried Dentists	Male Professional, Technical and Kindred Workers[b]	
1939	$ 3,263[a]		$ 1,809	$ 1,280
1947	8,744		—	2,612
1951	13,150		4,071	3,262
1955	16,107	$11,533	5,055	3,923
1963	25,050		7,182	5,349
1965	28,960		7,798	5,814
1967	34,740	22,850	8,882	6,307
1970	43,100	28,100	10,722	7,713
1972	46,780		12,097	8,760
1973	50,823		12,977	9,290
1974	54,140	30,500	13,391	9,991
1975	58,440		14,311	10,845
1976	62,799		—	11,623

SOURCE: Dyckman, 1978.

[a] For 1939 *Medical Economics* published an estimate of mean rather than median income. Median income is estimated by assuming that the ratio of median to mean income in 1939 is the same for *Medical Economics* data as it is for Department of Commerce data.

[b] Data on male professional workers are used since data for all professionals are not available for the entire time period.

REFERENCES

Abelson, Philip H., "Changing Climate for Medicine," *Science*, **188**:1888, 1975.

Acton, Jan, "Demand for Health Care Among the Urban Poor with Special Emphasis on the Role of Time," Memorandum R-1151—DEO/NYC, Rand Corporation, April 1973.

Altman, Stuart, and Eichenholz, Joseph, "Inflation in the Health Industry: Causes and Cures," in Zubkoff, Michael, Ed., *Health: a Victim or Cause of Inflation*, New York: Prodist, 1976.

Anderson, Odin W., *Blue Cross Since 1929: Accountability and the Public Trust*, Cambridge, Mass.: Ballinger, 1975.

Anderson, Odin W., personal communication, 1980.

Anderson, Odin W., and Neuhauser, Duncan, "Rising Costs are Inherent in Modern Health Care Systems," *Hospitals, Journal of the American Hospital Association*, **43** (February 16):50–73, 1969.

Arrow, Kenneth, "Uncertainty and the Welfare Economics of Medical Care," *American Economic Review*, **53**:941–973, 1963.

Auster, Richard, Levenson, Irving, and Sarachek, Deborah, "The Production of Health: An Exploratory Study,' *Journal of Human Resources*, **4**:411–436, 1969.

Benham, Lee, and Benham, Alexandra, "The Impact of Incremental Medical Services on Health Status, 1963–1970," in Andersen, R., Kravitz, J., and Anderson, O., Eds., *Equity in Health Services,* Cambridge, Mass.: Ballinger, 1975.

Berg, Robert L., Browning, Francis E., Hill, John G., and Wenkert, Walter, "Assessing the Health Care Needs of the Aged," *Health Services Research,* 4:36–59, 1970.

Berger, Laurence, and Sullivan, Paul, *Measuring Hospital Inflation,* Lexington, Mass.: Lexington Books, Heath, 1975.

Berki, Sylvester E., *Hospital Economics,* Lexington, Mass.: Heath, 1972.

Berry, Ralph E., "Cost and Efficiency in the Production of Hospital Services," *Milbank Memorial Fund Quarterly/Health and Society,* 52:291–313, 1974.

Blumberg, Mark S., "Rational Provider Prices: An Incentive for Improved Health Delivery," in Chacko, G. K., Ed., *Health Handbook,* Amsterdam: North Holland, 1978.

Boulding, Kenneth E., "The Concept of Need for Health Services," *Milbank Memorial Fund Quarterly,* 44(October, Part 2): 202–223, 1966.

Bunker, John P., "Surgical Manpower—A Comparison of Operations in the U.S. and in England and Wales," *New England Journal of Medicine,* 282:135–144, 1970.

Burney, Ira L., Schieber, George J., Blaxall, Martha O., and Gabel, J. R., "Geographic Variation in Physicians' Fees: Paying the Physician Under Medicare and Medicaid," *Journal of the American Medical Association,* 240:13(September 22), 1978.

Campbell, R. R., *Economics of Health and Public Policy,* Washington, D.C.: U.S. Department of Commerce, 1974.

Coase, R., "The Problem of Social Cost," *Journal of Law and Economics* (3) 1960.

Cochrane, A., *Effectiveness and Efficiency,* London: The Nuffield Provincial Hospitals Trust, 1971.

Colombotos, John, "Physicians and Medicare: A Before-After Study of the Effects of Legislation on Attitudes," *American Sociological Review,* 34:318–334, 1969.

Congressional Budget Office (CBO), Congressional Research Service, *Hospital Cost Containment—Update,* Washington, D.C.: U.S. Congress, 1979.

Cooper, Barbara S., and Gaus, Clifton R., "Controlling Health Technology," in Altman, Stuart, and Blendon, Robert, Eds., *Medical Technology: The Culprit Behind Health Care Costs?* Sun Valley Forum on National Health, Washington, D.C.: USDHEW (PHS) No. 79–3216, 1977.

Council on Wage and Price Stability (COWPS), *The Complex Puzzle of Rising Health Care Costs,* Washington, D.C.: Executive Office of the President, 1976.

Davis, Karen, "Community Hospital Expenses and Revenues: Pre-Medicare Inflation," *Social Security Bulletin,* 35(October):3, 1972.

Davis, Karen, "Theories of Hospital Inflation: Some Empirical Evidence," *Journal of Human Resources,* 8(Spring):181–201, 1973.

Davis, Karen, "Hospital Costs and the Medicare Program," *Social Security Bulletin,* 36 (August):18–36, 1973a.

Davis, Karen, and Russell, Louise, "The Substitution of Hospital Outpatient Care for Inpatient Care," *Review of Economics and Statistics,* 54:109–120, 1972.

Davis, Karen, Testimony before the Subcommittee on Health of the Ways and Means Committee, U.S. House of Representatives, Washington, D.C.: U.S. Congress, February 25, 1980.

Derzon, Robert, Administrator, Health Care Finance Administration, personal communication, 1978.

Dukakis, Hon. Michael, Governor of Massachusetts, Testimony before the Subcommittee on Health and Scientific Research, Human Resources Committee, U.S. Senate, May 24, 1977.

Dyckman, Zackary U., *A Study of Physician Fees*, Washington, D.C.: Council on Wage and Price Stability, 1978.

Evans, Robert G., "Supplier Induced Demand: Some Empirical Evidence and Implications," in Perlman, Mark, Ed., *The Economics of Health and Medical Care*, New York: Halsted, 1974.

Fein, Rashi, "Some Health Policy Issues: One Economist's View," *Public Health Reports*, 90:387, 1975.

Feldstein, Martin S., "The Rising Price of Physicians' Services," *The Review of Economics and Statistics*, 52(May):121–133, 1970.

Feldstein, Martin S., *The Rising Cost of Hospital Care*, Washington, D.C.: Information Resources Press, 1971.

Feldstein, Martin S., "Hospital Cost Inflation: A Study of Non-Profit Price Dynamics," *American Economic Review*, 61:861 (December), 1971a.

Feldstein, Martin S., "The Welfare Loss of Excess Health Insurance," *The Journal of Political Economy*, 81:251, 1973.

Feldstein, Martin S., "The High Cost of Hospitals—What To Do About It," *The Public Interest*, 48:40–54, 1977.

Feldstein, Martin S., and Taylor, Amy, *The Rapid Rise of Hospital Costs*, Washington, D.C.: Council on Wage and Price Stability, 1977.

Feldstein, Paul J., "Research on the Demand for Health Services," *Milbank Memorial Fund Quarterly*, 44(3, July, Part 2):128–165, 1966.

Feldstein, Paul J., *Health Care Economics*, New York: Wiley, 1979.

Feldstein, Paul, and Severson, R., "The Demand for Medical Care," in *Report of the Commission on the Cost of Medical Care*, Vol. 1, Chicago: American Medical Association, 1964, pp. 54–76.

Fineberg, Harvey V., "Clinical Chemistries: The High Cost of Low-cost Diagnostic Testing," in *Medical Technology: The Culprit Behind Health Care Costs?* Sun Valley Forum on National Health, Washington, D.C.: USDHEW (PHS) No. 79–3216, 1977.

Freeland, Mark S., Anderson, Gerard, and Schendler, Carol E., "National Hospital Input Price Index," *Health Care Financing Review* 1(1): 37–61, 1979.

Fuchs, Victor R., "The Contribution of Health Services to the American Economy," *Milbank Memorial Fund Quarterly*, 64(October, Part 2): 65–103, 1966.

Fuchs, Victor R., Ed., *Essays in the Economics of Health and Medical Care*, New York: Columbia University Press, 1972.

Fuchs, Victor R., "Health Care and the United States Economic System: An Essay in Abnormal Physiology," in McKinlay, John B., Ed., *Economic Aspects of Health Care*, New York: Prodist, 1973.

Fuchs, Victor R., *Who Shall Live?: Health, Economics, and Social Choice*, New York: Basic Books, 1974.

Fuchs, Victor R., "The Economics of Health in a Post-Industrial Society," *The Public Interest*, 56:3–20, 1979.

Fuchs, Victor, and Kramer, Marcia, *Determinants of Expenditures for Physicians Services in the United States, 1948–1968*, New York: National Bureau of Economic Research, Occasional Paper 117, 1973.

Gaus, Clifton R., "Biomedical Research and Health Care Costs," Testimony before the President's Biomedical Research Panel, September 29, 1975.

Gaus, Clifton R., et al., "Contrasts in HMO and Fee-for-Service Performance," *Social Security Bulletin*, May: 3, 1976.

Gibson, Robert M., "National Health Expenditures," *Health Care Financing Review*, 1(1):1–36, 1979.

Gibson, Robert M., and Fisher, C. R., "Age Differences in Health Care Spending, FY 1977," *Social Security Bulletin*, **42**(January):15, 1979.

Ginsburg, Daniel H., "Medical Care Services in the Consumer Price Index," *Monthly Labor Review*, August:36, 1978.

Grossman, Michael, "On the Concept of Health Capital and the Demand for Health," *Journal of Political Economy*, **80**:223, 1972.

Hardwick, C. Patrick, Shuman, Larry, and Barnoon, Shlomo, "Effect of Participatory Insurance on Hospital Utilization," *Health Services Research*, **7**:43–58, 1972.

Health Insurance Institute, *Health Insurance Fact Book: 1979*, Chicago, 1979.

Hetherington, Robert W., Hopkins, Carl E., and Roemer, Milton I., *Health Insurance Plans: Promise and Performance*, New York: Wiley-Interscience, 1975.

Holahan, J., Hadley, J., Scanlon, W., Lee, R., and Bluck, J., "Paying for Physician Services Under Medicare and Medicaid," *Milbank Memorial Fund Quarterly, Health and Society*, **57**(Spring):4, 1979.

Hughes, Edward F. X., Fuchs, Victor, Jacoby, John, and Lewit, Eugene, "Surgical Work Loads in a Community Practice," *Surgery*, **70**(March):315–327, 1972.

Institute of Medicine, *Medicare-Medicaid Reimbursement Policies*, Washington, D.C.: National Academy of Sciences, 1976.

Jacobs, P., "A Survey of Economic Models of Hospitals," *Inquiry*, **11**(June):83–97, 1974.

Jeffers, James R., Bognanno, Mario F., and Bartlett, John C., "On the Demand Versus Need for Medical Services and the Concepts of 'Shortage,' " *American Journal of Public Health*, **61**:47, 1971.

Joseph, Hyman, "Empirical Research on the Demand for Health Care," *Inquiry*, **8**:61–71, 1971.

Kelman, Sander, "Toward the Political Economy of Medical Care," *Inquiry*, **8**(3):30–38, 1971.

Kisch, A., "The Health Care System and Health: Some Thoughts on a Famous Misalliance," *Inquiry*, **11**:269, 1974.

Klarman, Herbert E., *The Economics of Health*, New York: Columbia University Press, 1965.

Klarman, Herbert E., "The Difference the Third Party Makes," *Journal of Risk and Insurance*, **36**:553, 1969.

Klarman, Herbert E., "Observations on Health Care Technology: Measurement, Analysis and Policy," in *Medical Technology: The Culprit Behind Health Care Costs?* Sun Valley Forum on National Health, Washington, D.C.: USDHEW (PHS) No. 79–3216, 1977.

Krizay, J., and Wilson, A., *The Patient as Consumer*, Lexington, Mass.: Heath, 1974.

Lee, M. L., "A Conspicuous Production Theory of Hospital Behavior," *Southern Economic Journal*, **38**:48–59, 1971.

Lees, Dennis, and Rice, Robert, "Uncertainty and the Welfare Economics of Medical Care: Comments," *American Economic Review*, March 1965.

Lewis, Charles E., "Variations in the Incidence of Surgery," *New England Journal of Medicine*, **281**:880, 1969.

Lipman, Aaron, and Sterne, Richard S., "Aging in the United States: Ascription of a Terminal Sick Role," *Sociology and Social Research*, **53**:194–203, 1969.

Luft, Harold S., "How do Health Maintenance Organizations Achieve Their 'Savings'?" *New England Journal of Medicine*, **298**:1336–1343, 1978.

Marcus, Glenn, "Group Health Insurance Premium Setting," Washington, D.C.: Congressional Research Service, 1980.

Marmor, Theodore, and Thomas, D., "The Politics of Paying Physicians: The Determinants of Government Payment Methods in England, Sweden and the United States," *International Journal of Health Services*, 1:71–78, 1971.

May, J. Joel, "Utilization of Health Services and Availability of Resources," in Anderson, Ron, et al., Eds., *Equity in Health Services*, Cambridge, Mass.: Ballinger, 1975.

McKeown, Thomas, and Lowe, C. R., *An Introduction to Social Medicine*, 2nd ed., Philadelphia: Lippincott, 1974.

McKinlay, John B., and McKinlay, Sonja M., "The Questionable Contribution of Medical Measures to the Decline of Mortality in the United States in the Twentieth Century," *Milbank Memorial Fund Quarterly*, 53(3):405–428, 1977.

McMahon, J. Alexander, Testimony before the Subcommittee on Health, Committee on Labor and Human Relations, U.S. Senate, March, 9, 1978.

Mellman, Richard, personal communication, 1980.

Monsma, George, "Marginal Revenue and Demand for Physicians' Services," in Klarman, H., Ed., *Empirical Studies in Health Economics*, Baltimore: Johns Hopkins University Press, 1970.

Newhouse, Joseph P., "Toward a Theory of Non-Profit Institutions: An Economic Model of a Hospital," *American Economic Review*, March 1970.

Newhouse, Joseph P., and Taylor, Vincent, "How Shall We Pay For Hospital Care?" *The Public Interest*, 23(Spring):78–92, 1971.

Newhouse, Joseph P., and Phelps, Charles, "New Estimates of Price Income Elasticities for Medical Services," in Rosett, Richard, Ed., *The Role of Health Insurance in the Health Services Sector*, New York: National Bureau of Economic Research, 1976.

Pauly, Mark V., "A Measure of the Welfare Cost of Health Insurance," *Health Services Research*, 4(Winter):281–292, 1969.

Pauly, Mark V., "The Welfare Economics of Community Rating," *Journal of Risk and Insurance*, September 1970.

Pauly, Mark V., and Redisch, M., "The Not-for-Profit Hospital as a Physicians' Cooperative," *American Economic Review*, 63:87–99, 1973.

Pauly, Mark V., "The Behavior of Non-Profit Hospital Monopolies: Alternative Models of the Hospital," in Havighurst, Clark, Ed., *Regulating Health Facilities Construction*, Washington, D.C.: American Enterprise Institute for Public Policy, 1974.

Phelps, Charles, and Newhouse, Joseph, "The Effect of Coinsurance: a Multivariate Analysis," *Social Security Bulletin*, June 1972.

Phelps, Charles, *Demand for Health Insurance: A Theoretical and Empirical Investigation*, Santa Monica: Rand Corporation, 1973.

Phelps, Charles, "The Effects of Insurance on Demand for Medical Care," in Anderson, Ron, et al., Eds., *Equity in Health Services*, Cambridge, Mass.: Ballinger, 1975.

Phelps, Charles E., "Public Sector Medicine: History and Analysis," in *New Directions in Public Health Care*, San Francisco: Institute for Contemporary Studies, 1976.

Phillip, P. Joseph, Jeffers, James, and Hai, Abdul, "Indexes of Factor Input Price, Service Intensity, and Productivity of the Hospital Industry," *The Nature of Hospital Costs: Three Studies*, Chicago: Hospital Research and Educational Trust, 1976, pp. 219–229.

Rayack, Elton, *Professional Power and American Medicine: The Economics of the American Medical Association*, Cleveland: World, 1967.

Reinhardt, Uwe E., "A Production Function for Physician Services," *Review of Economics and Statistics*, February: 63, 1972.

Reinhardt, Uwe E., *Physician Productivity and the Demand for Health Manpower*, Cambridge, Mass.: Ballinger, 1975.

Rettig, Richard A., "End-stage Renal Disease and The 'Cost' of Medical Technology," in *Medical Technology: The Culprit Behind Health Care Costs?* Sun Valley Forum on National Health, Washington, D.C.: USDHEW(PHS) No. 79-3216, 1979.

Rivlin, Alice M., *Social Policy: Alternate Strategies for the Federal Government,* Washington, D.C.: Brookings Institution, 1974.

Roemer, Milton J., "Bed Supply and Hospital Utilization: A Natural Experiment," *Hospitals, Journal of the American Hospital Association,* 35(November 1):36–42, 1961.

Roemer, Milton J., and Shain, Max, *Hospitalization Under Insurance,* Chicago: American Hospital Association, 1959.

Roemer, Milton I., et al., "Copayments for Ambulatory Care: Penny-Wise and Pound-Foolish," *Medical Care,* 13:457, 1975.

Rosenthal, Gerald, *The Demand for General Hospital Facilities,* Monograph No. 14, Chicago: American Hospital Association, 1964.

Rosenthal, Gerald, "Price Elasticity of Demand for Short-Term General Hospital Services," in Klarman, H., *Empirical Studies in Health Economics,* Baltimore: Johns Hopkins University Press, 1970.

Rossett, Richard, and Lien-fu, Huang, "The Effect of Health Insurance on the Demand for Medical Care," *Journal of Political Economy,* 81:281, 1973.

Salkever, David, "A Microeconomic Study of Hospital Cost Inflation," *Journal of Political Economy,* 80:1144–1166, 1972.

Schieber, George J., Burney, Ira L., Golden, J. B., and Knaus, W. J., "Physician Fee Patterns Under Medicare: A Descriptive Analysis," *New England Journal of Medicine,* 294:1089, 1976.

Schultze, Charles, Chairman, Council of Economic Advisors, Testimony before the Select Committee on Small Business, U.S. Senate, August 21, 1978.

Scitovsky, Anne A., and Snyder, Nelda M., "Effect of Coinsurance on Use of Physician Services," *Social Security Bulletin,* June 1972.

Scitovsky, Anne A., and McCall, Nelda, "Changes in the Costs of Treatment of Selected Illnesses, 1951–1971," Health Policy Discussion Paper, San Francisco: University of California School of Medicine, 1975.

Shain, Max, and Roemer, Milton, "Hospital Costs Relate to the Supply of Beds," *Modern Hospital,* 92(April):71–73, 1959.

Shanas, Ethel, Townsend, P., Wedderburn, D., Friis, H., Milhoj, P., and Stehouwer, J., *Old People in Three Industrial Societies,* New York: Atherton, 1968.

Shilit, S., "A Doctor-Hospital Cartel Theory," *Journal of Business,* January 1977.

Silver, Morris, "An Economic Analysis of Variations in Medical Expenses and Work Loss Rates," in Klarman, H., Ed., *Empirical Studies in Health Economics,* Baltimore: Johns Hopkins University Press, 1970.

Sloan, Frank, and Steinwald, B., "The Role of Health Insurance in the Physician Services Market," *Inquiry,* 12(December):275–299, 1975.

Somers, Herman M., and Somers, Anne R., *Doctors, Patients and Health Insurance,* Washington, D.C.: Brookings Institution, 1961.

Somers, Herman M., and Somers, Anne R., *Medicare and the Hospitals: Issues and Prospects,* Washington, D.C.: Brookings Institution, 1968.

Stevens, Rosemary, *American Medicine and the Public Interest,* New Haven: Yale University Press, 1971.

Stevens, Rosemary, and Vermeulen, Joan, *Foreign Trained Physicians and American Medicine,* Washington, D.C.: USDHEW(NIH) No. 73-325, 1972.

Stevens, Robert, and Stevens, Rosemary, *Welfare Medicine in America: A Case Study of Medicaid,* New York: Free Press, 1974.

Stewart, Charles T., Jr., "The Allocation of Resources to Health," *Journal of Human Resources* 6(Winter):1971.

Strickland, Stephen P., *Politics, Science, & Dread Disease: A Short History of United States Medical Research Policy,* Cambridge: Harvard University Press, 1972a.

Sunley, Emil M., Deputy Assistant Secretary of The Treasury, Statement before the Health Subcommittee of The Committee on Ways and Means, U.S. House of Representatives, 1980.

U.S. Bureau of The Census, *Statistical Abstract of the United States,* Washington, D.C.: Department of Commerce, 1979.

U.S. Comptroller General, *Health Costs Can Be Reduced by Millions of Dollars If Federal Agencies Fully Carry Out GAO Recommendations,* Washington, D.C.: General Accounting Office, 1980.

USDHEW, "Excess Hospital Beds," Washington, D.C.: USDHEW(PHS), Bureau of Health Planning, Health Resources Administration, 1978b.

USDHEW, "Capital Expenditures for Hospital Services," Washington, D.C.: USDHEW, Office of the Assistant Secretary for Planning and Evaluation, mimeo, 1977a.

USDHEW, *Health, United States, 1978,* Washington, D.C.: USDHEW(PHS), 78-1232, 1978.

USDHEW, *Health, United States, 1979,* Washington, D.C.: USDHEW, 79-1232, 1979.

USDHEW, "Hospital Cost Containment—Fact Sheet," Washington, D.C.: USDHEW, Office of the Assistant Secretary for Planning and Evaluation, mimeo, 1979a.

U.S. House of Representatives, Interstate and Foreign Commerce Committee, Subcommittee on Oversight and Investigations, "Getting Ready for National Health Insurance: Unnecessary Surgery," Hearings, July 15–18/September 3, 1975.

Vladeck, Bruce C., "Why Non-Profits Go Broke," *The Public Interest,* 42:86–11, 1976.

Wagner, Judith L., and Zubkoff, Michael, "Medical Technology and Hospital Costs," in Zubkoff, M., Ruskin, I., and Hanft, R., Eds., *Hospital Cost Containment: Selected Notes for Future Policy,* New York: Prodist, 1978.

Waldo, Daniel, "Implicit Price Deflation for Health Expenditures," *Health Care Financing Notes,* 1:1979.

Wildavsky, Aaron, *The Politics of the Budgetary Process,* Boston: Little, Brown, 1974.

CHAPTER THIRTEEN

The Structure of the Health Care Economy and Strategies for Containing Health Costs

There is widespread agreement among most experts in the field about the elements and nature of health cost escalation discussed in Chapter 12. As soon as the question turns to *which* of the causes should be the target for controlling costs, however, consensus disappears. Some argue that the key is the insurance system of health care financing which in effect forces consumers to purchase more sophisticated and expensive care than they actually want (M. Feldstein, 1977). Many studies (Federal Trade Commission, 1977) have demonstrated the lack of effective competition in the health care sector, and some economists pinpoint this as the critical cause of cost escalation (Enthoven, 1978). They contend that lack of competition results in excessive waste and inefficiency in the health industry which could be avoided without loss of quality by forcing providers to compete for patients. Some students of the health system argue that the perverse incentives built into the physician payment mechanisms are central in leading to unnecessary surgery, hospitalization, and other services, as well as inordinate physician fees (Blumberg, 1978; Dyckman, 1978). Similarly, many argue that the cost method of reimbursing hospitals for their services is crucial in creating incentives to increase their outlays unnecessarily and overuse resources (Altman & Eichenholz, 1976). Others contend that the uncontrolled growth of medical technology is the major driving force pushing up costs (Gaus, 1975). Advocates of health planning argue that the primary cause lies in excess hospital beds and duplication of expensive services or maldistribution of manpower and facilities.

This multiplicity of explanations for health care cost escalation and implied or explicit strategies for control suggests that there is no single dominant cause and no simple solution. The vehemence of the disagreement about the relative importance of the factors causing the increases in health care costs suggests that this is *not just an empirical question*. Underlying the arguments about the causes and control of costs escalation is an *implicit* dispute concerning the nature of the health care *market* itself. In question is what economic structure and what fiscal mechanisms *actually function* at present? More crucially, what structure and fiscal mechanisms *ought* to be furthered in order to attain a more effective and efficient health care system? This debate has ideological overtones rooted in the divergence of assumptions and value implications inherent in theoretical models and philosophical justifications for the different types of economic structures.

In our society three fundamentally different structural types of economies occur for different circumstances of production, financing, and consumption: (1) competitive (supply-demand controlled), so-called free markets; (2) publicly financed, budgeted, and planned public services; and (3) regulated utilities. These three economic types are all used successfully in certain sectors of the economy where the circumstances fit. They differ in the way that supply, allocation, price, demand, consumption, and financing relate to each other and to public policy decisions. Because of their basically different structures and control mechanisms, elements from the different types *do not mix well* in the same economic sector. The present health care economy in this country, however, represents just such a mixture of discordant elements and mechanisms from all three types. This mixture evolved when new methods of financing, such as health insurance and tax-supported care, were added to the original out-of-pocket, fee-for-service payment system. Increased government regulation parallel to the developing complexity and cost of the health system further exacerbated the mixture. These new characteristics are incongruent with certain original market features that have been retained. The resulting incompatibilities and mutual aberration of economic mechanisms account for much of the cost escalation, uneven allocation of services, and failure to meet the needs of patients.

In the following sections, we try to demonstrate certain key incongruencies among economic structures in the health care sector. First, we have come to pay for medical care predominantly with public money as if it were a public service. Yet individual providers are not publicly accountable or constrained in their budgeting and allocation of resource as is usually the case with public financing. Utilization is largely freed from control by price to the consumer. Providers, who control most utilization of care, are also freed from the usual economic constraints in producing services. They are not required to conserve on inputs or improve efficiency to be price competitive in order to sell their services. Thus the free market's "invisible hand" (Smith, 1776) of decentralized individual choices cannot serve to determine collectively an overall aggregate budget and its allocation. On the other hand, there is no mechanism for central prospective budgeting to control and allocate health care resources. Removing the free-market constraints on cost without substituting public budgeting explains much of the inability to control expenditures or improve cost effectiveness.

Second, we have eliminated price competition between providers as a means of forcing resource distribution to conform to consumer need. Yet the location of services is allowed to occur as if health care were a free-market commodity. Practice-location decisions take place at the choice of the physician without the limitation of demand in proportion to the population served. Providers can largely determine the demand for their own services and be assured of payment for the resulting consumption. Consequently there is little pressure to distribute their services in relation to the population. Public regulation of the health system is inconsistent. We limit supplier entry and some kinds of investment as if health care were a public utility, but we do not guarantee allocation of services by franchising. The health planning system is mandated to deal with distribution of services but does not apply to physicians or to institutional operating budgets, so that its influence is very limited.

Third, absence of financial mechanisms for rationing and apportioning services and the maldistribution of allocation lead to rationing of services by other (nonmonetary) barriers, such as difficult access, long waiting times, and the unpleasant conditions for care found in hospital outpatient departments. Yet these nonfinancial rationing methods do not allocate services in accord with "need" as assessed by expert opinion—as would be the case with a deliberate public service. Instead the mixture of public and private systems of financing services results in a two-class system of care, one for the rich and one for the poor, with the predictable inequities. This is especially ironic because both systems of care are, in effect, financed in large measure from public monies. The public system is financed directly from taxes by way of a budget that is clearly visible and open to constant criticism. The private system is financed through a hidden back-door system of quasi-public funding through tax writeoffs and cost pass-through by way of employment-related health benefits.

The incompatible mixture of economic mechanisms and structures makes it exceedingly difficult to plan rationally or to predict the impact of strategies to improve the economic function of the health care system. No composite economic model exists to analyze the effects of such a mixture of economy types. To explain economic responses of the health care sector, analysts must revert to one of the three standard economic models—whichever they believe is the best approximation of the situation—and then treat the features of the other economy types as *distortions*. There are ample characteristics of each economy type to justify using any as a starting point for analysis. Since each model is internally consistent and describes certain sectors adequately, there is no way to say, *a priori*, which model is most appropriate for analyzing the health care economy. The question is only which model proves most useful in providing insight to the nature of economic problems of the health sector and suggesting realistic approaches to their improvement. Therefore we analyze the health economy from each of the three perspectives to determine what insight it provides.

HEALTH CARE AS A FREE-MARKET COMMODITY

For so-called competitive, or free-market, commodities, the price, consumption, and total expenditures for particular goods and services are determined by the equilibrium of supply and demand. Certain small businesses, like clothing stores, represent the best remaining approximations to competitive markets, but government regulation and tax policy place considerable constraint on most economic sectors today (Galbraith, 1973). Supply and demand for a given commodity are expressions of the relative tradeoffs that suppliers and consumers make in budgeting their available resources between alternative goods and services at the going prices. Prices fluctuate in response to competition between suppliers and to varying demand from consumers. Price in turn alters supply and demand for each commodity until an equilibrium is reached. The price mechanism allows individual decentralized decisions to create an overall (composite) budget for each commodity or economic sector in accord with the aggregate wishes of the consumers and suppliers.

The practice of medicine in the United States did develop in the nineteenth century within a rather standard free-market for physician services in which fee-for-service payment created a framework for price competition. Today, however, little remains of a competitive market for health care but the trappings. The necessary mechanisms for such a market to function have long since eroded away. The modifications of that economy have been so incremental and seemingly within the free-market framework, however, that there was never an obvious break with that approach. Thus many think about the health sector as if its basic economic framework remained an unchanged (or slightly distorted) supply-demand determined market. Despite its largely fictitious nature, almost all discussions of health care costs and financing still start with the free-market framework.

If we use the free-market model to analyze the economics of health care, the primary reason for increased expenditures seems to be growth in demand.* In recent years both "price" (as measured by the medical care component of the CPI) and consumption of health care have grown more rapidly than for most major items in the economy. When both price and consumption of a commodity increase together—out of proportion to other goods and services available to the same consumers—microeconomic theory usually signifies this as a relative rise in "demand."

---

* The term "demand" is used here in the strict economic sense to designate the schedule of consumption in relation to price. Thus it represents neither an independently assessable objective "need" nor a psychological "desire" for a certain amount of service. It is simply a neutral (noncause-implying, statistical) description of the tendency to consume various amounts of a particular commodity as a function of the price. Thus it measures the relative readiness to sacrifice other goods and services in order to have this one.

A number of factors can be interpreted as contributors to a growth in demand for medical care: (1) increase in the portion of aged and chronically ill in the population requiring more service per capita; (2) growth of consumer expectations in regard to health services out of proportion to those for other commodities and services; (3) development and introduction of new technologies and services creating potential for consumption that was not previously possible; (4) changes in the financing mechanisms that enabled access for groups previously hindered by financial barriers, that increasingly earmarked funds specifically for health care, and that lowered the effective price to consumers.

Many economists add the category of "provider induced demand" as a means of explaining the fact that variables with a major influence on utilization and health expenditures are the density of physicians, hospital beds, and so on—even more than consumer decision factors like family income, price, and incidence of disease, as in most demand functions (Evans, 1974). This terminology represents the attempt to find a way of using the free-market framework to deal with a phenomenon that in fact has no place within standard supply-demand equilibrium theory. Provider rather than consumer control of consumption is a fundamental aberration of the competitive market that no free-market model can encompass. We treat it later in the context of discussing market distortions that change the basic structure of the health economy.

How well are the effects of these demand factors explained by a free-market model, and what do they tell us about the appropriateness of that model for analyzing the health economy? As we have seen, the increased percentage of aged and the increased prevalence of illness in the population account for only 6% of the growth in health expenditures (Table 12.8). Thus, although these factors work in a direction consistent with the free-market model, they explain a very small part of the increase. Consumer expectations for health care rising more rapidly than for other commodities could account for increased demand. There is no direct quantitative index of consumer expectations (or consumer initiated demand) like the percentage of aged and their relative utilization rates or the indicators of illness prevalence. We are, therefore, forced to assess the impact of consumer expectations on demand indirectly.

If health cost escalation were primarily a product of consumer initiated utilization, one would expect consumer initiated services to be rising rapidly and account for a large part of the growth in costs. Physician office visits are the service most under consumer control, but the per capita rate of physician visits (after age adjustment) has actually decreased over the last ten years. This occurred despite a 1% per year increase in illness prevalence and an almost 2% per year increase in the number of primary care physicians per 1000 population during this period (USDHEW, 1980). If consumer initiated demand were a major factor in cost escalation, we would also expect utilization to be more sensitive to price and income. In fact, as we have seen, both price and income elasticities of health care demand are quite low (Phelps, 1975). This is one reason that many analysts speak of health care utilization as determined by "need" rather than "demand" in the usual sense. From the free-market perspective, then, consumer demand does not seem to account for much of the growth in costs in any direct way. The indirect impact of consumer demand must be analyzed by way of its influence on supply and insurance.

The large portion of cost growth attributable to service intensity increases suggests that medical technology plays a major role in health cost escalation. On the other hand, providers have a legal monopoly over access to and utilization of medical technology. Therefore the sense in which technology "creates its own demand" is not in the usual market sense of consumer demand (Chapter 12). The presumed influence of rising consumer expectations on technology utilization must be explained by way of the political process, making funds available for its development (Strickland, 1972; P. Feldstein, 1977) and "demand" (e.g., collective bargaining) for insurance benefits that reimburse preferentially for high-technology services (Munts, 1967). As we have seen, the effect of insurance on health costs occurs to a very large extent by way of the influence of the reimbursement methods on provider revenues rather than by the price-lowering effect for consumers. The Medicare/Medicaid legislation of 1965 did enfranchise a large number of new beneficiaries, but the growth of new insurance beneficiaries since 1970 has been slow (Health Insurance Institute, 1979). In summary, then, none of the factors that would explain increased demand in the usual free-market sense accounts for very much of the growth in health expenditures within the framework of that model.

LIMITATIONS AND DISTORTIONS OF THE FREE MARKET FOR HEALTH CARE

Today, in fact, little remains of the free market in health care except certain entrepreneurial prerogatives without the corresponding competition, risks, or financial restrictions to encourage efficiency. For the free market to work selling health services on an item by item basis, a number of conditions would have to be met—none of which presently exists in the delivery of health services. Price competition, the essential basis of supply-demand equilibrium in a free market would require that:

1. Price would have to make a difference to the patient. He would have to pay an appreciable part of the bill himself and be ready to forego that service if the price is too high in relation to other commodities that he wants. The patient would need to participate in a significant way in the physician's decision to order various services.
2. Consumers would need an effective opportunity to comparison shop be-

tween various providers in regard to price and comparability of services. This would require much better information and knowledge for the patient to understand what he is getting for his medical care dollar and what similar services cost in different settings.

3. Physicians and other providers would have to compete in regard to price, attempting to lower prices through more efficient production (cost savings) and increasing supply as demand and price go up. This would require free entry of physicians and hospitals into the system.

None of these conditions for a competitive market is (or easily could be) met in regard to the health services economy today.* Free-market mechanisms do operate in relation to the consumption of some health services paid out-of-pocket, but very weakly and then only where the patient is in a position to make the decisions himself about the use of services, for example, purchase of over-the-counter drugs, the first physician visit in an episode of illness, or (unfortunately) whether to get needed preventive services. For the vast majority of health expenditures, the influences of price and consumer choice on utilization are overshadowed by other factors that place major restraints on the operation of a price-supply-demand market for control of consumption and allocation.

For hospital and physician services, which make up 60% of the health care budget, the insurance system of financing eliminates the essential mechanisms for a competitive market to function. For patients, the price is so highly subsidized and the rate of cost sharing so different for various kinds of care that the actual cost of producing the services makes little difference to the consumer (Pauly, 1968, 1969). If patients controlled utilization decisions, apparent price would have a perverse market effect because the most expensive services have the lowest out-of-pocket costs (Chapter 12). For physicians and hospitals, who do control most utilization decisions, the insurance reimbursement methods essentially guarantee adequate revenues without the need to be competitive in price in order to attract patients. Studies of physicians and of hospitals show rate and fee behavior that is exactly counter to the predictions of a competitive market. The greater the density of hospital beds or physicians in relation to the population (and thus supposedly the greater the competition for patients), the higher the prices charged (Blumberg, 1979; Anderson, 1980). The fee-for-service payment system may once have been the basis for competitive pricing, but the insurance mechanism of payment together with consumer dependence on providers in the face of technological complexity has long since removed all fee competi-

---

* The impossibility of restoring competition to the health care market at the individual service level does not mean that there are no opportunities for improving cost effectiveness through greater competition. As we have seen in our consideration of Health Maintenance Organizations (Chapter 10) and show in considering the Enthoven national health insurance plan (Chapter 14), whole systems of care can be put into competition with each other.

tion. Without competitive pricing and with almost 70% of physicians' fees paid by third parties, fee-for-service no longer provides a mechanism for supply-demand control of the health care market. Instead it allows physicians to obtain their "target incomes" and protects their central, controlling position in allocation of health services.*

Individual health services are seldom purchased in a free choice situation. They are usually sought when the patient is already sick and believes professional help is essential. Prices are not known in advance—what services will be necessary and the charges are determined after the fact. There is no opportunity for comparison shopping (Klarman, 1965). In some minor illnesses care may be postponed or foregone by the poor because of their inability to pay. Those with higher incomes may also defer obtaining care because of the time or inconvenience involved (opportunity costs). But if the illness is considered serious and care is believed necessary, patients seek care without regard to price. This decoupling of decisions to obtain health care from knowledge of cost precludes the "shopping" mechanism essential for a free-market to exercise any competitive constraint on prices or to determine utilization and allocation.

Physicians (and hospitals) operate in a market that has many features of a so-called natural monopoly. Entry into the health care market is severely restricted by licensure and technical expertise requirements. Because of the importance of licensure for consumer protection, no one seriously suggests decreasing that monopolistic nature of the market. Nevertheless, the limitation of supply would be a serious restriction on the potential for competition if the price mechanism were somehow reestablished—as it was for physicians prior to the rapid growth of insurance financing (Dyckman, 1978). The monopoly market, in combination with the high portion of fees covered by third-party payment, means that neither physicians nor hospitals face any of the competitive pressure in regard to price that is characteristic of free markets. The guild tradition makes overt competition among providers, such as advertising, nearly impossible. This monopoly situation is not balanced by the usual counterweights imposed on regulated utilities such as franchising. Once licensed, the physician has the right to establish practice wherever he wants (and until recently hospitals as well) with no associated franchise restrictions or market responsibilities. He has wide discretion in setting charges, with only minimal limitations (such as Medicaid fee schedules in some states), and is essentially unrestricted in collecting them save for moral pressure and community customs.

Unlike utilization of most commodities, the "demand" for health services (as well as the supply) is controlled to a large extent by the providers of

---

* This creates a powerful vested interest in the present payment system and buttresses physicians' ideological commitment to that system. Consequently great resistance arises to any suggestion of change in the medical economy that appears to threaten the supposedly free-market form of the health care industry—even when such changes are in the financial interest of physicians, as, for example, with health insurance and Medicare.

care (May, 1975). Except for the decision to seek primary care, most medical care utilization decisions are made by the physician rather than the patient. After the initial contact in an episode of illness, the physician largely determines what services will be utilized, whether the patient should be hospitalized (and at which hospital), what diagnostic tests, drugs, and treatments will be employed, how often the patient will return, whether or not surgery will be used. Insurance financing frees their utilization decisions regarding intensity of care. The patient can resist or delay in certain circumstances, but by and large he lacks the knowledge to evaluate the recommendations of the physician. Even if a patient has misgivings about a particular decision by his physician, he hesitates to question it or to seek another consultation for fear of "showing lack of confidence," particularly in a situation where finding a physician at all may be difficult.

The technical nature of medical knowledge is usually unfathomable to the layman. Professional prestige makes it possible to intimidate even the knowledgeable patient. Physicians have a legal monopoly to practice, which makes them gatekeepers to all medical services. The spectrum of health services generated by technological innovations, together with the rising consumer expectations and the lifting of financial barriers for patients, has created a situation of almost unlimited potential consumption of care (Fuchs, 1974). Physicians remain the only limiting factor in the actual utilization of services. As gatekeepers in this monopoly economy, physicians can effectively control the demand for their own services plus those of other health facilities and technicians.

Physicians' decisions are based on professional opinion about need, and are only minimally affected by the cost considerations from the perspective of consumers—in contrast to a normal free-market situation. If physicians take patients' financial interest into account at all, it is usually with regard to which services are covered by insurance, often leading to use of more expensive rather than less expensive services. The only effective restraints on provider control of utilization are the ethical ones embodied in their professional tradition and the limits of their own time. Provider rather than consumer or payer determination of consumption completely inverts the normal mechanisms necessary for the free market to control consumption and allocation (Fuchs, 1973).

THE HEALTH CARE SECTOR AS A PUBLIC SERVICE ECONOMY

Public services are supplied, financed, allocated, and consumed in a kind of economy quite different from that for free-market commodities. Examples of public services are the public schools, fire, police and public health departments, or the Defense and State Departments. Such services are financed by taxes or other public funds and are generally provided without appreciable direct cost to consumers. This mode of financing is usually established where the services are so-called public goods from which all may benefit or else have "externalities" from which many benefit when there is utilization by others (Musgrave, 1959).* Since the price mechanism is lacking for consumption control and allocation through consumer choice, other means are necessary to apportion utilization among those who want the services if they are limited (Klarman, 1965). Supply, allocation, and consumption are controlled largely through public decision making by means of the budgeting process. Publicly accountable officials decide how much will be spent on a particular service within a politically determined budget furnished by a given taxation level (Wildavsky, 1974). Availability of services to consumers and often individual utilization are largely controlled by expert opinion about "need." Thus individual consumption is based only in part on how much a consumer wants and not at all on how much he is able to purchase at a given price. This nonmonetary allocation of public services is the very point of such an economic structure. It is assumed that the public interest is better served by having the service where it is needed than where someone can afford to pay the most for it.

The health care system has taken on many of the characteristics of a public service. A kind of quasi-public national health insurance system has grown up piecemeal that pays for most medical care through collective financing rather than individual payment in exchange for services. The method of financing has almost completely uncoupled financial obligation from the individual's utilization of health services. Consumers pay in ways that seem quite unrelated to paying for health costs. Forty percent of health care expenditures is paid directly out of tax dollars. An additional 12% is paid through tax subsidies in the form of tax deductions for health insurance and medical expenses, which must be made up from other tax sources, making a total of 52% financed through the tax system (Sunley, 1980).

Voluntary health insurance, which pays for 37% of hospital care and physician services (more than one-third of this subsidized by tax writeoffs), has also become, in effect, back-door public financing for health care. Most voluntary health insurance is obtained on a group basis as a fringe benefit of

---

* "Public goods" are those, like national defense and public health surveillance of food and water supplies, where everyone benefits by the same resulting condition. In such cases there is no way to divide up the cost on the basis of consumption. Since all may benefit "equally," the usual way to pay for such "public" goods is by some kind of public financing. "Externalities" are advantages (or disadvantages) that accrue to others as a result of the action or consumption by a first consumer. If a person with tuberculosis receives treatment, he benefits, but the public also benefits by being protected from further contagion. Therefore, we subsidize the individual's treatment for the good of the general public. Similar, if less direct, externality reasoning is used to justify public financing of clinical services with a major preventive impact, such as maternal and child health programs. Disease not prevented in childhood is apt to force the individual to fall back on charity or publicly supported clinical care later when it is more costly. As discussed in Chapter 14, a new justification is used increasingly today for creating certain public services: ensuring access to basic life-needs as "human rights."

employment (USDHEW, 1980). Only 10% of the total dollar volume is sold on an individual basis. Today virtually all group health insurance is experience rated. As shown in Chapter 12, all three methods of experience rating effectively act as direct cost-pass-through mechanisms from providers to ultimate payers, the employers and employees. Consequently voluntary health insurance, like tax financing of care, offers a blank check to providers and exacts from subscribers whatever costs are thereby incurred. In this way beneficiaries' payments are completely disconnected from their own decisions in regard to use of services or choice of providers. Insurance carriers do not (and within the present system *probably can not*) bargain effectively with providers to obtain lower rates for their beneficiaries as a method of offering lower premiums to compete for subscribers (Marcus, 1980). Therefore employer (or employee) choice of carriers cannot act as a lever to produce any market constraint on provider charges (or costs) as a result of competition between underwriters. The only, even theoretical, market force on provider costs lies in cost-sharing required of patients at the time of using services. As we have seen, however, there is little evidence that this creates any effective constraint on provider charges (or costs) or on the intensity of services ordered in an episode of illness.

Employers (and employees to the extent they share premium costs) must absorb in their premiums whatever costs are generated by the utilization of their beneficiary group. They (in turn) are faced with the problem of how to finance the premium costs. Approximately 35% is subsidized by the income and payroll tax exclusions and in this way passed-through to the tax system. The remainder must be divided in some way between the employee and employer. Nationally on the average employers pay about 85% of the total premium burden for fringe benefit health insurance, employees pay about 15%. It remains unclear, however, to what extent the employer share represents benefits in lieu of wages foregone in the collective bargaining agreement. Whether the ultimate burden is born by employees in the form of lower wages or in the form of higher prices passed on by employers, financing health care through employment related insurance has economic effects that are virtually indistinguishable from financing it through payroll taxes (Chapter 12).

What are the characteristics of the public financing of services that ordinarily distinguish this method from the private financing of such services? In regard to their influence on the economy and the behavior of those involved, the most important characteristics of public financing are the *collective* nature of benefit policy making and financing, the *compulsory* nature of contribution, and the *dispersion* of the cost burden over the entire population rather than having the recipient of services bear it alone. In relation to these key features, there is little practical difference between private (fringe benefit) health insurance and public programs. Collective decisions determine what benefits are to be provided in both cases. The private benefit package is largely determined by collective bargaining agreements whereas public program benefits are determined by political bargaining, but for the individual beneficiary this difference has little effect. In both cases precedent plus the political and tax incentives make it virtually impossible to decrease benefits, and in both cases the coverage already includes a very large portion of the critical (and most costly) basic services. With the benefit package collectively set in either way, the individual beneficiary does not have the option to choose and pay only for the coverage he wants.*

For both public and private health insurance, benefits are collectively financed. Within the collective all contribute equally or according to the same rules, which are independent of the use made of the services. For tax supported insurance, the contribution is compulsory, and the amount is not under the control of the beneficiary or the payer. The employer's fringe benefit contribution is equally compulsory once a collective bargaining agreement on benefits is signed. Because of the experience rated premium system, the amount of the employer's contribution is also largely beyond his control. In its economic impact the employer's contribution is indistinguishable from an *employer payroll tax or excise tax*. The employee's insurance contribution is not strictly compulsory, but it is effectively enforced by the threat of losing the larger employer contribution if it is not paid. The contribution is withheld from his paycheck, and its economic effect is no different than an employee *payroll tax*. Insofar as it is taken in lieu of a higher wage settlement, the portion of premiums that employers agree to shoulder in the collective bargaining package is equally like a payroll tax on employees.

Like a tax, the premium is neither susceptible to market pressure on the insurance carriers nor can the employer exert any such pressure on the providers of care. An employer also cannot realistically negotiate with individual potential employees over fringe benefit premiums as he might over salary in a competitive labor market situation. The premiums tend to be much the same for all businesses of the same kind in an area, just like the local taxes. The benefits are relatively standard for an industry, and costs depend only on the area and his employee's actuarial characteristic. Therefore, as with taxes, there is little competitive pressure to absorb health fringe benefit costs as a loss from profits. Instead they are passed through as higher prices to consumers of the industry—just as payroll or excise taxes are.

Because of collective financing under both public and private systems, the cost burden of any utilization is spread over the entire participating collective. This dispersion of cost leads to the so-called "problem of the common" (Hiatt, 1975; Somers, 1971): Insofar as an advantage is gained by the use of such services, every member of the collective has a positive incentive to

---

* Some health financing reform proposals currently under consideration attempt to modify this situation partially by requiring that a low-benefit plan be offered as one option, with rebates to employees of the difference between its premium and the employer's contribution to the high-benefit insurance plan (Chapter 14). However, this multiple option system could equally well be applied to public health insurance programs so that it does not constitute a structural difference in the two routes of financing.

increase his share of utilization. What he gains from use accrues entirely to him, while the cost of that utilization is spread equally over the collective—its impact on the user is only his fraction of the whole. Any divergence from this collective financing in insured health care is a matter of co-insurance rates rather than whether it is routed through the public or the private sector. Provider control of utilization (in both the public and private systems) exacerbates the problem of the common. As an agent for his patient, as well as having a financial vested interest himself, each provider has the incentive to increase his share of utilization from the common pot of resources. Neither public nor private health insurance exerts any market pressure on providers to improve efficiency or hold down costs. From the provider perspective, whether one is paid by an insurance carrier for its private beneficiaries or by the same company acting as an intermediary for Medicare makes little difference. In either case the provider is assured payment requested with little restriction on the amount. The fact that the "underwriter" for tax supported programs is government and for voluntary insurance is private industry makes little difference since experience rating sets the "premium" in either case.

The only practical difference between public and private insurance financing, then, is how the reserves are used. But there is probably greater variation in reserve investment policies among private carriers than between the private sector as a whole and the Medicare Trust Fund. Moreover, these reserves tend to be very small relative to cash flow (in either case) compared to life insurance underwriting. The net result of this complex system of subsidies and pass-throughs of health costs is *that health care is to a very large extent collectively financed* in ways that are indistinguishable in their economic effects whether through the tax system or the private insurance industry.

The fact that such a large share of health care is collectively financed does not in itself convert the structure of the health economy into a public service. Government can purchase goods or services in a free market or from a utility, just as any other buyer, for example, food or electricity for the army. It can subsidize production of utilities to lower their price to consumers, as with subway transit fares. It can support the purchase of goods and services by consumers from a free market, as with rent subsidies to welfare recipients. Such government payments add to the demand for the particular commodity but do not in themselves necessarily convert its economy into a public service if other buyers compete in the same market. With hospital and physician services, however, government and insurance carriers are essentially the only buyers, and their payments constitute the major revenues for the providers (over 90% for hospitals and 67% for physicians). Thus provider budgets are completely dependent on the financing policy set by these collectively paid sources.

In hospital reimbursement, and to some extent in reimbursement for physicians, consumers are entirely bypassed, as with public services. The price mechanism for allocation and utilization control, which is essential for a free-market (or a regulated utility) economy to function, has been eliminated. Revenues and thus budgets depend primarily on the provider side of the equation rather than on consumer generated demand. With hospitals, the costs are simply prorated over the number of patient services provided. If utilization falls or rises (within limits), operating costs change very little. Therefore hospital income also remains virtually the same—since costs, not the utilization, determine revenues. Although physicians are not paid on a cost basis, within a wide range of patient availability, practitioners can control both the utilization of their services and the level of their fees. As a result, they can achieve "target incomes" (Blumberg, 1978; Evans, 1974) without having to attract more patients by effective price competition against other practitioners. For both physicians and hospitals, then, budgets are not only paid primarily by public or other collectively financed sources, but their revenues are also determined by how much and in what way the collective sources are made available to them, and are largely independent of consumer demand (Sloan & Feldman, 1978; Reinhardt, 1978, 1973).

Several other features of the health care system are also characteristic of public services rather than of free markets. Most health care utilization decisions are made by professionals on the basis of their expert appraisal of *need** rather than by consumers on the basis of choice (Boulding, 1966). Provider (professional) control of utilization is typical of public services but not of free markets. In the absence of the price mechanism, decisions about utilization and allocation of public services must be made on nonfinancial bases, usually according to objective criteria of need. Society ordinarily delegates the responsibility for that determination to persons who are considered experts in assessing such need. This control of utilization by experts is sanctioned in the belief that the benefit of such services is a matter of public as well as private concern.

The tradition of so-called welfare medicine is closely related to the principle of need as a basis of utilization and is likewise typical of public services (Fuchs, 1972; Pauly, 1971). Because access to care is seen as critical to well-being, health professionals have long felt compelled (in the public interest) to provide it whether the patient could pay or not. At first this was done as a charitable act, then as professional responsibility. But, increasingly, support of "welfare medicine" has been institutionalized, first by public and voluntary hospitals and then in part by insurance payment systems. Finally, under Medicaid (and other programs) government has as-

---

* Many economists object to differentiating between "want" and "need" in discussing demand and consumption of commodities or services because these are psychological concepts that are not distinguishable in terms of the usual economic variables. But the concept of "need" expresses not only the descriptive fact that the demand curve has very low price and income elasticities, but it also suggests the kind of things that are apt to influence utilization besides price, such as incidence of disease and physicians' beliefs about appropriate treatments.

sumed most of the responsibility for supporting it—thus recognizing at least last-resort financing of medical care as a necessary public service. This shift in the acknowledged responsibility for supporting welfare medicine makes up one part of an overall evolution in social attitudes about the public service nature of medical care. The combination, then, of public (and other collective) financing, provider control of utilization, "need" rather than "choice" determination of consumption, and public recognition of government responsibility to assure access to the service, creates an economy that is much more characteristic of a public service than a free market or a regulated utility.

LIMITS AND DEFECTS OF THE PUBLIC SERVICE ECONOMY FOR HEALTH CARE

Viewing health care as a public service, provides insights into the causes of its economic problems quite different from the free-market model. From the perspective of the public service model, the major defects of the system can be attributed to the incompleteness or distortions of the public budgeting, planning, and allocation processes. When the free-market (price) mechanisms for control of consumption, supply, and allocation of services are removed from any economic sector by public financing, public decision making becomes essential to replace them.

There are two traditional ways that public budgeting is normally implemented to control expenditures for public services—by prospective budgeting and by entitlement. First, with *prospectively* budgeted services, such as schools, fire departments, the Defense Department, and most preventive health services, the budget is fixed in advance. It is set on the basis of estimated need in relation to other needs that must be supplied from the same overall budget. The services enabled by this level of funding must be distributed among the beneficiaries and functions as effectively as possible—even if the need increases in the course of the year. If the need for services seems inadequately met by the allotted budget, the agency or representatives of its beneficiaries must convince the budgeting authority to increase their share the following year or to approve a supplemental appropriation. Such increases are not automatic. They must be fought out against proponents of other programs that would have to be cut back proportionately or against opposition of taxpayers who would have to pay more if equivalent cutbacks are not made elsewhere (Wildavsky, 1974). Second, for *entitlement* programs like Social Security, unemployment insurance, or other categorical public assistance, anyone meeting certain requirements is guaranteed the designated benefits. The benefit levels are fixed by public decision making, however. Thus entitlement program budgets are somewhat less controllable than prospective ones, but only to the extent that the number of persons who qualify may vary with changing conditions. Expenditures can be controlled if necessary—either by changing entitlement requirements (as with welfare) or by adjusting benefits (Singer, 1976).

Health care benefits fit neither of these categories of controllable public budgeting. First, although a very large portion of medical care is financed as if it were a public service, expenditures clearly are not controlled by prospective budgeting. There are no prospective constraints on outlays and no public decision making in regard to budgets or the allocation of such funds to various regions and services. The insurance reimbursement system for financing health care simply passes the cost burden through to payers who have no part in the utilization decisions and therefore cannot relate expenditures to the benefits received. This payment mechanism allows highly decentralized utilization decisions—primarily under the control of providers of care—which nevertheless obligate public (and other collective) funds. Budgeting for health takes place *retrospectively* and *by aggregation*. Medicare and other public programs mandate payment for whatever costs are incurred by beneficiaries for covered services. The taxpayer gets the bill after the fact. Because of the pass-through features, most private insurance premiums likewise simply reflect how much was paid out during the preceding year. Neither consumers nor governments are ever presented with direct choices between spending for health care and other goods and services, or the opportunity to control allocation of resources within the health sector (Campbell, 1974; U.S. Senate Finance Committee, 1970).

Second, the present system of Medicare and Medicaid (and voluntary insurance) benefits for health care ostensibly falls under the entitlement approach to control of public budgeting, yet it has proved incapable of containing costs. The number of beneficiaries can be controlled by entitlement requirements, as with other entitlement programs, but it is impossible to constrain the benefit costs per beneficiary, even in the aggregate. Health insurance entitlement guarantees not a fixed dollar amount of benefits but a specified set of service benefits to whatever extent these are needed. There is little or no limit on the dollar amounts to be paid out for these benefits for any beneficiary. This is, of course, the point of insurance: to protect each beneficiary from the risk of unanticipated major expenses brought on by illnesses that strike with very uneven incidence and cost burden.

If health care were an ordinary commodity used on the basis of consumer choice, the highly subsidized price of services to consumers would make it impossible to limit their utilization (and cost) by beneficiaries. But health care is not a commodity consumed by choice. Utilization would seem to be limited by need based on the incidence of illness. Primary care is used when the patient becomes ill, and secondary care is ordered according to need as judged by the physician after contact has been initiated. Although the need of any particular beneficiary is unpredictable, the incidence of disease in the population is rather constant, and therefore presumably the total need for care. Thus, even without dollar limits on individual benefits, medical expenditures seemingly ought to be constrained by the amount of sickness in society—and this has increased only slowly in recent years (Chapter 12).

The uncontrollability arises primarily from the fact that the *intensity* of care provided for the same illnesses is not set by public (or private insurance) budget policy. The types of services utilized in treating a given illness and their price are at the discretion of the provider who benefits by increasing either utilization, intensity, or price. Thus, the unsolved problem of controlling the *cost* of care from the entitlement approach is how to limit provider-controlled utilization of services and costs for the given amount of illness (and therefore provider budgets) (Cooper, 1975). Because of the system of open-ended, provider-controlled, retrospective, aggregate budgeting in our current system of health care financing, there is no way that Congress or any public agency can decide how much to spend for health, or how that money should be spent—even the major portion that is paid directly or indirectly out of public funds.*

HEALTH CARE AS A REGULATED PUBLIC UTILITY

The so-called regulated utility is a third type of economic structure, in some ways representing a kind of compromise between the free market and the public service structures. Utilities, like free markets, are financed by direct payments from consumers in relation to their consumption (price), but certain features of the supply-demand equilibrium mechanism are replaced by public (collective) decision making. Regulated utilities have most commonly been established for so-called natural monopolies, such as gas and electric companies, public transportation, and communication industries. For services of this kind, a regulated monopoly or franchise is sanctioned in order to assure provision of an essential service while avoiding the duplication and gross inefficiency that many competing suppliers might create.

As a result, however, the consumer is at the mercy of a single supplier for a commodity or service that is vital to his well-being. Therefore, such utilities must guarantee a supply that is adequate to meet expected demand. Plans for necessary expansion to meet this demand are publicly scrutinized periodically. Since competition is eliminated or seriously inhibited, the customer is forced to pay whatever price is asked or go without. Utility service rates are therefore set or at least sanctioned by a regulatory agency, usually on the basis of audited costs plus a reasonable return on equity. Public

---

* Public health services and other governmentally *organized* (as well as publicly financed) services do not have the same retrospective and decentralized budgeting as clinical services. They must compete prospectively for the limited funds of government budgets and consequently have systematically lost out in the allocation of resources in comparison with clinical medicine. See also Chapter 5.

hearings are commonly held when rate changes are requested to allow airing of consumers' arguments or complaints as well as the supplier's justifications before the regulatory agency. Thus supply and price are influenced by public decision making processes. Consumption and allocation, however, depend on the choice of the individual consumers within the constraints imposed by the established price per unit—that is, the tradeoffs he is willing to make with other items in his budget—as in a free market.

In some industries where competition exists potentially but the consumer is at the mercy of the provider because he lacks the information to evaluate the product, industries are also regulated—even though there is not a monopoly. Such consumer protection regulation does not necessarily convert an economic sector into a utility. In fact, one of the objectives of such regulation can be to maintain as free a market as possible by ensuring the maximum feasible degree of fair competition, for example, antitrust regulation by the Federal Trade Commission. In some cases the boundary line is blurred between the two types of regulation—protection against deceit in the face of inadequate information and against price exploitation because of noncompetitive markets. Banks, for example, are regulated primarily to ensure financial solvency for consumer protection, but some aspects of Federal Reserve regulation also have the effect of making them partially into public utilities to provide loans at reasonable rates and for the sake of controlling the money supply. Health care regulation similarly has features where it is difficult to separate the consumer protection aspects from the public utility aspects.

Certain types of regulation of the consumer protection kind are longstanding in health care and generally accepted as necessary for the public interest. Licensure of health professionals, accreditation of hospitals and other health institutions, approval of drugs and devices for safety and efficacy, epidemiological surveillance, and state regulation of the health insurance carriers for solvency were all instituted to ensure patient protection where inadequate information or knowledge might make it impossible for him to protect his own interests. The need for the regulatory functions of this first type is seldom questioned. But regulation of this kind also does not in itself give the health care economy the structure of a regulated utility (Ball, 1975).

The health care economy is also treated like a regulated utility in many ways, however, and seems to be moving steadily further in that direction. As the cost of medical care has risen so rapidly in recent years, several new forms of *fiscal* regulation have been added. Certificate-of-need legislation and required approval by the local health planning agency are used to regulate capital investment in health care. Utilization review by Professional Standards Review Organizations (PSROs) is increasingly seen as a means to help control operating costs—although these organizations were originally promoted as a means of quality control. A number of states have now established hospital budget and rate review commissions as a means of limiting increases in hospital operating costs.* These new forms of regulation can be interpreted as steps toward treating the health sector like a utility (or perhaps even like a public service). Consequently, they are the focus of heated debate about the proper role of regulation in the health industry.

There are many features of the health care industry that fit the usual justifications for treating an economic sector as a utility requiring public regulation (Noll, 1975). The moving force behind the new forms of regulation has been the apparently uncontrolled escalation of health care costs linked with the recognition that little effective price competition exists in the health care sector (Federal Trade Commission, 1978). Because the entry of new providers into the health care market is severely restricted by licensure and educational requirements, many argue that a natural monopoly exists in health care that justifies utility-type economic regulation. Yet a true monopoly situation exists only rarely in the case of primary health care— although the difficulty of access to care in some geographic areas or dependency on the outpatient departments and emergency room of a hospital can have a monopolylike impact on patients. Once a patient is under the care of a physician, however, and particularly if he is hospitalized, any effective choice passes out of his hands. The most important "monopoly" element of medical care is the exclusive gatekeeper control that the profession as a whole exercises over medical technology and access to most other health services. This gatekeeper function creates a powerful monopolylike control over the consumers.

Yet the financial vulnerability of the patient (and of the collective public that bears the cost through indirect financing) is more a consequence of the provider control of service utilization because of expertise rather than lack of competition in the usual sense. The lack of information or knowledge about medical services precludes a patient from making intelligent choices by himself between competing options. This characteristic of medical practice is used to justify licensure of professionals and accreditation of institutions as well as PSRO utilization review from a quality standpoint.

LIMITATIONS AND DEFECTS OF THE REGULATED UTILITY APPROACH TO THE HEALTH CARE ECONOMY

Viewing the health care sector as a utility to be controlled by public regulation reveals a number of problems that account for much of the difficulty in applying this approach. As a regulated utility, the health sector lacks key economic mechanisms that are essential to control allocation, utilization,

---

* Hospital budget and rate review, though having the format of regulation, is actually designed to be protection of the public purse through prospective budgeting (rather than the open-ended budgeting), and as such really represents a public service approach rather than utility regulation. Federal hospital cost containment legislation being considered by the Ninety-sixth Congress would attempt to extend the latter strategy to the entire country.

and therefore total cost of services consumed. To be sure, in an ordinary regulated utility *price* does not play the role of determining supply by attracting more firms into the market or commitment of more resources. Neither does it serve as a basis for competition between suppliers to promote efficiency or improved productivity. The utility model *does,* however, assume that consumer decisions based on price determine utilization and allocation of services. Effective absence of the price mechanism for the consumer at the time of procuring services and provider control of consumption constitute fatal flaws for the proper function of a regulated utility economy just as they do for a free market. The predominance of public and other collective financing is inconsistent with a regulated utility approach to controlling the health economy. The collective financing combined with the provider control of utilization without corresponding public control of budgeting—rather than the monopoly situation—is the major underlying cause of uncontrolled costs. The lack of effective competition is, in fact, a *consequence* of this financing system rather than of the monopolistic elements of the system (Ellwood, 1975).

Consequently, rate setting does not serve the same function in regard to health care that it does in a true public utility, such as electric power, where the consumer bears the cost directly. Rate setting in health care is an attempt to *control public outlays* for health by placing constraints on provider revenues paid out of collectively financed funds. Because providers largely control utilization of services, however, constraints through rate limits can be circumvented by simply increasing utilization. Therefore, protection of the total budget for health care also requires restraints on utilization. The problem of unnecessary utilization arises because consumers do not make the utilization decisions or have to pay for them in a direct way. This corresponds more to a public service situation rather than a utility. Restraints on utilization are attempted through utilization review (e.g., PSROs) and limitation of supply, such as certificate of need laws. These mechanisms (strategies) of regulation have no counterpart in the structure of ordinary utilities. The nature of the health care financing makes it very questionable whether increasing the regulatory apparatus can deal with the cost and financing problem of the health care market. We return to these questions under strategies of cost control.

Another deficiency of the health care sector from the perspective of the utility model is the incompleteness of franchising. Franchising is often used in utility regulation to prevent "ruinous competition," but at the same time to guarantee service to certain areas that are in themselves unprofitable. Some areas can only be served at a reasonable price through cross-subsidization using linked franchises, which give access to highly profitable areas in exchange for serving the unprofitable ones as well (Noll, 1975). Public transportation and mail service are examples. Franchising hospitals in exchange for guaranteeing ambulatory services to underserved areas has been suggested but never tried (Somers, 1969). Certificate of need and planning agency approval of new programs have the appearance of franchising, but are actually cost-control measures.

In summary, neither private (voluntary) nor governmental health insurance programs have succeeded in solving the problems of keeping the cost of providing health services within reasonable bounds. The underlying reason is the fundamental incompatibility between the elements of the financing system, similar to the mismatch between the structure of the delivery system and the pattern of diseases prevalent today. The effects of this discordant mixture are synergistic with the mismatch of health care technology and organization to the problems of post-clinical medicine. Together these two sets of mismatches largely account for the inappropriateness of cost and resource allocation for the health needs of today.

PROPOSALS FOR CONTROLLING HEALTH CARE COSTS

During the 1970s, a broad consensus emerged that health costs are rising at an unreasonably rapid rate (Chapter 12). This increase is out of proportion to other sectors of the economy, and there is little evidence that it contributes comparable improvement to the nation's health or the quality of life for the sick. There is also general agreement that health expenditures are somehow "out of control"—in the sense that none of the parties involved seems able to restrain them despite the consensus that we are spending too much (Anderson & Neuhauser, 1969). When it comes to explaining the *cause* of uncontrolled spending, however, there is much more dispute among health policy makers and analysts. As argued above, the reason for this multiplicity of conflicting explanations put forth by various analysts lies in the diverging interpretations of the incongruent mixture of economic mechanisms operating in the health sector. These mechanisms derive from elements of the three types of economic structure: free market, public service, and regulated utility. The strange mixture evolved stepwise over the years, primarily through the introduction of health insurance as a method of financing. The disagreements over the "primary cause" of rising costs are a result of the opposing ideological commitments to one or another of those types of economic structure as the ideal that should be sought by bringing the other elements into accord with it. Not surprisingly, the strategies suggested for dealing with the uncontrolled cost escalation also divide into groups following these ideological commitments with the goal of achieving one of the pure economic structural types.

FREE-MARKET STRATEGIES TO LIMIT HEALTH CARE COSTS

The present health care financing system retains little of the structure necessary for a free market to operate effectively. Yet, regardless of the obstacles, there is widespread philosophical allegiance to this approach to the health economy. Any strategy attempting to move in a free-market direction enjoys immediate broadly based political support. Because of this ideological predisposition to think in free-market terms and the gradual way that health insurance transformed the once competitive market, most policy makers and analysts until recently have simply assumed that the health economy has remained basically a free market. They looked for solutions to cost escalation through manipulation of standard market variables such as supply and demand. This traditional perspective, however, provided few clues to satisfactory strategies for controlling costs or rationalizing the allocation of resources in the health sector.

One of the striking developments in policy thinking in the late 1970s has been the growing recognition that the health economy is markedly different from traditional markets (Bromberg, 1980; Fuchs, 1973). Concern has centered particularly on the *lack of competition* with the resulting absence of provider incentives to improve efficiency and conserve on costs (Federal Trade Commission, 1978). Failure of the market mechanisms is now widely acknowledged as a major cause of overutilization and escalating prices. Much of this current analysis and strategies to remedy the problem have pointed to the role of health insurance (public and private) in financing care as the major factor responsible for eliminating competitive market forces (M. Feldstein, 1977). The most direct solution, eliminating health insurance or radically increasing the percentage of co-insurance to restore the price mechanism for controlling costs, has serious political, practical, and ethical limitations. Various strategies therefore attempt to achieve partial restoration of market mechanisms in more limited ways. Two aspects of the market failure problem must be considered: (1) the loss of provider incentives to compete through developing more efficient systems of producing care and (2) the loss of consumer restraints on the utilization and price of care. Both involve the role of insurance and tend to be mixed rather indiscriminately in the same analyses and the same remedial proposals. To clarify the resulting confusion, however, it is necessary to examine the two factors separately.

First, there is now widespread agreement that health maintenance organizations (HMOs) (including PGPs and IPAs; Chapter 10), as well as other alternative organizational forms of health care delivery, can achieve appreciable savings in providing care without sacrificing quality (Saward, 1970; Luft, 1978). Yet the growth of these alternative arrangements for health care has been slow, and public acceptance has been less than enthusiastic, despite the fact that they can reduce the total cost of care by 30 to 40%. One of the major reasons is the system of insurance financing that subverts the competitive advantage such plans should enjoy. Neither public insurance programs like Medicare and Medicaid nor most private insurance (obtained as a fringe benefit of employment) allows the consumer to benefit commensurately by choosing to join a more efficient delivery system. Medicare and most Medicaid programs pay costs for hospital care and fees (with certain limits and co-payments) for physician services independently of the hospital payments. Since the major savings of HMOs derive from reduction in hospitalization, almost the entire cost saving accrues to the government insurance program. There is little savings to the patient and thus little incentive to join (Ellwood & McClure, 1976).

A similar situation holds for most private employment health benefit programs. The employer often bears the full cost or a major share of whatever plan the employee chooses. Even where the employee pays a substantial part of the difference in cost between the various options, the fact that his contributions are income tax deductible reduces the apparent premium cost difference between options by whatever his marginal tax rate is. If Federal, state, and local income tax and payroll taxes are all considered, the average subsidy rate is almost 35% (Sunley, 1980). Moreover, HMO payments are almost entirely by way of the premium, while conventional plans usually include some cost-sharing at the time of utilization. As a result, the payroll premium deduction for HMOs may be as high or higher than for the fee-for-service plans. Since the employed population is, in general, young and reasonably healthy, there is often the inclination to gamble that no illness will occur and no out-of-pocket costs will be necessary. On the providers' side, there is little financial incentive to practice in cost-saving organizations. A large and growing share of fees are paid by insurance on a UCR reimbursement basis (Dyckman, 1978; Chapter 12). As a result of this method, physicians can hope for and often realize considerably greater income on a fee-for-service basis than in HMOs or other alternative systems of care where their earnings are limited, though on the average they are quite comparable with fee-for-service incomes.

As a strategy to improve the incentives for both consumers and physicians to join HMOs, many policy makers and analysts propose to increase the competitive advantage of alternative delivery systems by imposing certain restrictions and conditions on the insurance plans. Typical proposals would require all employers providing health insurance to their employees to offer multiple options including any HMOs in the area (Ullman, 1980; Martin, 1980). The employer's contribution to each plan would have to be the same so that the employee bears the full difference in the cost of the option selected.* In some plans the difference would be refunded in the form of a tax-free rebate to avoid unequal tax subsidy to the higher cost plans. Some proposals would also place a limit on the amount of employer contribution that can be excluded from taxation. Medicare has proposed instituting a similar scheme by paying HMOs on a capitation basis at 95% of the actuarial costs for its fee-for-service beneficiaries in the same area. The HMOs would be required to return the difference between costs (plus the usual profit margin)

---

* Multiple choice and equal employer contribution are already required for Federally certified HMOs in an area under the 1973 HMO Act.

and the capitation rate in the form of extra benefits and by eliminating the usual Medicare cost sharing. States would be encouraged to develop similar plans for Medicaid.

Many analysts believe that such schemes could be useful incentives to encourage the development of efficient alternative delivery systems (Ellwood, 1975; Ellwood & McClure, 1976; Enthoven, 1978). There is more scepticism, however, whether these strategies can have much effect on the overall cost of care in the near future. Only 4% of the nation's population is presently enrolled in HMOs (half of them in Kaiser-Permanente alone). Projections indicate that at a maximum it will only be possible to develop HMO capacity for 10% of the nation's population by 1990 (OHMO, 1980). Establishing new HMOs is a slow and costly undertaking. It is no longer as difficult to recruit physicians as in earlier times, but experienced managerial talent is scarce, and capital or start-up funds under the 1973 HMO act are limited. Thus it seems unlikely that a major portion of the population can be accommodated in HMOs in the short run. Consequently, the savings achieved by alternative delivery systems cannot serve as the primary means of arresting cost escalation in the near future—even if "equal contribution" were enforced immediately.

Note that the only well-established cost saving effect of this mode of organizing care is *within* an HMO—and here the savings are accomplished through prospective budgeting—a public service strategy. In today's political climate, however, HMO development is being promoted as a *competitive* strategy. Some advocates of HMOs maintain that a cost restraining effect can be attained beyond the savings for HMO enrollees themselves. They believe that where an appreciable portion of the population is enrolled, the competitive effect on providers may exercise a constraining effect even on the fees and costs of care provided in the residual fee-for-service market (Ellwood & McClure, 1976). Evidence on this hypothesis is mixed. Minneapolis and Hawaii, each having a fairly large portion of the population enrolled in HMOs, do have slower rates of increase in health costs than the rest of the nation. But San Francisco and Portland, which have equally high percentages of their populations in HMOs, do not show such effects (OHMO, 1980).

The second element of competitive strategies for constraining health costs focuses on the direct consumer aspect of demand. The growth in the amount of health insurance, particularly first-dollar coverage, is believed by many to be a major factor in increased demand for care because of the price-lowering effect and because of the earmarking or channeling (precommitment) of funds for use only to pay for health care (Fuchs, 1979). The high tax subsidy for employment-derived health plans is seen as the major driving force behind the overpurchase of insurance to such an extent that it becomes effectively total prepayment (Feldstein, 1971, 1973). Some proposals designed to remedy this element of the problem would eliminate the tax exemption subsidies unless the insurance plans include an appreciable portion of patient costs sharing (Jones, 1979). Currently, however, many think a politically more realistic approach is to encourage employees to choose low-premium (high cost sharing) insurance options by granting rebates (with or without tax exemption) of the difference between the high and low option plans (Ullman, 1980; Martin, 1980). By combining higher deductibles and co-insurance with a catastrophic limit on patients' direct expenditures for health care, these proposals would concentrate protection at the high end where it is most needed.

It is questionable how much unnecessary utilization could be eliminated by increasing cost sharing rates through tax incentives to select such plans. Estimates vary greatly since two uncertainties are involved: (1) how much utilization would be reduced by the additional out-of-pocket payment facing patients at the time of receiving services; and (2) how many more persons would be induced to choose a health plan with greater cost sharing as a result of the modified tax incentives. As discussed, evidence from studies that measure the impact of cost sharing on individual patients suggests that some utilization can be reduced through out-of-pocket payment barriers (Chapter 12). This approach seems more promising for physician services than for hospital care since at least first visits are largely under patient control.

There is *no* good evidence, however, that higher patient cost sharing leads to lowering of intensity or price of care through price competition induced among providers—yet intensity and price are the major factors accounting for increased health expenditures over time. Even if some saving can be realized through decreased utilization by those who face higher cost sharing, there is little reason to believe that this will decrease the total cost of services in an area. Because the cost reimbursement method of paying hospitals and the UCR method of paying physicians insulate them from price competition, intensity and price of care are largely under the arbitrary control of providers. Consequently, total revenues for both hospitals and physicians are to a considerable degree independent of even *total* utilization, let alone of consumer initiated demand. Since only a small part of utilization is determined by patient choice, simply adding cost sharing does little to restore free-market mechanisms of utilization constraint in the health care sector. The fundamental distortions of market structure on the provider side raise serious doubt about the efficacy of using the strategy of increased consumer payments to control costs.

It is even less clear whether cost sharing would selectively decrease *unnecessary* utilization. Besides serving to discourage some use of unnecessary services, co-payments can act as serious barriers to *needed* services (whose early use might prevent later need for more expensive care). Few studies disaggregate utilization effects by type of service, but those that do suggest that the major impact is on primary care and preventive services. For example, imposition of a $1 per visit co-payment as an experiment in the California Medicaid (Medi-Cal) program led to 6% reduction in primary care visits and 22% reduction in Pap smears (Roemer et al., 1975). If cost sharing leads to postponement of such services, the net effect may well be to increase total system costs. The California experiment, in fact, found some increase in hospital utilization beginning about three months after cost sharing was imposed. On the contrary, systems of care such as HMOs or other payment arrangements where the physician rather than the patient is at risk for unnecessary utilization *do* reduce total system costs for health care appreciably. Even on the provider side, there is some question whether *only unnecessary* utilization is reduced by economic incentives to limit costs (Luft, 1978). This unwanted effect is probably greater, however, the more directly the benefit of decreased utilization accrues to the individual provider and the less group pressure or peer review exists to encourage professional standards (Freidson, 1970).

Cost sharing also has the disadvantage that it strikes hardest those who are least able to pay (Aday, 1975). The utilization of services by the poor is more sentitive to out-of-pocket cost sharing than utilization by upper-income families. Therefore cost sharing as a means of utilization restraint is at variance with the social equity principle. It is especially prone to cause delay of needed early treatment unless the patient payment schedule is tapered off for those at the bottom of the income scale. This creates a difficult and costly administrative problem. Means testing (which is quite expensive to administer) would be required to ascertain the required level of payment. Records would be needed to cross-reference the various providers to the same patient for determining whether deductibles have been met and when catastrophic coverage should take effect (and stop). It would also be necessary to exempt certain kinds of services, such as prevention, from all cost sharing in order not to discourage their use. This would require further policing of claims to ensure that services were being appropriately reported and not billed under false labels in order to avoid cost sharing. Modeling of administrative costs for national health insurance plans indicates that a scheme using co-insurance, deductibles, and a catastrophic ceiling on out-of-pocket payments, all or partly graduated by income could add as much as 4% of total premiums to the expense of running the program (USDHEW, 1977a). This increment in administrative costs would probably outweigh the questionable savings through decreased utilization.

The second uncertainty factor in regard to the strategy of inhibiting utilization by encouraging higher cost sharing through tax incentives is the degree to which employees will be persuaded to select low-option plans. Under the Federal Employee's Health Benefit system, where equal government contributions are made to each plan, only 13% of employees choose low-option plans (Davis, 1980). The rest preferred to accept a greater payroll deduction rather than face higher co-payments at the time of utilization. Such incentives for increasing patient cost sharing also potentially entail certain adverse self-selection consequences. Those who are young and healthy have a greater incentive to opt for the low-premium plans because they are less likely to need care and to face cost sharing. This leaves a disproportion-ate percentage of the heavier users of care in the high-option plans which drives up the experience rated premiums for those options. The cross-subsidization of the less healthy by the younger and healthier is thereby decreased. This can make the payment of premiums a heavy burden for those who can least afford to pay (Pauly, 1970).

Another potential disadvantage is that low-income employees faced with the choice between a larger pay check or protection from possible future cost sharing are under particularly heavy pressure to choose the low-option plan despite their need for greater protection. As a result they may find themselves in serious financial difficulty later and be forced to fall back on some publicly supported system of care. Finally, mandating multiple choice of plans including low-option ones can lead to much higher administrative costs by breaking up employee groups, to losing the advantage of large-group experience rating and to discouraging self-insurance (Marcus, 1980). Despite these disadvantages and the questionable effectiveness in reducing utilization or total system cost, it seems likely that such strategies will remain politically popular because of their association with the free-market ideology.

PUBLIC SERVICE APPROACHES TO COST CONTAINMENT

As discussed, the present system of paying for health care (particularly hos-pitals and physician services) most closely resembles the financing of a public service. Taxes and tax subsidies pay for 52%; another 17% (beyond tax sub-sidies) is paid collectively through the insurance system with effects on the consumer, provider, and the general economy equivalent to payment through taxes (Sunley, 1980). For hospitals, collective financing makes up an even larger portion of the total—60% being paid by taxes and tax subsidies and another 30% (beyond tax subsidies) by way of the private insurance system. The logical cost containment strategy to match such extensive collective financing would be a system of public (or other collective) prospective bud-geting such as we usually institute for public services.

Health planning agencies have the mandate to undertake overall plan-ning and rationalization of the health care system in an area. One of their objectives is to limit health costs by allocating services more nearly in ac-cord with need. They would seem to offer a logical administrative frame-work for areawide prospective budgeting. Under present law and the existing insurance system of financing care, however, such planning agencies are es-sentially limited to restricting major new capital investment through project review and approval authority. By discouraging construction of unneeded services, which tend to generate unnecessary utilization, the planning pro-cess does have some restraining effect on health costs. But planning agencies have no authority to review (or influence) institutional *operating* budgets or to do anything about location of physician practices, fees, or utilization. As a consequence, the health planning system remains a very limited regulatory process rather than a means of imposing public budgeting on the financing of health care.

Given the present diffuse insurance system of financing medical care, there is no mechanism that could easily be used to establish publicly accountable overall prospective budgeting. In Chapter 14, we examine a proposal for national health insurance (Kennedy, 1979) that *would* provide the necessary framework and implement a binding nationwide budgeting process. Short of a major restructuring of the health financing system, however, public service strategies for containing costs are forced to use more limited and piecemeal approaches. The most effective method of limited prospective budgeting in clinical care at present is the health maintenance organization (Chapter 10). HMOs contract prospectively to provide all necessary health services to an enrolled population at a fixed annual premium. Their demonstrated ability to provide care more economically through decreased use of expensive hospitalization is due to the prospective budgeting for hospitals and medical groups within the plans and the consequent provider incentives imposed by the restricted budgets.

Another limited strategy of cost containment based on the public service model is so-called prudent buying. Under this concept the fiduciary responsibility of purchasers of services with public funds obligates them to negotiate or establish contract prices that are in the best interest of both the beneficiaries and the tax payers—as, for instance, with Defense Department or General Services Administration contracts. There are two basic methods of prudent buying: If there are multiple potential suppliers of the same good or service, the standard method is to solicit competitive bids and buy from the lowest bidder meeting the required standards for the desired product. If there is only a single producer available or capable of supplying the appropriate product, prudent buying requires negotiation by the government purchaser to establish a reasonable price on the basis of the necessary cost for *efficient* production of the product. Although there are multiple potential suppliers of medical services in most geographic areas, the principle of free choice of provider by the patient requires that each physician, hospital, and so on be regarded as a single-source supplier. Under the law and medical custom, providers cannot be asked to bid against each other for government or private* contracts to supply services to beneficiaries. The problem of prudent buying therefore becomes one of finding a means of determining reasonable cost for efficient production. There are several health cost containment measures and proposals that attempt to accomplish this for hospital and physician expenditures.

* There is no reason that the concept of prudent buying need be restricted to government purchasing. A private buyer with a fiduciary responsibility to its beneficiaries, such as an insurance carrier or a union welfare fund, is equally obligated, at least morally, to exercise prudent buying.

Because of the magnitude of hospital expenditure increases, their inflationary impact, and the heavy load placed on Federal and state budgets as
a result of the large portion of public money involved, many attempts are
being made to bring these cost escalations under better control. The most
direct way to control hospital costs would be to set operating budgets directly and prospectively (Hellinger, 1978). At present there is no authority
and no framework for doing this nationally. In response to the impact of
rising hospital costs on Medicaid budgets, however, a number of states have
enacted legislation giving mandatory authority to statewide hospital budget
review and rate setting commissions (Bauer, 1978; Cohen, 1975, 1978). New
York took the lead in 1969, followed by eight other states. (Colorado subse-
quently withdrew its commission's authority in 1979.) These programs vary
in the type of payers to which they apply and the method of calculating or
negotiating rates, but all establish binding prospective budgets or rate limits of some kind. They have been quite successful in slowing the overall rate
of hospital cost increases in those states. Beginning with annual cost increase rates in the same range as the rest of the nation, by 1978 these states
had slowed their growth rates of hospital costs to 65% of the rate in states
without such mandatory programs* (USDHEW, 1979a). A number of other
states have opted to establish voluntary hospital cost programs of one sort
or another, but there is no evidence to date that these have succeeded in
holding down hospital cost growth appreciably.

At the national level a number of measures have been tried for controlling hospital costs through restrictions on *rates alone*. As already noted, rate
setting only has the appearance of utility-type regulation. Because of the
absence of the consumer price mechanism due to collective financing, rate
setting for hospitals actually represents a "prudent buying" strategy to protect public budgets for those services. Because providers control most utilization, however, rate regulation alone cannot be expected to limit expenditures effectively. It is equally necessary to employ special methods to
curtail utilization—something that has no counterpart in ordinary utility
regulation. The combination of rate setting and utilization limitation then
becomes a means of constraining the total budget, a strategy actually corresponding to a public service approach to cost containment through overall
budget constraints.

From 1971 to 1974 hospitals were subject to *wage and price controls* as
part of the Nixon administration's Economic Stabilization Program. Just
prior to imposition of those controls, hospital budgets had been growing at
about 16 to 17% per year. The rise in hospital costs slowed to about 13%

---

* It has been argued that the basis for this success was the very high base rate of the costs
in the states that implemented such programs (Stockman & Gramm, 1979). And indeed,
on the average, per diem costs of the eight states were above the national average. On
the other hand, even those states, such as Washington, with base costs below the national
average were quite successful in slowing their rates of growth. Final judgment on the
efficacy of this state strategy must await more definitive studies of all the factors involved.

per year during the wage and price control program, but quickly jumped back with a bulge to 18.5% for the two years after controls were removed. Increases in cost per day slowed much more during the control program than total costs. Since controls were only applied to per diem costs, hospitals apparently could compensate to a considerable degree by increasing the number of patient days used (Lipscomb, Raskin & Eichenholz, 1978). The program was also plagued by the expectation that these controls were only temporary. The assumption that they would be lifted within one or two years allowed the hospitals just to defer many expenses for a short time. This probably accounts for much of the bulge in hospital costs that occurred in late 1974 and 1975 when the controls were lifted (Ginsburg, 1976, 1978; Berman, 1976).

Another strategy for limiting hospital costs is *utilization review* to discourage inappropriate admissions, unnecessary lengths of stay, and other utilization abuses (Lewin & Associates, 1975). The original Medicare law required hospitals and nursing homes to establish utilization review boards to monitor lengths of stay by diagnosis, notify patients and providers, and possibly withhold reimbursement. The 1972 Social Security Amendments mandated extension to Medicaid and established the more extensive Professional Standards Review Organization (PSRO) system of quality and utilization review, which has still to be fully implemented (Decker & Bonner, 1973). The impact of PSROs and Medicare/Medicaid utilization review has been minimal, however, compared with the 30 to 50% lower hospitalization rate found in HMOs. Providers are the decision makers in regard to utilization. Unless something changes their incentives, such as placing them at risk for excessive use of services, peer review can have little effect. Because of the highly judgmental nature of these decisions, review committees can challenge physician decisions only in the most flagrant cases.

In the 1972 Social Security Amendments, HEW was given broad authority to set reasonable limits on Medicare reimbursement rates for hospitals (Sec. 223 of PL 92–603) (Institute of Medicine, 1976). In 1975 regulations went into effect limiting the per diem payment for hospital routine costs. Because of the great variety of hospitals and the difficulty of establishing criteria for "reasonable" rates of reimbursement representing "efficient" production of services, the original regulations were minimally restrictive and led to less than 1% of reimbursable costs being disallowed. Only the so-called routine costs or hotel-type services were covered because these tend to be more comparable among institutions. So-called ancillary costs, including operating room, laboratories, and other special services, vary much more depending on the complexity of the cases treated by the hospitals. With increasing experience and a better data base for calculating limits, HEW has gradually increased the stringency of these limits in their annual updating of the regulations. A method has now been developed for appraising the average complexity of cases treated by each hospital, so-called diagnosis-related-group case-mix. This technique should make it possible to apply limits to total hospital costs per admission in the near future (Fetter et al., 1980).

In January 1977 the Carter administration came into office having campaigned on a platform of fiscal responsibility as well as improvement of social programs. New HEW officials were alarmed by the impact of hospital costs on Medicare budgets and by the difficulty in finding funds for new social programs, such as welfare reform, if Medicare increases continued to eat away potential budgetary leeway. A hospital cost containment bill was quickly developed and introduced attempting to avoid the pitfalls encountered by the Economic Stabilization Program controls (Dunn & Lefkowitz, 1978). The bill placed a limit on growth of hospital costs per admission* (somewhat less under the discretion of hospitals to manipulate than days of care). The allowed growth limit on reimbursement per admission was calculated on the basis of a formula (identical for all hospitals) indexed to inflation (the GNP deflator, a wage and price index) that would gradually slow cost growth from the existing level ($2\frac{1}{2}$ times the GNP deflator) to one approaching that index.

After initial favorable consideration by several Congressional committees, the resistance of the well-organized health industry lobbies stiffened. In December 1977 the hospital associations and the AMA established the Voluntary Effort (VE) to contain health costs through self-policing by the industry. Lobbyists convinced many Congressmen that it would be better to allow the industry to deal with the cost problem on their own rather than have government controls. After a protracted legislative fight, the bill was passed by the Senate in the last days of the Ninety-fifth Congress but allowed to die by the House. A similar bill was introduced in the early days of the Ninety-sixth Congress but badly defeated on the floor of the House of Representatives after another prolonged fight in committees. If eventually enacted, this public-service strategy of "prudent buying" could have a significant impact on hospital costs and would provide an interesting experiment in the use of a limited public-service budgeting strategy.

Similar strategies are being tried or suggested in regard to physician expenditures. The most commonly suggested "prudent buying" strategy for containing physician expenditures is control of physician fee schedules. Negotiated fee schedules have been used with considerable success in Canada and other nations (Lewin & Associates, 1976). Some states use such payment methods for their Medicaid programs. HEW has been studying the possibility of such a system for Medicare. Several national health insurance proposals include the use of such schedules. There are two major independent features to the fee schedule strategy, which can be used separately or in conjunction: (1) across-the-board restraint on the rate of increase in fees, and (2) readjustment of the relative fees paid for various services to improve incentives for more efficient delivery of care.

---

* To discourage hospitals from circumventing the limit by increasing admission rates, it allowed only a 50% marginal cost increase for each admission in excess of the previous year (beyond a narrow no-growth band).

The 1972 Medicare amendments (PL 92–603) authorized HEW to place a limitation on physician fees through the so-called prevailing test for reasonableness. The 75th percentile level of customary fees for any procedure in a given medical service area was originally defined as the "prevailing fee"—above which no fee would be considered "reasonable" for reimbursement under Medicare. Since 1975, however, "prevailing" has been redefined by regulation each year as the previous year's prevailing rate times an economic (inflation) index. Since customary fees have generally gone up faster than the economic index, most physicians' customary fees gradually rise to exceed that "prevailing" limit. Medicare reimbursement is then limited to the more slowly increasing prevailing rate. Thus areawide schedules of reimbursement limits are gradually being created that are proportional to historic prevailing rates for various fees (U.S. House of Representatives, 1978).

The major problem with this method is that it only limits Medicare's portion of the reimbursement. Unless the physician voluntarily agrees to accept this as his full payment (and be paid directly by Medicare), he can bill the patient whatever he believes is just, while the patient can only be reimbursed the maximum Medicare payment schedule (minus 20% coinsurance). Under present law the government saves money by this method, but the individual patient, who is least able to afford it, may find paying the difference a heavy burden. New legislation has been suggested to prevent this (so-called mandatory assignment of claims), but enactment seems very unlikely except in the context of a national health insurance plan. Even if enacted, mandatory assignment, limiting a physician's total reimbursement to the set fee schedule, could entail serious difficulties in making such a system work as intended. State experiences with Medicaid fee limits have shown that if these schedules are appreciably less than their non-Medicaid customary rates, physicians are reticent to accept Medicaid patients at all, and access to care for these beneficiaries can become difficult (Holahan et al., 1979).

Unless there is a carefully designed and audited system of defining the services provided, it is also easy for physicians to disaggregate their claims into bills for several services with a greater total or to inflate the definition of the service rendered and submit claims for more expensive categories of service than actually rendered. Since a large portion of utilization is under physician control, another means of circumventing fee limits is to increase the overall utilization rate. During the Economic Stabilization Program (1971 to 1974), limits were imposed on the rate of increase in physician fees (as for all wages and prices). The inflation in the physician services component of the CPI fell to half its former (and subsequent) rate. Yet, after only one year of slightly slower growth, physician income and total physician expenditures accelerated again to rise at almost the same rate as before, even while fee increases were still held in check. Apparently the utilization simply was increased sufficiently to make up the difference (Dyckman, 1978).

A second important fee schedule strategy would be to negotiate or assign by regulation the relative level of various fees (Crncich, 1976). The goal would be to achieve a more appropriate relationship between the amount and value of a physician's effort and the rate of payment (Blumberg, 1978). The rate of increase in fees for hospital visits, high-technology procedures, and specialist care would be slowed or reversed. The rate for rural, generalist, and hands-on care would be increased. This would not only create savings in the fastest-growing and most expensive items of physician expenditures, but it would also diminish the incentives for those procedures that generate the most additional (nonphysician) health care expenditures. Thus even without appreciably slowing the rate of physician income growth a considerable savings could be achieved for the system as a whole. Such fee rationalization could also provide incentives for gradually improving the geographic and specialty maldistribution (Burney et al., 1978). It is unlikely, however, that hospital cost containment or mandatory physician fee schedules would have as great an effect on reducing costs as do HMOs. Without an overall budget constraint, there is no tradeoff between hospitalization and physician expenditures and therefore no incentive for physicians to reduce utilization of hospital care (or other expensive service) for their patients.

Politically, any attempt to change the present system of physician reimbursement can be expected to meet very stubborn and effective resistance. The present fee-for-service, CPR, or UCR reimbursement system serves to guarantee physicians their "target incomes" and protects their central, controlling position in allocation of health services (Chapter 12; Blumberg, 1978). This creates a powerful vested interest in the present payment method and buttresses physicians' ideological commitment to that system. Consequently, great resistance arises to *any* suggestion of change in the medical market—even when such changes are in the financial interest of physicians, as, for example, with Medicare and national health insurance (Colombotos, 1968). All proposals for change in the payment system are immediately labeled as threats to the supposedly free-market form of the health care industry. Because of the concerted opposition of powerful interest groups, enactment of either hospital cost containment or physician fee legislation seems unlikely except in the context of national health insurance. In summary, then, the present structure of the health care financing system and the political strength of opponents make it improbable that limited prudent buying strategies can have much impact on health costs.

REGULATED UTILITY APPROACHES TO COST CONTAINMENT

Most regulation of the health industry is of the consumer protection variety rather than the typical rate regulation used in monopoly situations as a substitute for the competitive pricing mechanism of free markets (Chapter 12). As we have seen, when rate setting is imposed for health services, its function is actually quite different in most instances from that for ordinary utilities. Most regulated utilities, just as free markets, depend on the price barrier to consumers as the means to control utilization, total expenditures, and allocation among users. Public funding and insurance-mediated, collective financing of health care therefore make a standard public utility approach to control of the health economy ineffectual. Since the consumer price mechanism is absent, rate setting in health care is intended to limit total health outlays.

One "pure" regulatory strategy being suggested as a method of cost containment is medical technology assessment and restriction of reimbursement for cost-ineffective modes of care. Once technologies and services are in place, however, there is probably little that can be done, short of setting overall budgets prospectively, to limit costs incurred by their use. As discussed in Chapter 10, it should be possible to limit implementation and expenditures for new technologies that are not cost effective in regard to health outcomes by requiring prior assessment and approval of proposed modes of care before granting reimbursement authority or approving capital investment plans. Ineffective technologies already in use might be gradually phased out using similar methods.

The most widely used "pure" regulatory approach to health care cost control is the certificate-of-need requirement for new capital investment within the health planning process (Havighurst, 1973). The objective is to control operating expenditures through restriction of the supply of hospital beds and major capital equipment so that there simply are not more services to be used. The recognition that oversupply of hospital beds generates overutilization and that capital investment leads to increased operating costs stimulated strategies of controlling costs through limitation of new bed construction and other capital investments. A number of states, beginning with New York in 1963 passed certificate-of-need laws in the 1960s to deal with the excess bed problem. The 1973 Planning Amendments now mandate all states to legislate such certificate-of-need requirements. To date 39 states have done so, and the rest are in the process. The 1972 Medicare Amendments required review and approval of all hospital capital investments over $100,000, denying reimbursement for the costs attributable to interest and depreciation on unapproved projects. There are 950,000 community hospital beds in the United States, about 4.5 per 1000 population. Estimates based on differential occupancy rates, and lengths of stay in various parts of the country place the number of excess beds between 100,000 and 200,000. The National Health Planning Guidelines (promulgated under PL 93–641, The National Health Planning and Resources Development Act of 1973) set a goal of reducing the bed ratio to not more than 4 beds per 1000 (except in rural areas of low population density where greater underutilized capacity is necessary to allow for admission fluctuations and emergencies).

Considerable doubt is being raised, however, whether certificate-of-need laws alone can adequately deal with the problem of excess investment and overcapacity. Studies show that even where the rate of new bed construction has been slowed by such laws, the overall rate of hospital capital investment remains essentially unchanged (Salkever & Bice, 1978). Apparently limits on bed expansion merely channel the same investment resources into capacity for more intensive care of patients—perhaps with higher turnover per bed and shorter length of stay—but with little overall reduction in the rate of total capital or operating cost growth.

In recent years there has been growing dissatisfaction with the results of regulating industries as public utilities (Pressman & Wildavsky, 1973). Studies show that regulated industries increasingly come to control their regulatory agencies and legislative committees rather than the other way around. As a result, regulation seldom actually holds prices down (Noll, 1975). The reason for this so-called regulatory agency capture is the adversary process through which rate setting and other aspects of utility regulation take place. Industries can appeal unwanted decisions to the courts or to the legislative bodies that authorized the regulatory agencies. Such appeals are expensive and time-consuming, requiring perseverance and well-organized, well-financed campaigns. The industries have strong vested interests, powerful organizations, and adequate financing to carry this out. Few consumer groups opposing the industries have well enough focused interests or adequate organization and financing to win out over the long run. In trying to strike a fair balance, as most do, regulatory agencies are usually careful not to err in a direction detrimental to their industry. It is the prime interest of the agency that its industry thrives to provide the services demanded by the public even if this turns out to be more costly than absolutely necessary.

The legislative committees governing regulated industries are probably even more responsive to industry spokesmen than are the executive agencies. Legislators have to be reelected, and damage to an industry vital enough to be treated as a public utility would be severely punished by voters. Also, the industry lobbies can make major campaign contributions needed for reelection. In addition, the industries have access to influential constituents of the legislators—constituents who can exercise pressure on a committee member because they may influence many votes in his district.

Regulation tends to foster inefficiency in an industry. The allowable rate of profit is usually set as a percentage of capital invested ("return on equity") or, as with for-profit hospitals, a percentage of operating costs. The higher the costs, the higher the profits. Thus there is less incentive to economize on costs to attain higher profits than with competitive industries. With nonprofit hospitals higher operating costs make it possible to justify higher administrative salaries, more specialized services, and so on. In regulated industries price competition is eliminated. Competition for customers must take place by offering additional services or special amenities that customers often might be glad to forego in a price competitive industry in order to save money. These "extras" eventually must be adopted by everyone, increasing industry costs and hence price at the next rate review (Noll, 1975). Hospitals are almost completely unrestricted in their costs as a result of reimbursement methods and do not compete in price at all. They compete almost entirely by means of prestige or amenity incentives. These are aimed more at physicians than patients since patients come to them primarily by way of the physicians. Studies have shown that the more hospitals there are competing in an area, the higher their per diem costs tend to be (Salkever, 1979; Anderson, 1980).

Ironically, despite the disadvantages of the regulatory approach for controlling health costs, it seems probable that regulatory strategies will continue to be employed and extended. Politically, government regulation represents a kind of compromise between the two poles of the free-market and public services approach. Although increased regulation is championed by almost no political group, in the political process the emotional, mutual opposition of extremists often dictates a settlement somewhere in the middle. This compromise tends to be regulation—not by design, but by default. Because of their long experience with regulatory approaches Congressional committees tend to be comfortable with these solutions to sticky politically polarized problems (Scher, 1960). In a sense it allows them to defer decisions or at least keep them open for easy review and future adjustment. The authorizing committee to which the problem is initially referred will have jurisdiction over the regulatory agency they are creating or expanding. These committees also come to have a vested interest in that agency and its regulatory process. Thus the organization of the legislative process tends to favor regulation over other approaches.

REFERENCES

Aday, Lu Ann, "Economic and Noneconomic Barriers to the Use of Needed Medical Services," *Medical Care*, 13:447–456, 1975.

Altman, Stuart, and Eichenholz, Joseph, "Inflation in the Health Industry: Causes and Cures," in Zubkoff, Michael, Ed., *Health: a Victim or Cause of Inflation*, New York: Prodist, 1976.

Anderson, Gerard, personal communication, 1980.

Anderson, Odin W., *Blue Cross Since 1929: Accountability and the Public Trust*, Cambridge, Mass: Ballinger, 1975.

Anderson, Odin W., and Neuhauser, Duncan, "Rising Costs are Inherent in Modern Health Care Systems," *Hospitals, Journal of the American Hospital Association*, 43 (February 6): 50–73, 1969.

Arrow, Kenneth, "Uncertainty and the Welfare Economics of Medical Care," *American Economic Review*, 53:941–973, 1963.

Ball, Robert, "Background of Regulation in Health Care," in *Controls on Health Care*, Conference on Regulation in the Health Industry, Washington, D.C.: National Academy of Sciences, 1975.

Bauer, Katherine G., *Containing Costs of Health Services Through Incentive Reimbursement*, Boston: Harvard Center for Community Health and Medical Care, 1973.

Bauer, Katherine G., "Hospital Rate Setting—This Way to Salvation?" in Zubkoff, Michael,

Ruskin, I., and Hanft, R., Eds., *Hospital Cost Containment: Selected Notes for Future Policy*, New York: Prodist, 1978.

Bell, Daniel, *The Coming of Post-Industrial Society: A Venture in Social Forecasting*, New York: Basic Books, 1973.

Berman, Richard, "The Economic Stabilization Program of the United States: August 1971–April 1974," *World Hospitals*, **12**, 1976.

Bicknell, William, and Walsh, Diana, "Certification-of-Need: The Massachusetts Experience," *New England Journal of Medicine*, **292**:1054–1061, 1975.

Blumberg, Mark S., "Rational Provider Prices: An Incentive for Improved Health Delivery," in Chacko, G. K., Ed., *Health Handbook*, Amsterdam: North Holland Publishing, 1978.

Boulding, Kenneth E., "The Concept of Need for Health Services," *Milbank Memorial Fund Quarterly*, **44**(October, Part 2): 202–223, 1966.

Bromberg, Michael, "Hospital Cost Containment—Where Do We Go From Here?" address to the National Health Policy Forum, Washington, D.C.: 1980.

Bunker, John P., "Surgical Manpower—A Comparison of Operations in the U.S. and in England and Wales," *New England Journal of Medicine*, **282**:135–144, 1970.

Burney, Ira L., Schieber, George J., Blaxall, Martha O., and Gabel, J. R., "Geographic Variation in Physicians' Fees: Paying the Physician Under Medicare and Medicaid," *Journal of the American Association*, **240**(September 22): 13, 1978.

Campbell, R. R., *Economics of Health and Public Policy*, Washington, D.C.: U.S. Department of Commerce, 1974.

Cohen, Harold S., "Regulating Health Care Facilities: the Certificate-of-Need Process Re-examined," *Inquiry*, **10**:3, 1973.

Cohen, Harold S., "State Rate Regulation," in *Controls on Health Care*, Washington, D.C.: National Academy of Sciences, 1975.

Cohen, Harold, "Experiences of a State Cost Control Commission," in M. Zubkoff, I. Raskin, and R. Hanft, Eds., *Hospital Cost Containment*, New York: Prodist, 1978.

Colombotos, John, "Physicians' Attitudes Toward Medicare," *Medical Care*, **6**:320–331, 1968.

Congressional Quarterly, *The Washington Lobby*, Washington, D.C., 1974.

Cooper, Barbara S., and Gaus, Clifton R., "Controlling Health Technology," in Altman, Stuart, and Blendon, Robert, Eds., *Medical Technology: The Culprit Behind Health Care Costs?* Sun Valley Forums on National Health, Washington, D.C.: USDHEW (PHS) No. 79–3216, 1977.

Cooper, Michael H., *Rationing Health Care*, New York: Halsted, 1975.

Crncich, John, "The Making of the California Relative Value Studies: The Ideology and Administration of Pricing Policy in the Fee-for-Service Medical Market," Madison: Program in Health Administration, University of Wisconsin, 1976.

Davis, Karen, personal communication, 1980.

Decker, B., and Bonner, P., *PSRO: Organization for Regional Peer Review*, Cambridge, Mass.: Ballinger, 1973.

Dowling, William L., "Prospective Rate Setting: Concept and Practice," in Dowling, William L., Ed., *Prospective Rate Setting*, Germantown, Md.: Aspen, 1976.

Dunn, William L., and Lefkowitz, Bonnie, "The Hospital Cost Containment Act of 1977: An Analysis of the Administration's Proposal," in Zubkoff, Michael, Ruskin, I., and Hanft, R., Eds., *Hospital Cost Containment: Selected Notes for Future Policy*, New York: Prodist, 1978.

Durenberg, Sen. David F., "Health Incentives Reform Act (S. 1968)," *Congressional Record*, November 1, 1979.

Dyckman, Zackary U., *A Study of Physician Fees,* Washington, D.C.: Council on Wage and Price Stability, 1978.

Ellwood, Paul M., Jr., "Health Maintenance Strategy," *Medical Care,* **9**:291, 1971.

Ellwood, Paul M., Jr., "Alternatives to Regulation: Improving the Market," in *Controls on Health Care,* Conference on Regulation in the Health Industry, Washington, D.C.: National Academy of Sciences, 1975.

Ellwood, Paul M., Jr., and McClure, Walter, "Health Delivery Reform," Minneapolis: Interstudy, mimeo, November 17, 1976.

Enthoven, Alain C., "Consumer-Choice Health Plan," *New England Journal of Medicine,* **298**:650–658, 709–720, 1978.

Federal Trade Commission, *Competition in the Health Care Sector: Past, Present, and Future, Proceedings of a Conference,* Washington, D.C.: Federal Trade Commission, 1978.

Feldman, Paul, "Efficiency, Distribution, and the Role of Government in a Market Economy," *Journal of Political Economy,* **79**(3):508–526, 1971.

Feldstein, Martin S., *The Rising Cost of Hospital Care,* Washington, D.C.: Information Resources Press, 1971.

Feldstein, Martin S., "Hospital Cost Inflation: A Study of Non-Profit Price Dynamics," *American Economic Review,* **61**(December):861, 1971a.

Feldstein, Martin S., "The Welfare Loss of Excess Health Insurance," *Journal of Political Economy,* **81**:251, 1973.

Feldstein, Martin S., "The High Cost of Hospital—What To Do About It," *The Public Interest,* **48**:40–54, 1977.

Feldstein, Martin S., and Taylor, Amy, *The Rapid Rise of Hospital Costs,* Washington, D.C.: Council on Wage and Price Stability, 1977.

Feldstein, Paul J., *Health Associations and the Demand for Legislation: The Political Economy of Health,* Cambridge, Mass.: Ballinger, 1977.

Fennor, R., "The Internal Distribution of Influence: The House," in Truman, D., Ed., *The Congress and America's Future,* Englewood Cliffs, N.J.: Prentice-Hall, 1965.

Fennor, R., *Congressmen in Committees,* Boston: Little, Brown, 1973.

Fetter, Robert B., Shin, Youngsoo, Freeman, Jean L., Averill, Richard F., and Thompson, John D., "Case Mix Definition by Diagnosis-Related Groups," *Medical Care,* **18**(2, Suppl.):1–53, 1980.

Freidson, Eliot, *Professional Dominance: The Social Structure of Medical Care,* New York: Atherton, 1970.

Fried, Charles, "Equality and Rights in Medical Care," *Hastings Center Report,* **6**(February):29–34, 1976.

Fuchs, Victor R., Ed., *Essays in the Economics of Health and Medical Care,* New York: Columbia University Press, 1972.

Fuchs, Victor R., "Health Care and the United States Economic System: An Essay in Abnormal Physiology," in McKinlay, John B., Ed., *Economic Aspects of Health Care,* New York: Prodist, 1973.

Fuchs, Victor R., *Who Shall Live?: Health, Economics, and Social Choice,* New York, Basic Books, 1974.

Fuchs, Victor R., "The Economics of Health in a Post-Industrial Society," *The Public Interest,* **56**:3–20, 1979.

Galbraith, John K., *Economics and the Public Purpose,* Boston: Houghton Mifflin, 1973.

Gaus, Clifton R., "Biomedical Research and Health Care Costs," testimony before the President's Biomedical Research Panel, September 29, 1975.

Gaus, Clifton, and Hellinger, Fred, "Results of Hospital Prospective Reimbursement in the U.S.," International Conference on Policies for the Containment of Health Care Costs and Expenditures, Bethesda, Md.: The John E. Fogarty International Center, 1976.

Ginsburg, Paul B., "Inflation and the Economic Stabilization Program," in Zubkoff, Michael, Ed., *Health: A Victim or Cause of Inflation?*, New York: Prodist, 1976.

Ginsburg, Paul B., "Impact of the Economic Stabilization Program on Hospitals: An Analysis with Aggregate Data," in Zubkoff, Michael, Raskin, I., and Hanft, R., Eds., *Hospital Cost Containment*, New York: Prodist, 1978.

Havighurst, Clark C., "Regulation of Health Facilities and Services by Certificate of Need," *Virginia Law Review*, 59:1143–1242, 1973.

Havighurst, Clark C., "Regulation in the Health Care System," *Hospitals, Journal of the American Hospital Association*, 48:65, 1974.

Havighurst, Clark C., and Bovbjerg, Randall, "Professional Standards Review Organizations and Health Maintenance Organizations: Are They Compatible?" *Utah Law Review*, Summer: 41, 1975.

Havighurst, Clark C., "Regulation of Health Institutions," in *Controls on Health Care*, Washington, D.C.: National Academy of Sciences, 1975.

Health Insurance Institute, *Health Insurance Fact Book, 1979*, Chicago, 1979.

Hellinger, Fred J., "An Empirical Analysis of Several Prospective Reimbursement Systems," in Zubkoff, Michael, Ruskin, I., and Hanft, R., Eds., *Hospital Cost Containment: Selected Notes for Future Policy*, New York: Prodist, 1978.

Hiatt, Howard H., "Protecting the Medical Commons: Who is Responsible?" *New England Journal of Medicine*, 293:235, 1975.

Hofstadter, Richard, *The Age of Reform*, New York: Vintage, 1955.

Holahan, J., "Physician Availability, Medical Care Reimbursement, and Delivery of Physician Services: Some Evidence from the Medicaid Program," *Journal of Human Resources*, 10(Fall):3, 1975.

Holahan, J., Hadley, J., Scanlon, W., Lee, R., and Bluck, J., "Paying for Physician Services Under Medicare and Medicaid," *Milbank Memorial Fund Quarterly, Health and Society*, 57(Spring):4, 1979.

Huitt, R., "The Internal Distribution of Influence: The Senate," in Truman, D., Ed., *The Congress and America's Future*, Englewood Cliffs, N.J.: Prentice-Hall, 1965.

Institute of Medicine, *Medicare-Medicaid Reimbursement Policies*, Washington, D.C.: National Academy of Sciences, 1976.

Kelman, Sander, "Toward the Political Economy of Medical Care," *Inquiry*, 8:30–38, 1971.

Kennedy, Sen. Edward M., "Health Care for All Americans Act" (S. 1720), *Congressional Record*, September 6, 1979.

Kittredge, John, and Doyle, John, "A Public/Private Partnership for Effective Regulation of Hospital Costs," *Health Insurance Association of America Viewpoint*, December 1975.

Klarman, Herbert E., *The Economics of Health*, New York: Columbia University Press, 1965.

Krizay, J., and Wilson, A., *The Patient as Consumer*, Lexington, Mass.: Heath, 1974.

Leaf, Philip J., "The Medical Marketplace and Public Interest Law, Part 2," in Weisbrod, Burton, Ed., *Public Interest Law: An Economic and Institutional Analysis*, Berkeley: University of California Press, 1978.

Le Clair, M., "The Canadian Health Care System," in Andreopoulos, S., Ed., *National Health Insurance: Can We Learn From Canada?*, New York: Wiley, 1975.

Lewin and Associates, *Evaluation of the Effectiveness and Efficiency of the Section 1122 Review Process,* Washington, D.C.: Lewin and Associates, Inc., 1975.

Lewin and Associates, *Government Controls on the Health Care Systems: The Canadian Experience,* Washington, D.C.: HEW-OS-74-177, 1976.

Lindblom, Charles E., *The Intelligence of Democracy,* New York: Free Press, 1965.

Lipscomb, Joseph, Raskin, Ira, and Eichenholz, Joseph, "The Use of Marginal Cost Estimates in Hospital Cost-Containment Policy," in Zubkoff, Michael, Raskin, I., and Hanft, R., Eds., *Hospital Cost Containment,* New York: Prodist, 1978.

Luft, Harold S., "How Do Health Maintenance Organizations Achieve Their 'Savings'?" *New England Journal of Medicine,* 298:1336–1343, 1978.

Marcus, Glenn, "Group Health Insurance Premium Setting," Washington, D.C.: Congressional Research Service, 1980.

Martin, Rep. James G., and Jones, Rep. James R., "Medical Expense Tax Credit Act" (H.R. 3974), *Congressional Record,* May 7, 1979.

Martin, Rep. James G., "Medical Expense Protection Act" (H.R. 6405), *Congressional Record,* February 4, 1980.

May, J. Joel, "Utilization of Health Services and the Availability of Resources," in Andersen, R., Kravitz, J., and Anderson, O., Eds., *Equity in Health Services,* Cambridge, Mass: Ballinger, 1975.

Mayhew, D., *Congress: The Electoral Connection,* New Haven: Yale University Press, 1974.

Meeker, Edward, "Allocation of Resources to Health Revisited," *Journal of Human Resources,* 8(Spring):257–259, 1973.

McCarthy, C. M., "Incentive Reimbursement as an Impetus to Cost Containment," *Inquiry,* 12:320, 1975.

Munts, Raymond, *Bargaining for Health: Labor Unions, Health Insurance, and Medical Care,* Madison: University of Wisconsin Press, 1967.

Musgrave, Richard, *A Theory of Public Finance,* New York: McGraw-Hill, 1959.

Newhouse, Joseph P., and Taylor, Vincent, "How Shall We Pay For Hospital Care?" *The Public Interest,* 23:78–92, 1971.

Noll, Roger, "The Consequences of Public Utility Regulation of Hospitals," in *Controls on Health Care,* Washington, D.C.: National Academy of Sciences, 1975.

Office of Health Maintenance Organizations (OHMO), USPHS, *Projections for HMO Development, 1980–1990,* Washington, D.C.: USDHEW(PHS), 1980.

Pauly, Mark V., "A Measure of the Welfare Cost of Health Insurance," *Health Services Research,* 4(Winter):281–292, 1969.

Pauly, Mark V., "The Welfare Economics of Community Rating," *Journal of Risk and Insurance,* September 1970.

Pauly, Mark V., *Medical Care at Public Expense: A Study in Applied Welfare Economics,* New York: Praeger, 1971.

Phelps, Charles, *Demand for Health Insurance: A Theoretical and Empirical Investigation,* Santa Monica: Rand Corporation, 1973.

Phelps, Charles, "The Effects of Insurance on Demand for Medical Care," in Anderson, Ron, et al., Eds., *Equity in Health Services,* Cambridge, Mass.: Ballinger, 1975.

Perrott, George S., "The Federal Employees Health Benefits Program," Washington, D.C.: USDHEW, 1971.

Pressman, Jeffrey L., and Wildavsky, Aaron, *Implementations: How Great Expectations in Washington Are Dashed in Oakland, or, Why It's Amazing that Federal Programs Work at All. This Being a Saga of the Economic Development Administration as Told by Two Sympathetic Observers Who Seek to Build Morals on a Foundation of Ruined Hopes,* Berkeley: University of California Press, 1973.

Rafferty, John, "Enfranchisement and Rationing Effects of Medicare on Discretionary Hospital Use," *Health Services Research,* 10:51–62, 1975.

Reinhardt, Uwe E., "Proposed Changes in the Organization of Health Care Delivery: An Overview and Critique," *Milbank Memorial Fund Quarterly,* 51(Spring):169–222, 1973.

Reinhardt, Uwe E., "Alternative Methods of Reimbursing Non-Institutional Providers of Health Services," in *Controls on Health Care,* Washington, D.C.: National Academy of Sciences, 1975.

Reinhardt, Uwe E., "Comment on 'Competition Among Physicians' by Frank Sloan and Roger Feldman," in *Competition in the Health Care Sector: Past, Present, and Future, Proceedings of a Conference,* Washington, D.C.: Federal Trade Commission, 1978.

Rivlin, Alice M., *Social Policy: Alternate Strategies for the Federal Government,* Washington, D.C.: Brookings Institution, 1974.

Roemer, Milton I., et al., "Copayments for Ambulatory Care: Penny-Wise and Pound-Foolish," *Medical Care,* 13:457, 1975.

Sade, R. M., "Medical Care as a Right: A Refutation," *New England Journal of Medicine,* 285:1288, 1971.

Salkever, David, and Bice, Thomas, "Certificate-of-Need Legislation and Hospital Costs," in Zubkoff, Michael, Raskin, I., and Hanft, R., Eds., *Hospital Cost Containment,* New York: Prodist, 1978.

Salkever, David S., *Hospital Sector Inflation,* Lexington, Mass.: Heath, 1979.

Saward, Ernest W., "The Relevance of the Kaiser-Permanente Experience to the Health Services of the Eastern United States," *Bulletin of the New York Academy of Medicine,* 46(September):1970.

Scher, S., "Congressional Committee Members as Independent Agency Overseers: A Case Study," *American Political Science Review,* 54:911–920, 1960.

Singer, Neil, *Public Microeconomics: an Introduction to Government Finance,* 2nd ed., Boston: Little, Brown, 1976.

Sloan, Frank, and Feldman, Roger, "Competition Among Physicians," in *Competition in the Health Care Sector: Past, Present, and Future, Proceedings of a Conference,* Washington, D.C.: Federal Trade Commission, 1978.

Smith, Adam, *Inquiry into the Nature and Causes of the Wealth of Nations,* Edinburgh, 1776.

Somers, Anne R., *Health Care in Transition,* Chicago: Hospital and Education Research Trust, 1971.

Somers, Anne R., *Hospital Regulation: The Dilemma of Public Policy,* Princeton, N.J.: Princeton University Press, 1969.

Somers, Herman M., and Somers, Anne R., *Doctors, Patients and Health Insurance,* Washington, D.C.: Brookings Institution, 1961.

Somers, Herman M., and Somers, Anne R., *Medicare and the Hospitals: Issues and Prospects,* Washington, D.C.: Brookings Institution, 1968.

Stewart, Charles T., Jr., "The Allocation of Resources to Health," *Journal of Human Resources,* 6(Winter):103–122, 1971.

Stockman, Rep., David, and Gramm, Rep., Phillip, *The Administration's Hospital Cost Containment Act: A Critical Analysis,* Washington, D.C.: U.S. House of Representatives, mimeo, 1979.

Strickland, Stephen P., *Politics, Science, & Dread Disease: A Short History of United States Medical Research Policy*, Cambridge: Harvard University Press, 1972.

Sunley, Emil M., Deputy Assistant Secretary of the Treasury, statement before the Health Subcommittee of The Committee on Ways and Means, U.S. House of Representatives, 1980.

Titmus, Richard M., *Social Policy: An Introduction*, New York: Pantheon Books, 1974.

Ullman, Rep. Al, "Health Cost Restraint Act" (H.R. 5740), *Congressional Records*, October 30, 1979.

USDHEW, "Patient Cost Sharing," Washington, D.C.: USDHEW, Assistant Secretary for Planning and Evaluation, mimeo, 1978a.

USDHEW, "Hospital Cost Containment—Fact Sheet," Washington, D.C.: USDHEW, Assistant Secretary for Planning and Evaluation, mimeo, 1979a.

U.S. House of Representatives, Ways and Means Committee, Subcommittee on Health, *Proposed Amendments to the Medicare Program*, Washington, D.C.: Ninety-fifth Congress, 2nd Session, Committee Print No. 95–92, 1978.

U.S. Senate, Finance Committee, *Medicare and Medicaid: Problems, Issues, and Alternatives, Report of the Staff*, Washington, D.C.: U.S. Congress, 1970.

White, R., *Right to Health: The Evolution of an Idea*, Ames: University of Iowa Press, 1971.

Wildavsky, Aaron, *The Politics of the Budgetary Process*, Boston: Little, Brown, 1974.

CHAPTER FOURTEEN

Options Toward a National Health Financing Policy

THE NEW DEBATE OVER A NATIONAL HEALTH INSURANCE PLAN

Enactment of Medicare and Medicaid in 1965 took away much of the pressure toward national health insurance for several years. The two largest groups previously without adequate coverage had finally been assured financial access to health care: 24 million elderly and 20 million of the poorest in society. Yet, in 1978 23 million Americans still had neither health insurance, Medicare, Medicaid, nor access to a system of free care like that of the Veterans Administration. Eight million of these had incomes below the poverty level but were ineligible for Medicaid because of requirements in their states (Davis, 1980). Another 19 million—mostly poor and not receiving group health insurance benefits from employment—had only inadequate, costly, individually purchased health insurance policies. Even those with apparently adequate health insurance for most circumstances can drastically exceed their benefit limits in cases of especially serious illness. It is estimated that 40% of Americans do not have sufficient coverage for these so-called catastrophic illness expenses (Davis, 1980). As a result of the rapid rise in health care costs, the Medicare co-payments, additional billings beyond the allowable Medicare fee, and other out-of-pocket health expenses have increased so rapidly that the elderly are paying a larger share of their incomes for medical expenses today than prior to the Medicare legislation (though they also receive more care). The unevenness among states of Medicaid benefits and eligibilities, plus the high cost and poor administration has caused widespread disillusionment with that program. Thus, although it was a major step toward assuring access to adequate health care for all, Medicare/Medicaid legislation left many gaps and problems to be resolved (Davis, 1975, 1976).

Increasing awareness that problems like these continued to exist after 1965, plus the growing alarm about the cost of the Medicare and Medicaid programs, led to a new series of proposals for national health insurance. Organized labor (especially the United Auto Workers), acting in part from a long-standing ideological commitment and in part in response to the increasing bite that health fringe benefits are taking in collective-bargaining settlements, organized the Committee (of 100) for National Health Insurance to push for more definitive and comprehensive legislation (Falk, 1977). The group drafted the Health Security Bill, first introduced by Sen. Edward Kennedy (Dem., Mass.) and Rep. Martha Griffiths (Dem., Mich.) in 1970. In response, virtually every health interest group also developed and sponsored bills—including the Nixon Administration and the AMA, which had until then been a staunch opponent of any national health insurance legislation (Hyde & Wolfe, 1954; Colombotos et al., 1975). Extended committee hearings were held in both the Senate and House of Representatives. Experienced Congress watchers were predicting that national health insurance was finally just around the corner (Burns, 1971; Eilers, 1971). Yet, despite the disappearance of outright opposition, the plethora of proposed approaches and the inability to arrive at workable compromise solutions served to block legislation just as effectively as the AMA and Ways and Means Committee opposition of the 1950s and early 1960s did.

The old philosophical conflict over the role of government in regard to welfare versus social insurance still continued, but this was gradually submerged by two new overriding issues that began to dominate the discussion: (1) how to control the escalating costs, which national health insurance would surely push higher as Medicare and Medicaid had done; and (2) to what extent and how national health insurance should be used to restructure the system of health care delivery, which many experts (for varying reasons) agreed was in need of reform. It had become clear to most policy makers that national health insurance could no longer be just a way to pay medical bills, but there the agreement ended. The competing legislative proposals mirrored fundamental differences in philosophies about the "proper" nature of economic and organizational controls to be imposed on the health system (Chapter 13).

Philosophical differences were seldom expressed directly in such terms; instead they constituted implicit starting points that shaped positions on more specific issues. This makes it difficult to identify the fundamental issues that are often the true basis for disagreement, but it avoids ideological polarization.* The debate centered around the detailed structure of the proposals, especially payment mechanisms: How much of the financing should funnel through the Federal payment system and show up as part of the Federal budget? What financing source should be used? How much additional cov-

* This is not to imply that the other more explicit issues are no longer important, but only that the role they play in the debate can be better understood in the light of the underlying philosophical perspectives. Such specific issues also would be more amenable to compromise and technical solutions if certain of the underlying dilemmas could be resolved. The reader can find an excellent summary of the detailed issues in Davis (1975).

erage should be incorporated? Some called for just catastrophic reinsurance and filling the existing gaps in Medicaid and Medicare as add-ons to the present pluralistic system. Others demanded a uniform, compulsory, comprehensive benefit system for all. Thus, despite the optimism that national health insurance was an idea whose time had come, any workable compromise eluded the Congress (Bodenheimer, 1972).

On the other hand, it should also be noted that this debate was taking place within a surprising degree of *consensus* in regard to certain basic principles, goals, and assumptions, which had emerged since 1965. This unvoiced framework of agreement continues to serve as the context of debate and can be expected to shape any broad national health care policy initiative that eventually comes to fruition out of the current Congressional fight.

First, in 1965 health care was already widely acknowledged as a basic necessity of life, alongside of food, clothing, and shelter. Yet government's role in assuring health care was considered limited to a residual welfare function (as guarantor of last resort or at most as expediter of participatory social insurance). Fourteen years' experience with massive government involvement in financing health care has accustomed people to the idea of government as a major payer of health benefits (Burns, 1974). Despite problems of administration and costs that have far outstripped original estimates, few seriously question the indispensability of Federal health insurance programs today (U.S. Senate Finance Committee, 1970). The precedent of government as the guarantor of financial access to health care is now well-established (White, 1971). The remaining question today is *how* this responsibility should be exercised.

There is increasing agreement that universal coverage is needed that assures *all* residents of protection against serious financial consequences of illness without distinctions in regard to welfare or contributory status of the beneficiary (Woodcock, 1975). Fear of financial ruin from catastrophic illnesses has reached the middle class. Although virtually all middle-class Americans have some form of health insurance, many do not have adequate catastrophic coverage. Even with supposedly adequate health insurance, very prolonged or expensive periods of illness can overrun the insurance coverage and force a family into bankruptcy. Because of their dramatic impact, these cases—though infrequent in occurrence—have been highly publicized. In 1977, 7 million Americans experienced uninsured out-of-pocket medical expenditures that exceeded 15% of their income, a common definition of catastrophic expenses (USDHEW, 1979). The growing fear of such illness-induced financial catastrophies is one of the driving forces behind the movement for national health insurance legislation.

With the extension of concern to the middle class, the issue of social insurance (entitlement by contribution) versus residual welfare has receded. Recent major increases in the Social Security tax and discussion of bolstering the solvency of the Trust Fund with general revenues have also blurred the distinction between contributory entitlement and welfare programs involving income transfer. Today Social Security and Medicare have *de facto* come to entail an appreciable element of income transfer from one generation to another. The old ideological debate at center stage during enactment of Medicare and Medicaid has given way to a new one about the "proper" structure to be sought for the health care economy.

The second major area of consensus concerns rising costs and the need for reform of the health care delivery and financing system to improve efficiency and appropriateness of services. In 1965 most policy makers still saw the cost problem only in relation to the patient. The central economic issue was to provide financial access to the mainstream of medical care and to protect individuals from heavy cost burdens imposed by illness (Anderson, 1972). It merely seemed necessary to spread the risk of this cost by using the insurance mechanism. Government's role in regard to costs was simply to provide equivalent public insurance protection for those who did not have private insurance through employment and could not afford to purchase it individually. The burden of rising systemwide expenditures was too remote to concern most people. Except for a few economists and other critical students of the health care system, few noticed the trend of rising total health system costs, which actually began to accelerate immediately after World War II (Davis, 1972).

With the assumption of a large share of payment by the Federal government, however, the growth of health care costs became highly visible through their impact on the Federal budget. The tremendous rate of increase in expenditures for Medicare and Medicaid, from $4.5 billion in 1967 to $48 billion in fiscal year 1980, began to alarm Administration budget makers, then the Congress, and finally the general public, as the tax significance became apparent (Falk, 1977). The necessity of raising Social Security payroll taxes to protect the solvency of the Trust Funds focused public attention primarily on the rising cost of pensions. Yet it also illustrated the burden that Medicare was imposing on the Federal tax system. The increasing percentage of income that the elderly are forced to pay for health care in spite of Medicare made the rising cost more evident to this increasingly vocal segment of the population. Recently many studies of health care cost, waste, and inefficiency have come to public notice. The realization has spread that health care costs are escalating faster than other parts of the economy and out of proportion to the additional benefits received.

In the early 1960s the affluence of American society and the strength of the economy made it seem that endless sums could be committed for social programs including health care. The past decade of continued high inflation, loss of world economic dominance, and public revolts against growth of taxation to finance government expenditures have changed the attitudes of policy makers. The public is asking for firmer assurances that additional tax dollars will be spent efficiently to produce outcomes commensurate with the resources invested. The scandals of fraud and abuse in regard to government payments for health care have shaken the faith that taxpayers are getting a fair value for what they pay into these programs. Congress is demanding fiscal accountability (Eckhardt, 1980). Agreement has emerged among policy makers that any national health insurance program must include methods to control the problem of rising costs and use the leverage of any new public funding to improve the efficiency of the health care system.

A third, more tenuous unspoken consensus has evolved in regard to certain principles of social justice to be incorporated in any new national social programs. Agreements about social equity have gradually crystallized through the political process into a set of tacit rules concerning the implementation of new benefit programs. Social justice has come to mean that access to services that are necessities of life should be a function of need, not the ability to pay (Fried, 1976). The burden of payment for such services, on the other hand, ought to be more a function of ability to pay. Consequently, financing of the programs should preferably be from a progressive source, and any cost sharing by individuals ought to be graduated to prevent serious burden on those least able to pay (Rivlin, 1974).

This means that national health insurance will in effect also be an income transfer program—as Medicare and Medicaid are today (Berki, 1971). Certain tacit rules of "redistributional justice" have grown out of the legislative tradition derived from the political compromises necessary to secure enactment of laws that have an income redistributive impact. The burden of financing (and benefits) must be such that no one (and no political entity) will be placed *directly* in a worse position under the new legislation than before (the so-called "hold-harmless" rule). In following this rule it is usually necessary to finance a larger share of the payments through the (progressively financed) Federal budget than before. This is never the explicit objective of program proponents. In fact, it flies in the face of the widely and strongly held political goal of restricting growth of the Federal budget (and may therefore preclude enactment). Yet only in this way can more benefits go to those who previously had less without taking away directly from those who previously had more. The cost is diluted over the entire Federal tax base, while the new benefits are concentrated on the few who have been deprived before. Thus the many seem to be held "relatively harmless," while the few who were most in need obtain visible benefit.

The converse of the "hold-harmless" rule is the prohibition of "windfall gains" under a new law. Increased benefits for those who did not have them are not considered windfall, but no one should reap the "unearned" advantage of being able to decrease his present effort (level of contribution) appreciably. A final rule of redistributional justice seems at first glance to be a direct contradiction or exception to the antiwindfall precept. This is the rule of "fiscal relief" for states that have taken the lead in providing the same kind of benefits to their own citizens. States are considered to deserve fiscal relief (with some maintenance of effort requirement as an antiwindfall counterbalance) if their taxpayers come under an increasingly heavy financial burden as the cost of the benefits grow and/or because the state has a proportionately larger concentration of beneficiaries for the program than the nation as a whole.

Obviously it is impossible to satisfy all the redistributional justice rules at once in any strict sense. There can be no redistribution if no one is "harmed" and no one receives a windfall, for example, an unpaid-for new benefit. But these rules are the parameters within which the bargaining over the details of financing such programs is worked out. A compromise formula must be found between "fiscal relief" and "maintenance of effort" by each state, which still minimizes the new impact on the Federal budget. Similarly, compromise formulas must be found between the hold-harmless rule and the antiwindfall rule that preserve justice between those employers (and their workers) who have provided very adequate health insurance benefits in the past and those who have not. Employers not providing health benefits often have many low-wage employees and might suffer economic dislocations requiring layoffs if they are required to shoulder abruptly a burden of payment for health benefits equivalent to those paid today by most. Thus maintenance of effort and equity of contribution and benefit would have to be tempered by subsidies to some employers.

THE POLITICAL CONTEXT OF THE NEW DEBATE

These basic areas of consensus establish the goals and framework for the development of a new national health care policy. Within this framework of consensus, however, some very fundamental disagreements exist over *how* to achieve the agreed objectives. These controversies may make enactment of a national health insurance program just as difficult as the Medicare/Medicaid legislation was. The issues today are different from those in 1965—in part because public attitudes and political climates have changed radically. Many factors in the present political and public opinion environment pose serious potential barriers to enactment of any major new social initiative and limit the acceptable options for a national health insurance plan.

The most serious obstacle for the 1980s is probably the economic situation. The long-standing American belief in the growth of economic affluence and the political will for using it to improve society has been shaken by events of recent years. The weakening position of the American economy, continuing high inflation despite two recessions, and chronically high unemployment rates have created a new fiscal conservatism. This leaves little budgetary leeway for major new public program expenditures such as national health insurance. The "Great Society" optimism of the 1960s has given way to a more pessimistic appraisal of government's potential and the country's economic capability for solving social problems. The skeptical evaluations of some programs in relation to the monies spent and the turmoil of social change in the 1960s have discouraged many from attempts to correct injustice through Federal intervention or to undertake any changes in existing social and economic organizations. This public reticence is reflected in the more conservative complexion of the Congresses they elect.

The same reaction has fostered a strong antigovernment, antiregulatory attitude in the country and the Congress. The increased regulation of the health industry, which national health insurance would almost inevitably require, also constrains enthusiasm for such a program. The long devisive struggle over the Vietnam war and the political trauma of Watergate added to the suspicion of government and hesistancy to initiate new programs that increase its power over institutions and private lives.

This reaction also has included wholesale rejection of the traditional means of exercising political power within both the executive and legislative branches of government (Inglehart, 1975). The Congressional "freshman class" of 1974 elected in the Watergate backlash challenged the traditional power structure of seniority, committee chairmen's prerogatives, and other methods by which the Congressional and White House leadership exerted party discipline in the Congress (Fennor, 1973, 1965). Congressmen became much more dependent for reelection on satisfying the special interests of their local constituencies and less dependent on favors through traditional party channels (Mayhew, 1974). To a large extent, the new Congressmen were all "Washington outsiders" who gained election by campaigning against the "mess in Washington," that is, the traditional power structure. This palace revolt made the Congress more democratic but also made it much easier for any interest group to block action on legislation that threatens their vested interests (Congressional Quarterly, 1974). A legislative coalition needed to pass a compromise bill can more easily be broken by targeting on a few key members of particular committees and influencing them through public leaders in their home districts. As a consequence, it has become much more difficult to enact public interest legislation that is opposed by any well-organized special interest group.

REMAINING CONTROVERSIAL ISSUES—STRUCTURING THE HEALTH CARE ECONOMY

The divisions underlying the debates over individual issues of national health insurance plans are more basic and less amenable to compromise than the specific disagreements make it seem. They are deeply imbedded in the fundamental philosophical and political schisms of the country concerning the role of government and methods of *controlling* the economy. The single most fundamental decision in establishing any national health insurance plan is the choice of its basic economic structure for controlling the supply, distribution, utilization, cost, and allocation of services. This choice of economic structure is closely tied to the choice of the method for financing care. Many of the decisions on other issues and options flow quite naturally from this major choice—at least the remaining options are considerably narrowed. As analyzed in Chapter 13, there are three basically different types of economic structure within which goods or services can be produced and consumed: free (competitive) markets, public services, and regulated utilities. Any one of these structural types *can* work effectively, but the present structure of the health economy does not fit any of the three models. The financing system has created an incongruent mixture of economic mechanisms from all three types.

To review briefly, health care is largely collectively financed like a public service (either directly through the tax system or indirectly through the insurance cost-pass-through mechanism), but there is no corresponding public budgeting process to limit overall expenditures or determine distribution and allocation in accord with need. Supply and distribution decisions are made by providers as in a free market, but there is no price mechanism to restrain consumption or determine allocation in accord with consumer demand. Moreover, utilization decisions are primarily made by providers so that the entire consumer-dependent constraint side of the market equilibrium is missing. Market entry is limited as in a utility of the monopoly type, but distribution is not controlled by franchising. The missing control of utilization and allocation by the constraints of price and consumer demand is just as necessary for a utility economy to function effectively as for a free-market. These distortions, mismatches, and incompletenesses of economic structures account for much of the cost escalation, inefficiency, and misallocation of resources in the health care system.

Since characteristics of all three economic structural types exist in the present system, there are potential justifications for using any of the types for health care financing. It is not a foregone conclusion which of the three models would be the most suitable for a more consistent and effective economic framework toward which a national health insurance program should move. Since 1960, health care financing practice and public attitudes about health care as a human right have edged toward making the health system more like a public service (Mechanic, 1975). Many choices concerning objectives, financing mechanisms, economic structures, and decision making processes were reached almost by default, however, as the present system evolved stepwise without any overall plan. These questions are now being reopened for explicit decisions in the context of the current national health insurance debate. Legislating a national health insurance plan presents a chance to reassess the advantages and disadvantages of each economic structural type for achieving the agreed goals of our health care system. It presents the greatest opportunity we are apt to have for establishing a more rational and internally consistent financing structure for efficient function of the system.

Many options have been foreclosed in the course of history by other decisions or institutions established. But certain key choices do remain open that can profoundly influence the future organization and cost of health care: (1) We could seriously pursue the ideological commitment to the free-market approach and move toward a system where individual providers and consumers are placed at financial risk for their utilization and budgeting decisions without the protection of hidden subsidies and cost pass-throughs. (2) We could acknowledge the *de facto* public service financing with the corresponding social justice commitments and bring the rest of the system into congruence by establishing an effective public budgeting and allocation process. (3) We could patch up the present incongruent mixed system by filling the gaps in coverage through additional public programs while trying to control the open-ended, insurance-financed budget system by increased regulation.

There is a fervent ideological and political constituency for each of these strategies. Thus it is not surprising that each of the major contending plans for national health insurance represents one of the major economic structural approaches. Each of these fundamental options has different problems to solve, different limitations as a consequence of existing institutions and fiscal arrangements, a different distribution of the financial burden, and different new economic and administrative complexities. Each approach provides different advantages and disadvantages for solving the key problems and reaching the key objectives on which there is widespread consensus—cost control, systems reform for greater efficiency and responsiveness to patient needs, equity of access, and equity of burden. Each approach builds on a different ideological base, which evokes different political loyalties and support of different interest groups. Each will face different barriers to enactment. The final political choice among these options—or the choice to do nothing—will be a product both of weighing the relative pragmatic advantages and disadvantages of each approach and of the public and Congressional opinion influenced by the competing ideologies. We first examine the basic structures of the three competing approaches, then the options for financing and administering them, and finally analyze the specific proposed plans in detail.

The Free-Market Approach

Using the free-market approach to economic problems is an article of faith in this country. Politically, major weight can be added to an argument simply by showing that it uses the free-market philosophy. It is widely accepted as the best way to encourage efficiency, flexibility, and innovation in any economic sector. Free-market proponents believe that the more government involves itself in any economic activity, the less efficient and less adaptive to consumer needs the sector will be. They assume that the most effective way to bring about adaptive change is through the financial influence exercised by payment in accord with consumer choice between competing options. Such selective financial demand forces an industry to offer the quality and form of services most desired by consumers in proportion to price. It limits total expenditures, production, and consumption in accord with the amount consumers are willing to budget for that product as opposed to other goods and services they also want. This "invisible hand" of the market is the most flexible and accurate means to steer production into conformity with consumers' needs. Any government interference can only distort those mechanisms and detract from the optimum outcome. From the free-market perspective, the major defect of the health care economy today is the *absence of the price mechanism* through which consumers can exercise control using their selective demand to exert influence over the form of services provided (Campbell, 1974; Newhouse et al., 1974).

Yet, because of the unavoidable provider control of utilization due to lack of consumer knowledge about needed services, there is no practical way that a price-competitive market could be reestablished for health care at the individual-service level of consumption (Chapter 13). One national health insurance proposal, however, would attempt to recreate an effective competitive market between complete comprehensive systems of care (Enthoven, 1978). Insurers would arrange with providers to offer such packages of services available under prespecified conditions. To make competition work, even at this level of aggregation, it would be necessary to impose certain restrictions on the insurance system and its financing so that both consumers and providers are placed at risk for their decisions. The difficulty is to have a constrained source of financing while still guaranteeing everyone financial access to care. This would be accomplished by providing an actuarially equivalent subsidy to each beneficiary, allowing him to shop between competing comprehensive care packages, and requiring him to pay any premium in excess of the subsidy out of his own pocket. Providers would be at risk in their contracts with insurers to provide all necessary services to enrollees at the preagreed total payment rate. Insurers would be at risk to consumers to guarantee that the comprehensive service is made available for the preagreed premium. Insurers would compete in regard to premiums and the package of services offered to consumers (beyond the mandated minimum standards) on the basis of agreements they could obtain in their provider contracts. Thus the necessary basic elements and conditions for a competitive market would again be met (Ellwood, 1974; Ellwood & McClure, 1976).

The Public Service Approach

Proponents of the public service approach assume that access to health care has become a basic human right because of its indispensable nature and because of the externalities associated with the health of the populace.* Con-

* The traditional justifications for creating a public service and removing the consumer-payment control of consumption for a commodity have been situations entailing what economists call "public goods" or "externalities" (see Chapter 12 for examples). The necessity for public financing of public goods and individual services with important externalities has seldom been seriously questioned in modern times. Public financing of clinical

sequently government has the responsibility to assure access to care as payer of last resort where there are gaps in coverage (White, 1971; Sade, 1971). It also must provide or expedite a social insurance program to create the necessary mechanisms for making satisfactory and efficient financial access to services available to all. The combination of direct tax financing, indirect tax subsidies through income tax deductions for health expenses, and collective financing through fringe benefits has already converted the financing of health care into a public service model (Chapter 13). Government therefore has the fiduciary responsibility to protect expenditures of those public and other collective funds in the best interest of beneficiaries and payers.

From the public service perspective, the major shortcoming of the present system is the absence of a process for public budgeting and allocation of services in accord with consumer need to match the existing situation of public and collective financing (Chapter 13). Another deficiency is the lack of uniform universal entitlement to ensure that access is on the basis of need rather than ability to pay. The present two-class system of care is rejected as inherently inequitable. The national health insurance proposals following the public service model would deal with this problem by establishing universal entitlement with fixed areawide health care budgets (Falk, 1973; Kennedy, 1979). Provider groups and insurers would negotiate the distribution of this budget to assure comprehensive health services to all beneficiaries in the area. This approach carries to a logical conclusion the commitment of making access to health care a human right, which Medicare/Medicaid legislation in effect established in 1965. It adds the essential corresponding public decision making processes to enable implementing this commitment efficiently and equitably.

The Regulated Utility Approach

Proponents of the regulated utility approach to health care financing believe that any plan should disturb the present financing system as little as possible—both to minimize the economic impact and to minimize the political resistance to enactment of the legislation. They assume, in agreement with proponents of the free-market, that the private sector can generally

---

care, however, remained much more controversial. For the indigent it was classically justified as a means of preventing social unrest and keeping "undesirables" under control even where they presented no direct danger to the public health (Chapter 3). In more recent times this pragmatic argument became less respectable and was cloaked in the mantle of charity. Today even the charity argument has become publicly unacceptable. A newer justification for public financing of clinical services is as a "human right," or "government responsibility for the basic needs of individuals" (White, 1971). Other public services commonly justified by this third type of reasoning include welfare programs such as minimum-income maintenance. This argument remains controversial because "human rights" reasoning, unlike the traditional justifications, is not primarily economic, but rather humanitarian and ethical. Such arguments arouse highly emotional, political sentiments and divisions.

provide a service more efficiently and be more responsive to consumer needs than government can. Therefore, they strive to keep in place as much as possible of the private organization and financing of health services. They recognize, nevertheless, that certain unique characteristics of the health care economy, such as insurance financing and provider control of demand, impose unavoidable limitations on the function of the market. Consequently, consumer and taxpayer protection require countervailing regulation of the private sector. They also acknowledge that the inherent economic inequities of society would leave some members without access to vital services unless appropriate subsidies are provided to assure social justice.

Unlike the free-market approach, the regulatory strategy assumes that the private sector cannot always deal with these shortcomings on its own. Government has the responsibility to protect consumers and ensure their right of access to care—more in line with the public service philosophy. Where limitations of the market subvert the ordinary mechanisms to control cost and allocation of services, government has the fiduciary obligation to impose whatever controls are necessary to protect patients and taxpayers from inordinate costs—but only to the extent absolutely required. Government should not replace the market mechanisms where these are able to do the job. Similarly, where economic inequity bars some members of society from services, government has the responsibility to subsidize their care using tax resources as necessary. But government should not preempt the prerogatives of the private sector by financing services for those who are capable of doing so on their own through the use of private mechanisms like insurance.

Like proponents of the public service and free-market approaches, advocates of the regulatory strategy see the principal defects of the present system as (1) the gaps in coverage between where Medicare/Medicaid financing ends and where employment derived health insurance takes over and (2) failure of the market forces to control runaway costs because of the distortion resulting from insurance financing. Unlike them, however, they do not believe that fundamental changes in the financing system are necessary—only a little tinkering at the edges. Their solution would consist of extending Medicare/Medicaid coverage to those who are now excluded and imposing piecemeal cost controls where there is greatest abuse. They would also attempt to slow cost growth by encouraging HMO development but do not see this as a means to make major changes in the financing system in the foreseeable future. They propose to maintain the present mixed public-private approach to the financing and provision of care and merely to fill the gaps in order to achieve universal entitlement of some kind. Cost control and system reform should be incremental and targeted through such methods as hospital cost containment legislation and community-based health planning, rather than any major shift to overall public budgeting.

Each of the three fundamental approaches to structuring the health care economy requires a number of more specific decisions about particular elements necessary to implement the plan. These elements, such as the method of financing, program administration, economic market structure, reimbursement systems, underwriting, and cost control measures are theoretically all independent parameters of a national health insurance program. In practice, however, they are closely linked by traditional rules of operation, economic ideologies, and existing institutions. Consequently, certain choices in regard to one feature limit the realistic options for choices in regard to other features of the system. For example, mandating employer premium payments fits naturally together with the continued role of private insurance carriers as underwriters and traditional reimbursement mechanisms. Before analyzing the legislative proposals corresponding to the various economic structural approaches in more detail, we first examine the options for each of these elements and to what extent the choice of fundamental economic framework influences those options.

FINANCING METHODS FOR NATIONAL HEALTH INSURANCE

A major issue of any national health insurance debate is the method of financing because it determines the distribution of the burden of payment. In the final analysis, of course, the total cost always falls on consumers in some way, no matter what the route of financing. But the financing method determines how directly the burden will be felt and the extent to which various segments of the population participate in sharing the costs. For example, progressive financing methods, such as the income tax, place a larger share of the burden on the rich, while regressive financing methods, such as patient cost sharing and employee premium payments, place a larger share of the burden on the poor, relative to their incomes. The method of financing is also important because it is closely tied to the type of economic structure established, which in turn influences how costs can be controlled and what leverage is available for encouraging reform of the delivery system. Consequently there are strong political and ideological undertones to the financing debate intermixed with the purely economic ones. The choice of fiscal mechanisms for *controlling* the flow of funds from original payers to the final providers of care is as hotly debated as the method of raising the revenues. Like financing, fiscal mechanisms are closely related to the type of economic structure established.

In order to avoid major financial dislocations in the transition to any new national health insurance plan, it is likely that the present distribution of the financial burden among payers will be maintained as nearly as possible. This does not necessarily mean that the *methods* of financing must remain the same, however. There are several potential methods of assessing revenue under consideration for financing national health insurance: (1) direct patient payments (cost sharing); (2) premiums (employer, employee, or individually paid); (3) payroll taxes; (4) general revenues (either directly or as tax credits and vouchers). They are all used to varying degrees at present and are not mutually exclusive. Each has a different impact on the distribution of payment burden and therefore on the redistribution of income. Each fits more naturally with a different type of economic structure.

Off-Budget Versus On-Budget Financing

Besides the variety of revenue sources for financing, there are different ways that the funds can be collected from these sources and disbursed to providers. In designing a national health insurance plan, these mechanisms are just as controversial as the sources because the routing plays a key role in determining who controls the financing and reimbursement system. A central question is whether the funding should pass through the Federal budget or whether the contributions should only be mandated by law but be paid through other channels so that the monies do not appear in the Federal budget (so-called off-budget financing). Patient cost sharing is the most obvious method of off-budget financing. However, any of the potential revenue sources can be tapped in either an on-budget or off-budget mode. Patient cost sharing, for instance, could be collected by the program instead of by the providers and disbursed to them through the program budget. Premiums can be collected by a Federal insurance program as well as by private carriers. Earmarked payroll taxes can be collected directly by private carriers (so-called "income related premiums"). General revenues financing can be kept off-budget by using tax credits, which require equivalent increases in tax rates to offset the revenue lost. Thus the question of on-budget versus off-budget financing must be considered as an issue independent of the revenue source. All methods of off-budget financing have a number of advantages and disadvantages in common beyond the effect of how the particular revenue source influences the distribution of the cost burden.

Our present system of health care financing includes a great deal of off-budget financing (though some is simply by precedent, not by law)—12% through tax credits in the form of exclusions and deductions (Sunley, 1980); 15% through employer and consumer paid premiums beyond the tax credits; 30% through direct out-of-pocket payments. One of the arguments for including off-budget financing in the funding package for any national health insurance plan, therefore, is to disturb the present system of financing and the distribution of payment burden as little as possible. The greater the shifts in that pattern, the more difficult it will be to find a formula for the new method of payment that maintains the present distribution of burden in an acceptable way. How funding flows is also an important ideological and political issue because of the concern with preserving the role of the private sector in the health care financing system (see section, Administration, this chapter). Continuing the present modes of off-budget financing makes it easy to maintain the present pattern of fiscal management including the role of insurance companies. Thus keeping the funding off-budget appears to diminish the Federal involvement in the program. This could be important in minimizing the opposition from powerful vested interests.

Another apparent advantage of off-budget financing is the political appeal of keeping down the size of the Federal budget. This maintains the *illusion* that less money is being spent for the program than is actually the case. Because the size of the Federal budget is apparently not increased, lawmakers can avoid the onus of having raised Federal spending. It is easier to disregard the effects of off-budget program costs on individuals and the economic system than the effects of additional taxation and government expenditures. This entails the danger of burdening the economy far more than anticipated because of the self-deception employed in hiding the actual costs by not having them appear on the budget for public scrutiny. With the tax credit route, the total revenues *collected* do not appear to increase so policy makers can talk as if taxes had not increased to pay for the new programs. With patient cost sharing and mandated premium payments, even tax increases seem to be avoided. Yet other taxes must rise to offset the loss, which is reflected in the same tax bite out of the paycheck as before despite the tax credit that is supposed to offset the additional personal outlay for the new program. Thus if individuals are given tax credits that are usable only for the purchase of health insurance, the net effect on all parties and the economy is no different than if the same amount were collected as taxes and disbursed as subsidies to reduce the cost of purchasing insurance. Similarly, if employers are required by law to pay a given amount for insurance premiums for their employees, the impact on production costs is essentially the same as if the government would collect the identical amount from them as a tax and in turn purchase insurance for their employees through government outlays. Off-budget financing makes it *seem* that additional money is not being spent for government programs, but rather for private sector programs. In fact, however, the net effect on the economy is little different whether the funds are collected as revenue and disbursed through the present system of insurance carriers or collected by insurers directly (Chapter 13).*

---

* There are, indeed, certain differences in the economic effects of off-budget as opposed to on-budget routes for each financing source. All are minor, however, compared to the major differences that seem to be promised by the gross increments in the apparent (direct) program budgets one way in contrast to the other: First, administrative costs may differ slightly using the two routes. For instance, two steps are involved if taxes are collected first and then passed on to private carriers as intermediaries. There is only one step if the carrier collects the premiums directly. On the other hand, the tax collection system exists anyway and is much less costly per dollar collected than can be expected for insurance carriers because of economies of scale. Administrative studies indicate that, as a result, the tax route is actually less expensive despite the two steps (USDHEW, 1978a). In either direction the differences would only amount to a small fraction of a percent of total costs.

Second, reserve investment policies for the Trust Fund and private insurance may have

Thus the advantages of off-budget financing are primarily political (and ideological) rather than economic. All other things being equal, there would be no appreciable economic difference one way or the other. But this neglects the important politico-economic danger of the illusion involved in off-budget financing. As we have seen (Chapters 12 and 13), one of the major reasons for the uncontrolled nature of health cost escalation is the hidden indirect way we pay for care. Off-budget methods of financing are a major factor in this self-deception about what health care is really costing each of us and in our inability to have any control over those costs. The low visibility of back-door financing, together with the illusion that it is not public spending, lessens the public reaction to growth in the cost of health care. By avoiding the public outcry, which the rapid growth in health costs should have created, Congressional action to deal with these costs has been delayed. If additional health costs remain equally hidden, there will be little public constituency to counterbalance the provider interest groups and generate the necessary political pressure for effective cost containment. Insofar as new off-budget financing flows through existing fiscal channels, it will continue to enter the system in the same diffuse manner as today, primarily under provider control.

The reimbursement methods for hospital and physician services are pri-

---

somewhat different secondary economic effects. In either case the amounts involved are small compared to the cash flow. Trust Fund policy is more sensitive to the economic needs of the public interest. Private reserve investment is more sensitive to business needs. The difference in net economic impact is probably minimal.

Third, it is sometimes argued that the impact of on-budget financing is different from that of off-budget because government funds have a macroeconomic "multiplier" effect different from that of private funds. This is true for government expenditures as a whole because of the pattern of spending. But for any particular kind of spending, the multiplier is unchanged since it depends on the pattern of *respending* (saving versus consumption and type of consumption) of those dollars by the recipients (Samuelson, 1967). Once reinjected into the general economy, government-routed funds are no different from any other.

Fourth, one route as opposed to the other may have rather different income redistribution effects. The present system of tax exclusions and deductions is quite regressive. Those with the highest income receive the highest marginal rate of benefit from the reduced taxable income and also tend to have the highest values of premiums that are excludable. A tax supported system would almost certainly be more progressive, requiring a higher rate of contribution from those with higher incomes instead of the higher deductions. The net macroeconomic effect would only depend on the marginal differences in the propensities to save (invest) versus consume between the higher-income and lower-income groups.

These differences in economic effect due to income redistribution are not really a consequence of on-budget versus off-budget financing alone, but rather a result of the degree of progressivity versus regressivity of the financing sources chosen. These are theoretically—if not always practically—independent of the off-budget versus on-budget decision. For example, much of the redistribution effect in substituting the payroll tax route for present employer/employee premiums would already occur simply by eliminating the tax exclusion for employer paid health benefits.

With the exception of these minor modifications, then, the net reduction of otherwise disposable consumer income (cash flow out) and net channeling as input into the health sector would be no different by one route than by the other.

marily responsible for their uncontrolled costs. Allowing the funding to remain off-budget makes it very difficult to reform payment mechanisms. Control over the flow of financing provides some immediate control over expenditures and more political leverage to bring about the necessary long-range reimbursement and organizational reforms of the health care system. To the extent that new financing remains off-budget, potential financial leverage is lost that might be used to bring about improved efficiency and responsiveness to consumer needs. Attempts at health system reform will have to be imposed through superstructures such as planning agencies, cost containment legislation, and regulation of various sorts—none of which have been very successful until now. Congress and the Administration feel much more responsibility for financing that appears directly on the Federal budget. They are more inclined to face their fiduciary responsibility in regard to it and to insist on efficient, responsible, and consumer-responsive operation.

Cost Sharing By Patients

The most direct method of financing is patient cost sharing, that is, out-of-pocket payments linked to utilization of services. There is a wide spectrum of options concerning the extent and way that patients receiving services might share in their cost through deductibles and co-insurance (or co-payments). Cost sharing is a very regressive method of raising revenue. It not only strikes the lowest-income groups hardest but also those who are sick and, as a consequence, often least able to pay. For this reason no major national health insurance plan proposes using patient cost sharing for more than a small part of the total funding. Yet even a modest degree of cost sharing can create a significant burden for low-income patients (Roemer et al., 1975). Consequently, most national health insurance proposals would place a limit on total out-of-pocket payments graduated in relation to income.

Cost sharing has been a feature of most private health insurance and of Medicare. Therefore, minimizing change in the present burden of payments is one implicit argument for incorporating cost sharing in a national health insurance plan. Conversely, however, because of the "hold-harmless" political rule, any plan that appreciably increased the patients' burden of payment for those already insured would encounter serious opposition. Since the gaps in coverage are mostly among the poor, decisions about cost sharing for new entitlement under national health insurance would primarily affect them. Consequently, from a social justice perspective, any national health insurance program that requires a higher cost sharing rate for new entitlement than the present norm would seem to be unacceptable.

Two principal arguments are commonly used explicitly in favor of including appreciable patient cost sharing in the financing of any national health insurance plan: (1) to discourage utilization of services by forcing the patient to face out-of-pocket payment when seeking care; and (2) to reduce the apparent program cost by having consumers pay a portion of it directly rather than collecting it as revenues and paying it out from the program for the benefits—that is, by off-budget financing.

First, as argued in Chapter 13, it is doubtful whether appreciable overall health system savings can be realized by imposing patient cost sharing to reduce utilization (Phelps, 1975). If barriers to primary care for the low-income population and to preventive care are to be avoided, the co-payment rates must be graduated to prevent undesired underutilization effects on needed services. Any saving to the system by eliminating unnecessary utilization would be largely balanced by the additional administrative costs. Hospital utilization and provider-determined utilization in general is much less influenced by cost sharing. Since this makes up almost 80% of total system costs, the actual saving that can be achieved is probably very small (Blumberg, 1978). Because of patients' lack of knowledge about what is really needed and provider control of most medical decisions, major reduction of unnecessary utilization must occur through provider incentives rather than from financial barriers to care for the patients (Falk, 1977; Jonas, 1977). Thus the only valid justification for cost sharing must be keeping that portion of the real system costs off the direct program budget.

Even if off-budget financing is desired for its political advantages, it is questionable whether cost sharing is the best means of incorporating such financing into a national health insurance plan. Mandated premiums or tax credits achieve the same goal, are less regressive, and require less administrative expense to implement. Cost sharing is often suggested in schemes that attempt to create incentives to improve the efficiency of the health care system by increasing competition. Yet it actually detracts from the incentive to join more cost-efficient HMOs and other alternative organizations of care by encouraging younger healthier people to self-select the low-premium plans with higher cost sharing—gambling that they will not need health care. This leaves the higher risks in the comprehensive coverage plans, which are then *less* able to compete under the equal contributions requirement (Chapter 13). The net effect is more total healthy system costs rather than less.

Cost sharing as a means of off-budget financing makes it more difficult to use the leverage of new financing to get physicians to take a fixed fee schedule as full payment (so-called assignment). They are faced with the administrative problem of collecting additional fees in any case. The alternative of having the government (or private insurer) program collect the cost sharing from the patient after paying the physician in full (to act as an inducement to accept assignment) is more costly administratively. It also puts the financing back on-budget if the government program acts as the paying agent either directly or through a fiscal intermediary. On the contrary, using mandatory employer premiums or tax credits (and vouchers) to purchase private insurance as the method of off-budget financing is more appealing to insurance carriers and more apt to provide leverage to demand reimbursement reforms from them as a quid pro quo.

Despite these major drawbacks and lack of any significant advantage, the political attractiveness of patient cost sharing persists. It is linked with the ideological belief that patients *ought* to participate in the cost of their care in order to remain aware of their share of the responsibility in properly using it. Cost sharing is seen as the only vestige of the free market that remains. Thus even though there is no empirical evidence that competition among providers is increased by patient charges, the hypothetical link between cost sharing and competition remains politically influential. Ideologically, the trappings of a free-market economy seem to be important as a symbol even though the actual mechanisms of such a market do not function.

Mandated Premiums

A large share of health care financing at present comes from insurance premiums. The major part of premium costs is paid by employers as fringe benefits. Although these premium payments are not government mandated, they are enforced by collective bargaining contracts or their precedent. Adding to the same system by mandating additional employer contribution would minimize disturbance of the present system. It is generally assumed that these new payments would flow through the same fiscal mechanism and payers as at present. This assures maintaining the role of insurance companies in the financing system. The precedent, plus the fact that premium payment directly to insurance carriers is an easy way to keep financing off-budget, makes the idea of mandating employer premium contributions very attractive politically. It requires a minimum of change in the present administrative mechanisms. It maintains the ideological and political illusion that health care is being financed as a private sector, free-market economy because private businesses are paying to private insurers who reimburse private providers of care. However, as long as the present tax subsidy to such premiums remains, employer and employee premium financing includes a major element of back-door public financing for health care (Chapter 12). Moreover, the group experience-rating system and the degree to which the premiums are included as production costs in the prices of goods and services means that health costs financed in this way are simply passed through and diffused over the general economy. This form of collective financing has economic effects that are equivalent to payroll or excise taxes (Chapter 13).

Premiums are a very regressive method of financing. The employer contribution for each employee is the same regardless of income. Thus the percentage of total income contributed varies inversely with the income level. To the extent that they are subsidized through tax exemptions, the effect of the income tax savings for the employees receiving the fringe benefit is even more regressive (see preceding footnote).

Mandating employer premium contributions can have a serious impact on employment opportunities particularly for low-wage jobs. Businesses with many minimum-wage employees are less likely to provide fringe benefits today for health care. Consequently, a mandated minimum level of premium contribution requires a large relative (percentage) increase in payroll costs. The same premium amount constitutes a larger percentage of a low wage. Moreover, merely catching up to the contribution level of other employers (already paying such benefits) would require a large increment. In many instances mandating premium payments could require a total payroll increase of 5 to 10% (USDHEW, 1979). Such businesses might either have to close or cut back on the number of employees. Mitchell and Phelps (1974) predict that a mandated employer contribution of $750 per year would decrease employment by 1.4%. Subsidies would be necessary to help such employers over the transition in order to avoid such an impact on employment. This would in effect constitute introducing an equivalent amount of general revenue financing. Such a subsidy also presents a problem of social equity to avoid giving windfalls to those who had simply avoided health fringe benefits by exploiting a hard-pressed labor market—while protecting employers operating in a truly marginal position because of difficult competition.

A final problem with mandatory premium financing is that it would probably be channeled through the present uncontrolled insurance reimbursement mechanisms. Unless reform of the physician and hospital reimbursement mechanism is required as part of the package, additional money will flow into the system, driving up costs; yet the major opportunity will be missed to use the leverage provided by new financing to achieve reimbursement and organizational reform. Mandated premium financing through existing insurance carrier arrangements is also apt to perpetuate the present two-class system of care. Unless mandatory reimbursement restriction is established for all payers, the present open-ended financing of care would remain for the employed. Meanwhile public budgetary constraints will undoubtedly force greater stringency through regulation for reimbursement rates under the tax financed parts of the system.

Despite the lack of cost control and leverage for system reform in the present insurance payment system, employer premium contributions are likely to be a major means of financing national health insurance. The popular political fiction that it is not really additional "taxation" makes it easier to justify forcing an employer by law to contribute more for health care as long as it is not paid directly to the government. The mandated premium approach gains support from the ideological and political belief that health care financing *ought to* remain within the private sector as far as possible—regardless of the extent to which public and other collectively paid funds are used to finance it.

PAYROLL TAXES AND TRUST FUNDS

The Social Security payroll tax is a well established and generally accepted method of financing health benefits through the Medicare program. It is proportional to earnings but only up to $22,900 (in 1980). This is a more progressive tax formula than patient cost sharing or premium financing, though less progressive than the income tax. Since property and capital earnings are not taxed, wage earners shoulder a disproportionate share of the burden. For minimum-wage earners a payroll tax increase, as with mandatory employer premiums, can lead to layoffs or slower growth in new jobs. This effect is less than in the case of employer premium contributions, however, since the impact is only incremental (never starting from zero). The impact is also distributed more uniformly over the entire lower to middle-income payroll, not weighed so disproportionately on the lowest-wage groups.

There is no necessary reason for preserving the present payroll tax formula except for its operational simplicity. It would be possible to devise rate structures that are more progressive, but it is never apt to be as progressive as general revenues taxation because it does not apply to unearned income or corporate income. Nevertheless, there has been a strong political appeal to using the payroll tax for health insurance financing because of the tradition established by Medicare. The trust fund mechanism for earmarking these contributions provides the ideological underpinnings for the politically important perception of this financing method as "social insurance" rather than "welfare." The major political drawback to using the payroll tax for financing national health insurance is the recent series of Social Security tax increases which have been necessary to ensure the solvency of the Trust Fund. Since these increases have been achieved largely by raising the maximum taxable income base, they have been felt sharply by middle-income groups. These groups constitute powerful political constituencies. There is great resistance among them to any further payroll tax increases and in fact a growing pressure to roll back some of the recent increases. Use of a more progressive payroll tax formula would be one way to raise more revenues from this source without increasing the burden on the lower-income groups.

General Revenue Financing

Over 90% of Federal general revenues come from personal and corporate income taxes. Together these constitute the most progressive method of raising revenue available to government today. Although they have many loopholes and inequities because of the pressure of special interest groups, the overall structure that has emerged from the political process over the years reflects negotiated equity of burden more closely than other taxes.

This is the tax base generally accepted politically for financing public services, where all citizens share in the advantages occurring from having those services assured by government.

Many influential groups, however, oppose financing health care as a public service. Financing mechanisms other than general revenues (even off-budget methods that in end effect amount to general revenue financing) help maintain the image that health care is primarily a private-sector, free-market economy—where government's role is only to subsidize and expedite it for those parts of the population where the private sector can not do the job. Another political problem with general revenue financing is the extent of income redistribution that it engenders. Because general revenue spending is clearly visible "on-budget," it is more difficult to hide the program costs through off-budget financing. Even direct tax credits are listed in the consolidated budget as Federal costs. Thus despite avoiding an equivalent increase in the total Federal budget, this route is clearly identifiable as a program cost. Because financing through general revenues creates much more political pressure for control of health budgets and reform of the health care system, providers generally resist direct general revenue funding of national health insurance. Subsidies to marginal-wage employers to compensate for premium payments or increased payroll taxes do amount to general revenue financing through a less obvious back door.

Special Health Care Related Methods of Financing

From the viewpoint of social justice, an interesting proposal for financing health care costs is the use of excise taxes on goods and activities that increase the incidence of illness and medical costs, such as cigarette smoking and alcohol consumption. A 20-cent per pack increase in the Federal excise tax on cigarettes would raise $5 billion in new revenues per year. It would also increase the average price by about 35% and thereby decrease utilization to some extent, particularly among teenagers, where it would be most important. Similarly, doubling the tax on alcoholic beverages could raise $5 billion per year (USDHEW, 1978a). An ethical argument against such excise taxes is their regressive nature, but this is balanced by the fact that only those who indulge in the activity that increases medical costs have to pay the tax. From a political pespective, however, powerful special vested interests opposing such taxes would probably make it impossible to enact any national health plan that included them as part of its financing scheme.

RELATIONS BETWEEN FINANCING METHODS
AND THE ECONOMIC STRUCTURAL TYPES

Financing methods not only differ in their income redistribution effects and the ease with which they can be established using on-budget or off-budget routes, but they are also accompanied by strong differing ideological and political sentiments. A major reason for these sentiments is the close traditional and practical association of certain financing methods with one or another of the economic structural types. Those who believe it is desirable and possible to reestablish a *competitive market* at the *individual service* level of consumption decisions in the health economy assume that this requires reintroducing an effective price mechanism. The only apparent means of doing this is through patient cost sharing. Therefore, proponents of increased competition as the means to control costs, decrease utilization, and provide incentives for system responsiveness to patients' needs consider greater cost sharing as an essential means of financing.

Competition at the *comprehensive system* level requires financing that gives HMOs and other efficient alternative delivery systems a fair market opportunity to underbid fee-for-service practice. Equal contribution to all plans is the sine qua non. To provide a maximum competitive advantage to HMOs, however, cost sharing in fee-for-service plans should be discouraged as far as possible. Theoretically almost any combination of financing could be used to pay for insurance premium vouchers. Administratively, however, the easiest method is simply to provide tax credits equivalent to the uniform premium contribution for most of the population and only to give actual vouchers to those paying no income tax. This is equivalent to (off-budget) general revenue financing and would result in the loss of massive amounts of revenue for the Treasury needing to be made up by equivalent new taxes. For equity in maintenance of effort, a large part of this tax loss would probably be recovered through an employer payroll tax approximating the present average rate of employer contribution to fringe benefits premiums.

An alternative method of financing that funnels less of the cost through the Federal budget would be simply to mandate equal employer contributions to all employee health plans and to tax any employer payment above the contribution equal to the premium subsidy envisaged in the first form of the plan. Tax supported vouchers and mandatory minimum employer contributions would have to be added in order to achieve universal entitlement. Such a system offers less control than the direct tax-credit system and encourages low-option plans with high cost sharing—to the detriment of HMOs. Politically, however, it is more feasible because it manages to keep much more of the funding off-budget.

The logical financing method to match a *public service* approach would be direct general revenue financing. However, this would entail major dislocations of the present system, appreciable income redistribution, and great difficulty in finding ways to ensure maintenance of effort (avoid windfalls). Thus general revenues are more likely to be used only to finance increased Medicare and low-income premiums. An employer and employee payroll tax roughly equivalent to their present premium contributions could be used as the major source of financing. In order to keep this off-budget, one plan would have it collected directly by insurance carriers as a so-called income related premium. Cost sharing would be rejected by the public service approach as inequitable and as an uncontrollable total system cost.

A major goal of the *utility* approach is to make as little change as possible in the present financing system. Therefore the present mixture of cost sharing, employer/employee premiums, payroll taxes, and general revenues would probably be maintained. Gaps in coverage would be filled for the employed by mandating employer premiums (subsidized by general revenues in cases of hardship) and by general revenue financing through a Medicare-like public plan for the residual low-income population. Cost sharing would be maintained for public plans and new entitlements as a means of keeping the addition to the Federal budget as low as possible.

ADMINISTRATION AND REIMBURSEMENT ORGANIZATION

There are only a limited number of organizational structures with the necessary administrative capacity for setting policy and channeling the payments needed to operate a national health insurance plan: a Federal government agency (DHEW), state governments, private insurance (and/or health care delivery) organizations, and specially created quasi-governmental public-benefit corporations. The possible combinations and linkages between such organizations are also fairly limited.

A Federal agency could assume complete responsibility for policy setting, management of the program, and disbursement to providers or even direct provision of services. Direct Federal services are provided today for certain special populations such as the military, veterans, Indians on reservations, and other wards of the government. However, there is too much political resistance to the idea of so-called socialized medicine to make extension of direct provision of services a realistic option in this country.* Direct Federal management and disbursement to providers would have the advantage of easy and effective enforcement of policy decisions, especially those aimed at controlling costs or reforming the structure of the health care delivery system. However, it would require major enlargement of the Federal bureaucracy accompanied by an equivalent dismantling of the existing reimbursement system in the private health insurance carriers. Such a proposal would meet serious political resistance because of the disruption of the present system. It would also encounter the widespread suspicion of growth in Federal bureaucracies.

The most likely and politically acceptable role for the Federal government would be continuation and extension of its present role in the

---

* The Dellums national health insurance bill does propose creation of a national health service similar to the pattern established in England, and this idea has been endorsed by the American Public Health Association, but few political analysts give it any real chance of enactment.

Medicare system. This includes policy making and receipt of tax funds but delegation of disbursement to insurance carriers operating as fiscal intermediaries. This has most of the same advantages found in the direct operating role of a Federal agency, uniformity of policy and control over reimbursement mechanisms necessary to enforce cost containment or system reforms. The disadvantage is that a second (regulatory) bureaucracy is needed to exercise surveillance over the fiscal intermediaries and the disbursement process—to ensure that established policy is actually carried out and that waste, fraud, and abuse are minimized. To the extent that there is growth in the portion of payments through either direct Federal management or Federal financing through fiscal intermediaries, there will be growth of "on-budget" health costs. This has the disadvantage of requiring increases in the Federal budget and in taxes of some kind. In today's atmosphere of fiscal conservatism, this is a decided impediment to enactment.

In order to give the impression of avoiding this increase in the Federal budget while maintaining the control, some plans have suggested establishing a quasi-independent, public benefit corporation to receive and disburse payments and administer the program. Although this has political appeal, the economic effect would be identical, and the degree of control could be weakened. As the case of the Federal Trade Commission has shown, such semi-independent status has certain tactical advantages and disadvantages but does not make it fundamentally different than other Federal agencies.

State operation of policy making has been advocated in the past by the American Hospital Association and other providers as well as by some state governments. The general dissatisfaction with the Medicaid program, however, makes it unlikely that any national health insurance plan will markedly increase the role of states in administration. The demand for fiscal relief means states will have less responsibility for payment and would therefore be less accountable for policy decisions and operating efficiency. One of the major goals of national health insurance is to do away with the social inequities caused by the major differences in Medicaid policy among states. Thus, although states will probably retain their traditional responsibility in regard to regulation, licensing, and so on, it is unlikely that their financial responsibility will be increased. Under one plan being considered for catastrophic health insurance, states would take on some additional responsibility for regulation of reinsurance "pools" for high-risk groups unable to obtain coverage from individual private carriers.

Insurance carriers might play a number of roles under different national health insurance plans: (1) continued marketing and underwriting roughly as today; (2) acting as fiscal intermediaries to pay claims for Federal or state financing systems; (3) organizing groups of providers to furnish a complete system of care to enrolled consumers; or (4) operating in pools (consortia) to share the risk of insuring catastrophic coverage or the care of various groups that are difficult to insure for health, social, and financial reasons.

If private insurers were given no role, 84,000 employees of the 70 Blue

Cross/Blue Shield plans would be out of jobs. A large part of them could probably be taken up by the new Federal reimbursement bureaucracy, which would have to be built up to replace them, but this probably would require relocation and many other adjustments. A significant reduction would also be necessary in the 160,000 agents of commercial insurers who earn part of their commissions from health policies (USDHEW, 1978a). Because of this large trained work force and the expertise of the organizations, which would be necessary in some form in any national health insurance program, most plans would retain the use of the insurance carriers at least as fiscal intermediaries. This is highly favored by providers of care. Providers see the insurers, with whom they have grown accustomed to working over the years, as "buffers" between themselves and the Federal bureaucracy, which they distrust.

The insurance companies, of course, hope to continue their marketing and underwriting roles as well. A large share of insurance companies' net incomes derives not from administration or premiums in excess of actuarial risk. It comes from investment of the reserves they are required to hold as underwriters to assure that they can meet their fluctuating obligations. Insurers argue that their marketing role introduces competition into the health care industry. In the present open-ended, experience-rated financing system for health care, competition between carriers makes little difference in benefit costs—at best in administrative costs (Chapter 12). Under national health insurance plans with areawide budget limits or equal premium contributions (Kennedy or Enthoven; see sections that follow), however, competition in regard to benefit costs could become a significant factor. Under these circumstances insurance carriers might play a true market role in putting together provider packages or negotiating with provider organizations to obtain coverage offerings that could represent significant savings to enrollees.

MAJOR NATIONAL HEALTH PLANS UNDER CONSIDERATION BY CONGRESS

The Consumer Choice ("Competition") Proposal for National Health Insurance

Because of the insurance cost-pass-through system of financing and the control of consumption by providers, there is no realistic way that the conditions for an effective price-competitive market can be reintroduced into the health care economy at the individual service level. A scheme has been suggested, however, for creating the necessary requirements for a competitive market at the insurance level of aggregation. The "consumer choice health plan" (Enthoven, 1978) would create a competitive choice between comprehensive packages of care by providing each beneficiary with an equal subsidy contribution to any plan he chooses. Price competition between plans would be effective because the consumer would have to pay the difference in cost with resources that have to be traded off against other goods and services he might want. (The Ullman and Martin and Durenberger plans for cost containment through competition use only this element of the Enthoven approach without the national health insurance element of a Federal subsidy.)

Consumers would be able to comparison shop in a situation where price and known quality of services make a difference. Some agency would conduct ongoing studies of out-of-pocket expenses in each plan, assessment of quality of care, waiting times, and consumer satisfaction. It would provide the results and interpretation to consumers, who could then make informed choices based on evaluation regarding effectiveness, cost, and satisfaction, as well as reports from acquaintances or patients who have tried them. Premiums for all plans would be community rated, and open enrollment would be required at least annually. Thus enrollees would be guaranteed easy opportunity to move from one plan to another if they were dissatisfied. This would enable consumers to shop knowledgeably for the cheapest plan appropriate for their needs. By setting the subsidy below the actuarial cost, the consumer would be forced to decide how much *more* of his total budgetary resources he is willing to commit to health insurance in tradeoff for the other things he would have to give up. Providers would depend on consumer choice to finance their production of supply and be forced to compete in price and quality of services to sell their product to consumers. Total revenues, and therefore potential supply expenditures, would be a function of how much consumers in the aggregate are willing to spend vis-à-vis other goods and services. In this way resources available in an area would also depend on the number of consumers (and their perceived need for medical care) in the area. This would limit (flexibly) the budget available for all health services.

Employers could continue contributions to their employees' health insurance costs, but any contributions would be considered as taxable income so it would be no different than additional salary. Individual tax deductions for out-of-pocket health expenses would also be discontinued. Thus the hidden tax-support for voluntary health insurance would disappear. An explicit tax subsidy would be substituted—financed by a combination of general revenues, payroll taxes, and business taxes structured to achieve equity and as little change in the present distribution of burdens as possible. This subsidy would provide an equal contribution to any plan selected so that the employee would have to bear the full difference in cost between various plans out of his own pocket. The Enthoven plan is modeled after a similar system of subsidizing health insurance for beneficiaries used by the Federal Employees Health Benefit Program. This program has worked effectively and efficiently and is well liked by beneficiaries and providers. The Federal government would provide the subsidy as tax credits or vouchers (for the poor not paying taxes) usable only for the limited purpose of purchasing health insurance coverage. The subsidy level necessary to preserve equity with existing arrangements is estimated to be about 60% of the actuarial value of the community-rated premium for each risk group (except for the poor, who would be subsidized up to 100%).

The credit or vouchers could be used for any approved plan. Such certified plans would have to provide (1) "catastrophic coverage" and specified minimum standards for the benefit package; (2) annual open enrollment with the same (community) rating for anyone in a specified health risk group; and (3) at least one low-option package limited to the minimum benefits. The catastrophic coverage is necessary to guarantee that enrollees would not fall back on some other public welfare system of health care in times of serious illness. The open individual enrollment and required community rating would make it possible for individuals to shop effectively in the market of competing health plans to find the least expensive and most appropriate one for their own needs.

Employees would pay income tax on the employer health insurance contributions but in turn would receive a tax credit for 60% of the actuarial value of health services (not necessarily 60% of the present contribution). Since overall tax rates would have to rise to pay for the tax credits, those employees who are presently in a tax bracket with higher marginal rates or who are currently receiving very high levels of contributions to their health benefits would be net losers. Employees in low tax brackets or with low current health fringe benefits would be net gainers. Employers would experience a smaller fiscal impact. What was previously fringe benefit cost would now be ordinary payroll cost—both excludable from net business income but the latter subject to a 6% Social Security tax. Of course, if part of the extra financing were levied in the form of higher corporate income tax rates or higher employer payroll taxes, this could impact more heavily on employers.

The major appeal of the idea is its use of competition (between health insurance plans) to create pressure toward health system reform and efficiency for saving costs. Private insurance companies could continue their present roles, but would have to compete on equal terms with HMOs and other innovative prepayment plans. Such plans might well be able to provide complete health services at very little additional cost to the consumer beyond the 60% of the community average paid by the tax credit. Some HMOs, for example, currently come close to doing this (Luft, 1978). On the other hand, with catastrophic coverage guaranteed, some individuals might want to buy minimal insurance coverage and take the risk of paying out-of-pocket for health costs up to the catastrophic-cutoff level. The potential unfairness of self-selection according to known health risk could be counterbalanced by making the subsidy dependent on the actuarial value of the consumers risk group and allowing insurance companies or health plans to graduate their premiums in the same way.

Physicians and hospitals would be only indirectly affected by the plan.

Nothing would legally prevent them from continuing to collect customary fees from Blue Shield or hospital cost reimbursement from Blue Cross. Enthoven's assumption is that HMOs, which decrease unnecessary utilization, or other insurance schemes that restrict fee schedules and reimbursement rates could underbid other premiums and gradually lure subscribers away from the open-ended cost plans. As a result physicians and hospitals would eventually have to sign up with more restrictive insurance plans in order to have enough patients. It might be necessary to narrow their patient market drastically, however, before this would begin to cut appreciably into physicians' target incomes. Meanwhile, the patients in the less expensive plans would be served by far fewer physicians. Under these pressures, a stratified class system of care could evolve in which accommodations, waiting times, and intensity of care would depend on which insurance plan was paying the bill.

Many employees presently receive fringe benefits of almost 100% coverage no matter what health plan they join. Being forced to pay a considerable portion of the premium themselves would create a considerable incentive to shop for the cheaper systems of care. On the other hand, even with the incentive of tax deductions gone, habit and preference for risk avoidance and desire to maintain existing physician relationships would probably induce most employees to continue using their employer contributions to pay the premiums of their present plans. For most, the new tax credits would almost cover their additional taxes. Few would feel severe financial pressure to switch to low-option plans in order to save the marginal differences. Experience with the Federal Employee Health Benefit Plan shows that 87% of its beneficiaries choose high-option plans. If significant competitive pressures do develop to provide lower-premium plans, insurers probably would not create them by negotiating harder with providers to obtain lower fee schedules or developing alternative delivery systems, but simply by offering plans with higher patient cost sharing. This keeps the premiums low (competitive with HMOs), but does not appreciably lower the amount of money flowing into the health care sector. Probably the only way to create an appreciably improved competitive position for HMOs in such a scheme would be to prohibit cost sharing entirely for all required benefits. The consumer would then be forced to face the real actuarial cost of one plan versus another in his prepayment rates.

There are a number of serious difficulties with the Enthoven plan that make it unlikely to be enacted as proposed—although some of its features may well be incorporated into other plans:

First, the Enthoven plan would dramatically change the current funding patterns for health care. Regardless of the system of taxation used to finance it, many workers who presently receive low fringe benefits and the self-employed would experience major gains. Workers who have bargained for higher fringes rather than wages would be major loosers under the plan. Special provisions might be included to recapture losses as compensatory salary increases or to reopen collective bargaining, but this would be diffi-cult politically and practically. Similarly, states like New York and Califor-nia that have massive Medicaid programs would experience windfall savings unless they were forced to contribute equivalent amounts to the Federal program (which might be constitutionally impossible). These amounts would have to be made up directly or indirectly by taxpayers in all states.

This radical change in funding patterns would create a serious barrier to enactment. USDHEW actuaries estimate that the tax subsidy level neces-sary for the Enthoven plan would require funneling an additional $60 bil-lion per year through the Federal tax system to pay for vouchers and tax credits (USDHEW, 1978b)! This is two to three times the estimate for the other major national health insurance plans to be discussed. Actually, only $21 billion more per year in *new* health expenditures would be created by the plan compared to continuing the present system. Yet a much larger share of "old" as well as "new" funding would have to occur by way of the Federal budget. The reason for this much higher portion of tax dollars re-quired by the plan is the need for control to ensure equal contributions to all plans. The same effect could probably be accomplished without the po-litically unpopular feature of channeling to much through the tax system. But, this would require a complicated system of mandating employer pay-ments and taxing only contributions above the 60% of actuarial cost level. The details or implications of such variations have not yet been worked out in regard to its income redistribution and tax burden effects—nor of the original Enthoven plan itself.

Second, to make the scheme work effectively, competitive alternative health plans, such as HMOs, would have to be widely available in order to provide real options for comparison shopping. At present only 8 million Americans are covered by such plans. It is estimated that even with rapid expansion subsidized by the government only 10% of the population can be served in such plans by 1990 (OHMO, 1980). With so little effective com-petition, there would be scant pressure for either system reform or cost con-tainment. It would probably require 20 to 30 years before sufficient effective competition could be generated to slow the escalation of health care costs significantly. By this time, health care expenditures would again have dou-bled their share of the GNP.

Third, in itself, the Consumer Choice Health Plan would offer no direct leverage to remedy the basic mismatch between health system and health needs. The only direct system reform objective of the plan is cost reduction through competitive market pressure. Any organizational or utilization re-form of the health system would have to occur through innovation by the insurance plans seeking to improve operating efficiency in order to under-sell their competitors. Only HMOs in the area would provide any significant leverage to distribute resources and manpower more effectively. Only HMOs devote much effort to improving preventive care (and often more for ideo-logical than pragmatic reasons) because the cost-savings payoff is so far removed from the additional investment. Thus independent government efforts would continue to be necessary to improve prevention under this plan. Similarly with long-term care, even within HMOs little has been done to rationalize or improve the use and function of nursing homes and home care or to introduce other alternative methods of extended care. Again, separate government initiatives would probably be needed for system reform or cost saving in this service area. Such reforms as technology assessment and management of dissemination or quality control would still have to be implemented through a separate regulatory process.

The appeal of a free-market, competitive approach to financing health care has been growing since its proposal by Enthoven in 1977. A number of Senators and Congressmen have introduced partial forms of the proposal (Ullman, 1979; Durenberger, 1979; Martin, 1980), although no one has seriously suggested the original form.* The same group that would support it for its principle of using competitive market mechanisms to control costs would find the idea of increasing taxes by $60 billion completely unacceptable—even if most of it would simply be returned in tax credits. These internal ideological contradictions make it very unlikely as a serious contender for enactment. Some of its elements, however, will certainly be used as arguments against other plans and/or incorporated piecemeal where they can be fitted in.

No major interest group has come out in support of the plan in its original form, although many like certain aspects of the idea. Labor opposes it because it would penalize those workers who have been able to secure the best fringe benefit settlements in the past. Business supports the ideological basis but is hesitant because it would transfer control away from employee benefit plans (which lend some stability to employee relations) to a Federally controlled plan. Physicians and hospitals oppose it because it would favor HMOs and threaten the status quo in health care generally. Insurance companies oppose it because it would intensify competition and destroy the group benefit plan system which assures them a stable market. The Carter Administration opposes it because its constituents do and because it would require major tax increases (to offset the tax credits), create potentially major economic dislocations, and make regulation of the health industry more difficult.

The Public Service Approach to National Health Insurance

There are two national health insurance plans that build on the public service approach to economic markets. One, introduced by Rep. Ronald Dellums (Dem., Cal.), would go furthest in this direction. The Committee for a National Health Service, established in 1976, proposes eliminating the en-

* As this book goes to press, a proposal much closer to Enthoven's original plan has been introduced by Rep. Richard Gephardt (Dem., Mo.) and Rep. David Stockman (Rep., Mich.).

tire insurance system for health care financing and substituting direct own-
ership and operation of health facilities by government—or else contracting
with institutions and individual practitioners to provide services on a non-
fee-for-service basis. Thus it would create a National Health Service, somewhat along British lines, run as a public service supported entirely by taxes.
This scheme is too radical a departure from the present system to have any
realistic chance of enactment. Too many vested interests in the status quo
would be threatened, and the underlying philosophy is too far removed
from majority economic ideologies to be acceptable.

The Health Care for All Americans Act, developed by the Committee for
National Health Insurance and introduced by Sen. Edward Kennedy (Dem.,
Mass.) and Rep. Henry Waxman (Dem., Cal.), would maintain the present
private delivery system while moving economic and organizational control
toward the public service model. It would establish universal coverage with
uniform standard benefits, complete control of the total health care budget,
and top-down planning to reform the delivery system. The plan would be
operated by a Federally chartered (and controlled) public benefit corporation, the National Health Board. It would make use of Blue Cross, Blue
Shield, and the private health insurance companies as carriers in a limited
underwriting role, within the budget negotiated with the Board.* The plan
would place major emphasis on developing HMOs as a source of economy
and for rational planning at the service delivery point. Individual practitioners and hospitals would be allowed to continue practice on a fee-
for-service or other individual basis if desired, but they would be subject to
much tighter reimbursement constraints than at present.

The growth of the total national health care budget would be legally
limited to parity with the growth of the GNP. The national budget would
be allocated to the states by the National Health Board on the basis of proposed state health budgets to make fiscal and resource planning effective
and equitable. Present maldistribution of resources and budgets among
states would be corrected gradually to prevent major dislocations of services
or serious hardships on providers presently in practice. Misallocations of
resources for inappropriate services (the mismatch between needs and services provided) could be corrected more rapidly.

Budgets would be further allocated within each state through annual negotiations with consortia of insurers. There would be one consortium for
each of the major systems for payment: prepaid group HMOs, independent
practice association HMOs ("Foundations for Medical Care"), Blue Cross/
Blue Shield plans, commercial carriers, and self-insurers. State health boards
would negotiate with the consortia to set fair statewide (or areawide) community rates for individual and family premiums. Negotiated to stay within
the total state health budgets, these premiums would cover all costs (with-

---

* This greater role of the insurance carriers is the principal difference from the original
Health Security Act (Kennedy-Griffiths and Kennedy-Corman bills).

out patient cost sharing) for the complete package of required benefits. The consortia would then negotiate budgets with hospitals and fee schedules with physicians that would allow them to provide all necessary services to patients within the established community premium rates. Consortia (and individual insurance plans within them) would be at risk for remaining within their budgets. Individual providers would also be at risk in relation to the consortia who could pro-rate fees if overutilization threatens to cause budget overruns and could require hospitals to absorb costs beyond their budgets. Further efficiencies and cost saving would be encouraged by allowing insurers to compete for enrollees by offering incentives to their beneficiaries in the form of rebates or extra services. This would be accomplished by making special arrangements with their providers to pay less than communitywide negotiated rates in order to attract more patients (Kennedy, 1979).

Financing of the plan would be through a nationally uniform percentage payroll and unearned-income tax rate paid at least 65% by the employer and not more than 35% by the employee (described as an "income-related premium"). All patient cost sharing would be eliminated. Revenues would be collected directly as a premium by the insurance consortia from employer/employee payroll deductions to keep these payments off the Federal budget. The maximum that any individual could be assessed would be his actual community-rated premium. Many businesses now pay more than the 65% of employee health premiums called for by the plan, but the total premium and tax load on most businesses would increase considerably. Smaller, low-wage firms where employer contributions have been much less would receive subsidies in order not to create an undue hardship or force layoffs of marginal workers. In order to enable arrangements for the special needs of the aged and disabled, Medicare would continue as a separate program but would be expanded to all persons over 65 and would discontinue all cost sharing. Special financing by state and Federal premiums would purchase care for welfare beneficiaries and the unemployed through the regular insurance plans and consortia.

The plan has the typical advantages of a public service program. Total budget and allocation are controlled by public decision making—allowing explicit consideration of the tradeoffs being made with other budget items. Because of this direct control, it would be the least costly approach for the total economy in the long run. This is the only approach to cost control that can have a significant retarding effect on the systemwide growth of unnecessary health care expenditures without radically restructuring the existing institutions and organization of the system (Chapters 12 and 13). Intraregional allocation and planning would be largely controlled by the quasi-public health system agencies—but within fixed overall budgets instead of the present open-ended situation that pits consumers and providers together against payers (Chapter 10). The plan could ensure that everyone who needs medical service would have both financial and physical access. Based on recommendations of the local and state agencies, the National and State Health Boards would use their authority to provide incentives and/or start-up assistance through grants from the Health Resources Distribution Fund to develop resources in areas of scarcity and limit them in areas of excess. Thus the plan would provide maximum leverage for health care system organizational reform. This public planning and budgeting approach represents the logical consequence of the commitment to the precept of health care as a basic human right, which public attitudes in this country have been moving toward since the 1950s.

The elimination of patient cost sharing as a means of financing and controlling utilization is also consistent with the concept of health care as a human right—as well as recognition that it is an inefficient means of eliminating unnecessary utilization. By placing providers rather than patients at risk for excessive utilization within binding negotiated budgets, it lays the burden of decision on those who are in a position to allocate resources and effort most effectively within the system. If the patient bears the burden, on the contrary, he may be forced because of financial pressure to choose between obtaining health care, whose efficacy he cannot assess, and having some other necessity of life. Placing the financial risk on providers structures the incentives for cost savings in a way that can do the most to improve efficiency rather than the most damage by delaying needed care and prevention.

The major objection raised to most public service programs is the potential inefficiency, unresponsiveness, and lack of innovation in government operated services. The plan attempts to avoid these problems by contracting for services rather than owning and operating them with government employees. Some of the competition found in the Enthoven plan is also incorporated in the Kennedy plan. HMOs (paid on a capitation basis) would compete for patients with the fee-for-service plans. HMOs or other innovative organizational schemes could offer premium rebates or extra services, such as drug coverage, as inducements to increase their market share. Operating efficiency and hospital utilization savings could thus be used to attract patients by lower premiums or better services and amenities. Bonuses to providers based on cost savings to the plan, as in HMOs at present, could also be used as incentives for efficiency. Thus the areawide budgeting approach has the same effect of creating a competitive framework as does the Enthoven strategy of restructuring total available funds by limiting subsidies to each consumer. In either case providers are forced to improve efficiency and compete for patients in order to increase their market share. In this feature, both plans stand together in contrast to the present open-ended financing system.

The major drawback to the plan is its high cost in the early years of the program. In the first year of operation it would cost $40 billion more than present law ($28 billion more to the Federal budget alone) and $16 billion more than the Carter Administration proposal. The major new Federal cost would be the assumption of present out-of-pocket payments borne by the hard-pressed elderly. Because of its greater control of program budgets, it is estimated (by independent actuaries) that after four years the plan would cost less than present law. If it went into effect in 1983, the saving in 1988 would be $38 billion (in 1980 dollars).

Even using the existing expertise of the insurance companies, some experts fear that planning and administering a $200 billion health system would be an awesome task. In particular, administrative and political analysts foresee serious difficulties in carrying out the negotiations necessary to determine and allocate areawide prospective budgets. Data, experience, and political precedent needed to implement this process are all lacking, but experience from other countries could be drawn upon. The gradual rate of adjustment in state budgets from present levels should allow acquisition of more adequate data and more sophisticated methods of budget setting by the time negotiations have to deal with more subtle inequities between states. Other analysts argue that the proposed system of premium collection and budget allocation to providers by the insurance consortia would be an administrative nightmare. On the other hand, if a consensus emerges that these procedures will create a serious problem, administrative mechanisms can be and often are modified on the basis of hearings during the Congressional enactment process for legislation. Whether administration of the plan would actually be so difficult or not, fear of such a major break with tradition will create political resistance to federalizing such a large economic sector.

Interest group positions in regard to the proposal are quite predictable. The proposal has the strong backing of labor, the aged, consumer groups, and many health advocacy groups such as the American Public Health Association. On the other hand, the insurance industry opposes strenuously. Even though their role would be a more active one than the fiscal intermediary status proposed under the original Kennedy-Corman ("Health-Security") bill, their opportunities for profit would be more limited than today. The business community has reservations because of its philosophical opposition to any increased Federal role in control of an economic sector and because of the fairly marked income redistribution effect—as well as the high cost to them in taxes and mandated premium payments. The medical profession and hospitals oppose the plan because they would be placed under much tighter fiscal constraints.

The Regulated Utility Approach

Unlike competitive market and public service approaches to national health insurance, plans using a regulated utility approach do not attempt to restructure the financing system as a means of controlling costs. Neither do they concern themselves primarily with changing the organization of the delivery system to improve efficiency and appropriateness of care. The more limited objectives of these plans are to fill the present gaps in coverage and to take steps to remedy the most grievous areas of cost escalation through regulation. This makes it easier to implement such plans piecemeal and opens the question of which gaps in coverage and which areas of cost control should be dealt with—or how they should be phased in. These questions are less easy to deal with in the other approaches.

From the perspective of the middle-class majority in this country, the major gap in coverage to be remedied by any national health insurance program is protection from the financial burden of catastrophic illness. Owing to the lack of any uniform reinsurance system or method of pooling risks among carriers, 40% of the population does not have adequate protection for extremely high-cost illnesses. In order to remain competitive in bargaining for major employer contracts, most insurance carriers offer a basic policy with an upper limit on reimbursement. The incidence of illnesses that exceed these limits is very small. For this reason it is difficult for all but the largest companies to average out the potentially very high cost of individual cases over enough policy holders to make the risk insurable at affordable premiums. Yet it is fear of just such occurrences that underlies much of the push among middle-class Americans for a national health insurance program. Most persons in this group have adequate coverage for the great majority of illnesses.

A national health insurance program that only fills this catastrophic coverage gap is very attractive politically because the cost is quite low compared to more comprehensive programs. Senator Russell Long (Dem., La.), Chairman of the Senate Finance Committee, has been a proponent of this approach for some time (Waldman, 1976). Current estimates are that adding catastrophic coverage (or reinsurance) to protect every family for out-of-pocket expenses above $3500 per year (beyond current insurance) would cost only $7 to $12 billion per year. The most conservative estimates for a comprehensive plan that would bring the level of coverage for all Americans up to the level enjoyed by those employed in major industries today are on the order of $30 billion per year. For just this reason, advocates of comprehensive national health insurance fear that enactment of so-called catastrophic-only insurance would remove the political pressure emanating from the major constituency. This could make later enactment of a complete national health insurance program impossible because of the high cost in the face of an increasingly tight budgetary situation for new social programs.

To gain support from liberals who would oppose catastrophic-only, Sen. Long and Sen. Abraham Ribicoff (Dem., Conn.) have suggested a compromise plan that would combine catastrophic coverage financed by employer-mandated premiums with some means of providing at least minimal protection for low-income groups currently without basic coverage. One form of the proposal would federalize the Medicaid program and bring benefits and coverage in all states up to minimum standards. Other possibilities for providing low-income coverage are also being explored. Besides the low cost, a major attraction to many supporters of these bills is the minimal disturbance they would create for the present system of financing and organization of care. It would merely add another layer of insurance for the present carriers. The Long-Ribicoff plan would simply fill a gap in the existing system with no changes in the present provider organizational or fiscal relationships. Insurance companies and providers of care would be undisturbed.

However, many policy makers see establishing a national health insurance program as the principal opportunity to require financing and delivery system changes to improve efficiency and make the system more responsive to the needs of consumers. They consider this avoidance of disturbing the system as a major defect. For them, pouring 9 billion additional dollars per year into the present system without using that leverage to force reform seems like a serious political mistake. In the Long-Ribicoff plan, any cost containment legislation or system reform would have to be enacted independently. Even if certain reforms could be secured as a quid pro quo for passage, there would be no ongoing leverage to gain further reform. The additional funding would simply be channeled through the existing uncontrolled diffuse, open-ended system of payments (Chapters 12 and 13). Thus opponents believe the plan would worsen the trend toward cost escalation and inappropriate organization of care (Falk, 1977).

The National Health Plan (NHP) proposed by the Carter Administration is the most fully worked out proposal following the fill-the-gaps and regulate approach (USDHEW, 1979b). It would maintain the present dual system of health care financing: a public plan financed primarily through the payroll tax; a private plan leaving the employer/employee fringe benefit system essentially untouched except to mandate universal catastrophic coverage for all. Competitive underwriting would be preserved for the private insurers, but in a more tightly regulated (utility type) market. Individuals and employee groups would have the option of either continuing their present (or similar) private plans or joining the public plan at the actuarial rate (subsidized in part by general revenues). Tax credits would be provided for employers of low-income or high-risk workers to cushion potential adverse economic impact.

The private plans would have to meet certain Federal standards. The benefit package would have to include at least those in the current Medicare plan. Employers would be required to pay at least 75% of the private premiums, and those now paying a higher percentage would have to maintain their present level of contributions. The maximum allowable out-of-pocket expenditure required of patients (deductible plus co-insurance payments) would be $2500 per family per year. Private plans or self-insurers could participate in a Federal catastrophic-risk reinsurance program to help equalize premiums for employee groups with different risk profiles. Except for the $2500 out-of-pocket catastrophic ceiling, however, there would be no limitation on the patient cost sharing which could be imposed for most services. Prenatal, postnatal, delivery, and infant care for the first year of life would be required free of any cost sharing. This is looked upon as only "Phase One" of an overall plan, however, which would gradually require lowering of the cost sharing for all services.

The public plan, called "HealthCare," would be a uniform national program for all Federal health beneficiaries (presently Medicare, Medicaid, etc.) and those who join it voluntarily in preference to a private plan, for example, groups who are presently uninsured or marginally insured. This public plan would maintain the present organizational and fiscal structure used for Medicare, employing private fiscal intermediaries as payment conduits. HealthCare would collect premiums from the self-employed and from employed groups that choose not to use a private carrier—75% from employer, 25% from employees. Premiums would be subsidized up to 100% of the beneficiary's share for low-income families (below 55% of poverty level or those who spend down to that level as a result of health costs). A 20% co-insurance would be collected from all beneficiaries for each service up to the $2500 per family annual ceiling where the "catastrophic limit" would initiate 100% coverage. Beneficiaries aged 65 and over would face a maximum annual deductible of $160 (adjusted for inflation) for hospital and physician services, and 20% co-insurance for physician fees only. There would be a cap of $1250 per beneficiary on total out-of-pocket medical expenses, at which point Medicare would begin to pay 100%.

Financing of the public plan, besides employer and employee contributions, would be from a combination of general revenues and Social Security funds. Since HealthCare would simply be a parallel (subsidized) payment conduit and not a public service contracting body, the public plan, in effect, would also be part of a single regulated utility—half publicly financed, half privately financed (but still partially subsidized by tax deductions). Physician reimbursement under the public plan would be according to a mandatory fee schedule prohibiting additional changes to the patient. Hospitals would be paid on a cost basis but with the restrictions foreseen in the Administration's present hospital cost containment proposal (Chapter 13).

The major political advantage of the Carter National Health Plan is that it requires the least change in the existing system. It consolidates Medicare and Medicaid (and certain other Federal health insurance systems) into a single program and increases regulation of the present private health insurance process. Allowing the private insurers to continue their underwriting role minimizes the amount of "new money" flowing through the Federal budget or through a highly visible quasi-public insurance plan as in the Kennedy bill.

The major disadvantage of the NHP is the inherent weakness of any regulatory strategy in controlling costs. It does not introduce the degree of competition between provider groups that would be provided by the Enthoven or Kennedy plans or the control over budgets and planning of a public service approach. The NHP incorporates a separate bill to improve the incentives for Medicare beneficiaries to join HMOs, which would improve competition for this group. Except for the "dual-choice" requirement already in the HMO Act, however, most employees would remain locked into their group health plans because of the "experience-rating" advantage. The hospital cost containment programs for both capital investment and operating costs incorporated into the bill would apply to private as well as public payers. Some additional leverage over the private element of health financing would be gained through the potential competition of the public plan if it underbids the private plans. Because the plan leaves so much of the payment flowing through multiple private channels, there is no firm framework for linking financing, planning, and development on a regionalized basis. Therefore, little new leverage is gained for system reform. The mutually reinforcing interaction between health care organization, medical technology, and reimbursement practices can continue to perpetuate the costly mismatch between health services and health care needs.

Of the *comprehensive* national health insurance plans presently being seriously considered by Congress, the Carter NHP seems the most likely compromise candidate. It makes the least threat of change in the present system while dealing with some of the most serious gaps in coverage and cost control. In spite of the disadvantages of the public utility approach, regulation represents a popular political compromise (by default) because it requires the least disruption of the existing industry structure while affording some protection of the public interest. Thus it is least threatening to existing vested interests and therefore politically most feasible. It is the path of least resistance for legislation to take—perhaps the only possible path as a first step.

By the same token, NHP would leave the present incoherent mixed-market financing system intact with its inherently inefficient, uncontrolled, inflationary dynamic. As we have seen, health services are produced and consumed in a system with highly decentralized supply and utilization decisions as if there were a free market, but with no effective competition and no effective budgetary constraint. They are financed much like a public service but with only retrospective, nonpublicly controlled budgeting.

This mismatch of economic mechanisms severely affects cost effectiveness of the system. The shift of the predominant disease pattern from acute curable diseases to chronic disorders requiring long-term maintenance and new approaches to prevention has accentuated the incongruence and unplanability of paying for services as we now do. What to do about these incongruencies is the tacit issue behind the current debates over medical care financing through national health insurance. Yet the question is seldom raised explicitly whether medical care should be treated as a *commodity* purchased by individuals (according to their relative choice in relation to alternative goods)—or as a *public service* financed and planned primarily to meet public needs—or as a *utility* left as far as possible to follow its own profit and prestige motives and only restrained by regulation where the public interest is seriously threatened. The Medicare legislation took a major step in the direction of public service financing of health care but stopped short of setting up the concomitant public fiscal and budget allocation mechanisms because of the political compromises that were necessary to secure passage of the law. As the national health insurance debate takes form, it might be wiser to face these difficult political issues squarely. We are likely to have to live with the product of that legislation for a long time to come. Yet the nature of the political process in this country makes it doubtful whether such fundamental policy direction questions can be debated and decided in such a way that implementation is allowed to follow the logical consequences of the basic decision.

POLITICAL PROCESS CONSIDERATIONS

Political decision making in this country has traditionally taken place through so-called incrementalism—solutions of major problems occurring in many small steps, each tested by its effects before going on to the next. The checks and balances on political power established in the Constitution favor such an approach, and by and large it has served us well. By favoring the safer middle ground between extreme options, it avoids radical new policy directions before they can be adequately assessed.

Yet piecemeal, middle-of-the-road incrementalism has serious drawbacks for dealing with certain of today's problems like energy policy and health care reform, which have become much more urgent in the face of growing limitations on resources. In the face of runaway inflation, limited economic growth, and increasing need for services failure to grapple with long-range, total-system problems may force us to cut back on other equally needed services because of budgetary constraints. Incrementalism has traditionally transformed systems gradually by adding on new components as a system grows, rather than by restructuring it within existing parameters. Incrementalism precludes intricate solutions to problems where a consistent new system (e.g., for health care financing and budgeting) must be introduced as a whole to make individual parts work efficiently. When interrelationships between the various parts of an economic sector are relatively simple, it is possible to deal with one part at a time. With complex systems, however, comprehensive legislative packages and systemwide effects must be considered in order to minimize adverse consequences in some parts of the system when improvements are made in other parts.

Incrementalism tends to minimize the restrictions imposed on the free development of interests in the economy because only as much is done at any stage as seems absolutely necessary to correct a problematic situation. This is advantageous in an expanding economy by allowing uninhibited exploitation of opportunities as rapidly and as completely as possible. On the other hand, incremental decision making makes it difficult to negotiate tradeoffs in which one thing must be sacrificed in order to make something else possible. For example, it is difficult to secure separate enactment of restrictions on hospital expenditure growth—although it would be a necessary tradeoff to have sufficient resources for better long-term maintenance or improved environmental health. Only if the legislation is considered as a total package, can the ultimate fairness of the tradeoffs be assessed. Politically, it may only be possible to gain the leverage for budget and financing reform if they are considered in a context where new benefits are used as tradeoffs to gain the desired system reform.

A stepwise approach embodied in incrementalism makes it very difficult to achieve long-term goals without exorbitant costs in the face of short-term pressures from vested interests. Without the entire long-range plan being agreed to in advance, all parties concerned will demand to be "held harmless" (to suffer no unilateral disadvantage) at each step of the way. This means the only steps possible are those that *add* advantages to all. The net gain of the end product cannot be used as a bargaining chip for intermediate sacrifices or for bearing short-term disruptions. Whatever already exists must be taken up in the new system at each stage. This makes arriving at the same goal incrementally more expensive than doing so in a single plan— or may make it impossible altogether.

Decisions arrived at incrementally have a number of characteristics that create barriers to rationalizing the incoherent, mismatched health system that has evolved in this country. Incrementalism means responding to problems or symptoms when they are serious or obvious enough to move a coalition to counteraction, and then only to the extent absolutely necessary. Therefore the actions tend to be patchups and stand little chance of changing the fundamental momentum of the underlying forces creating the problems. The compromises necessary to achieve legislation prevent seriously threatening any of the vested interests involved. Solutions that hold all vested interests harmless tend to be very expensive. Not wanting to confront taxpayers and consumers with this fact, there is a strong tendency toward public and self-deception through hiding the true cost to the economy by using such gimmicks as off-budget financing. This entails the danger that more resources are committed to unproductive use than would be the case if the decisions were arrived at explicitly—perhaps more than we can afford in a situation where lack of productivity growth already stagnates our economic life. As long as we were in a consistently expanding economy, the added cost of incrementalism was no great problem. One part of the budget might expand more rapidly than another in any given year, but no one really had to cut back.

The test of democratic process in the 1980s will be the ability of the Congress to face the real implications and tradeoffs of allocating limited budgets and resources in the face of opposition from powerful vested interests. We will also need a new degree of realism in assessing the nature of problems and options for solving them by demanding greater internal consistency of the economic (and organizational) mechanisms employed. In the past, compromises between various ideological approaches to a given problem have consisted of a gesture to each of the parties—a little public service financing for defenders of the poor, a little regulation and tax subsidy for protection of the middle class, a little more unrestricted entrepreneurial freedom for providers (in the name of the "competitive market"), and a lot of hiding of real costs in the name of fiscal responsibility for the taxpayer— with no regard to how these fail to fit together as a functioning economy. This method of compromising through inconsistent patchwork must be replaced by compromise through fair sharing of the burden within a consistent framework. Realism of this kind is particularly difficult because the payoff for the nation is years ahead while the payoff for political expediency is at the ever imminent next election. The question is whether our political system, at the mercy of short-range pressures, is capable of the broad reform and long-term vision necessary to create a more rational health care system for the era we are entering. In the absence of a clear consensus about long-range goals, we will be forced to develop our national health policy along the path of least resistance. Unless it is possible to break out of the present pattern of inconsistencies in our financing and service organization, we will continue to pour far more resources into the health system than the marginal benefit justifies and in a way that does little for the new health needs of the nation.

EPILOGUE

The reader may be disappointed that at the end of this odyssey no sweeping solutions are offered to cope with the problems we have uncovered along the way. Given the historical trend of the financing system the most logical strategy for health care reform would seem to be public budgeting to match the existing pattern of public (and other collective) financing. This would provide maximal leverage to reshape the delivery system for greater efficiency and for better adaptation to the needs for care. Politically, however, the special interests and the cautious, easily blocked dynamics of the legislative process make enactment of such sweeping reform of the health care financing and governance system very unlikely. Likewise, radically restructuring the health system by using a forced competition approach along the lines of the Enthoven (consumer choice) health plan is equally improbable. Too many parties would suffer major losses from their present situation and therefore would oppose enactment. Attempting to compensate these losses by increasing benefit levels or by other special provisions to make the plan politically acceptable would be a very complicated and expensive proposition. Budgetary considerations would weigh heavily against such a strategy. In sum, abrupt fundamental structural change toward either more consistent economic model seems out of the question in the foreseeable future.

Thus the present self-perpetuating mismatch of the health system to current health problems will most likely continue to exact its toll in costs and in failure to meet society's needs.

The frustration over this state of affairs prompts many to call for simplistic solutions such as "deregulating the health industry," "eliminating the tax exemptions for health insurance," "introducing competition to improve efficiency," "making health care a human right," or similar ideological prescriptions. Yet the thing that has become most apparent from the analysis in this book is the interrelatedness and mutually reinforcing nature of the social, institutional, political, and economic forces driving the health system in its present direction. The organization of health care and its financing evolved stepwise. The public and private decisions shaping it were arrived at incrementally with no overall plan. As a result the present system is fragmented and riddled with incongruencies. But this does not mean it could easily be moved incrementally in a new direction to overcome the existing problems. Many with vested interests are happy with the system as it is and will strongly resist attempts to restructure it. Although there was no master plan behind the design of the present system, each step in its evolution occurred under the influence of strong political, social, economic, and professional interests, which in turn were strengthened by each of those steps. Thus the health care system may be fragmented and its financing mechanisms incongruent, but the constellation of forces that undergirds the momentum of that system is anything but incoherent. This is the reason for the often observed paradox that "the health care sector looks like a non-system until you try to change it."

Because of this internal dynamic, only a coordinated strategy aimed from many directions at fundamental elements of the underlying causes can have an appreciable impact on current problems. Short of a radical shift in financing and governance, our pluralistic system of health care requires an integrated pluralistic approach to solving its problems. This may sound much like the "incrementalism" we have just criticized as inadequate for the highly interdependent world of today, but there is a significant difference. Like incrementalism, "coordinated pluralism" recognizes that our system of government and the structure of our economy preclude radical solutions that fundamentally reorganize industries and economic sectors or abruptly shift the locus of control. Unlike incrementalism, however, a coordinated pluralistic approach recognizes that a greater degree of integrated social planning will be necessary. This would focus the multifaceted approach so that the net impact on the underlying problems is cumulative in the desired direction. This calls for two new ingredients: First, some national planning and coordinating council for health is needed, accountable to the political process but independent enough of the day to day political problems and shielded from the immediate pressure of special interests so that needed actions can be taken despite short-range political opposition. A possible prototype could be the Federal Reserve Board, which has certain independent powers to enforce unpopular but necessary decisions in the short run and advisory functions with decisive influence on the legislative and executive process in the long run. Such a council would have to command enough prestige, independence and authority to ensure its effectiveness. It would speak for the public interest but would also include adequate representation of the various special interests to make its decisions acceptable.

Second, planning strategies for reform must work from an understanding of the constellation of interrelated forces acting in the system. Such strategies must recognize the key internal dynamics, and devise a coordinated approach using whatever leverage can be realistically applied to overcome countervailing forces. This will require a readiness to face the difficulty and complexity of the problems, and to avoid simplistic, ideological solutions and self-deceptive gimmicks like off-budget cost shifting. It will necessitate accepting unpleasant tradeoffs and persisting with plans long enough and with adequate resources to make them work. A National Health Council could serve as the bulwark for such persistence and avoidance of self-deception. This book itself is meant to be a base-line description and analysis of the health system of the kind needed to formulate such a plan.

REFERENCES

Aday, Lu Ann, "Economic and Noneconomic Barriers to the Use of Needed Medical Services," *Medical Care*, 13:447–456, 1975.

Alford, Robert R., *Health Care Politics: Ideological and Interest Group Barriers to Reform*, Chicago: University of Chicago Press, 1975.

Anderson, Odin W., *The Uneasy Equilibrium*, New Haven: College and University Press, 1968.

Anderson, Odin W., "The Politics of Universal Health Insurance in the United States," *International Journal of Health Services*, 2:577–582, 1972.

Anderson, Odin W., *Blue Cross Since 1929: Accountability and the Public Trust*, Cambridge, Mass.: Ballinger, 1975.

Bell, Daniel, *The Coming of Post-Industrial Society: A Venture in Social Forecasting*, New York: Basic Books, 1973.

Berki, Sylvester E., "Economic Effects of National Health Insurance," *Inquiry*, 7(June): 37–55, 1971.

Blumberg, Mark S., "Rational Provider Prices: An Incentive for Improved Health Delivery," in Chacko, G. K., Ed., *Health Handbook*, Amsterdam: North Holland, 1978.

Bodenheimer, Thomas, et al., "The Hoax of National Health Insurance," *American Journal of Public Health*, 62:1324, 1972.

Burns, Evelyn M., "Health Insurance: Not If, or When, But What Kind?" *American Journal of Public Health*, 61:2164, 1971.

Burns, Evelyn M., *Health Services for Tomorrow*, New York: Dunnellen, 1974.

Campbell, R. R., *Economics of Health and Public Policy*, Washington, D.C.: U.S. Department of Commerce, 1974.

Cochrane, A., *Effectiveness and Efficiency*, London: The Nuffield Provincial Hospitals Trust, 1971.

Colombotos, John, Kirchner, Corinne, and Millman, Michael, "Physicians View National Health Insurance—a National Study," *Medical Care*, 13:369–396, 1975.

Congressional Quarterly, *The Washington Lobby*, Washington, D.C., 1974.

Cooper, Michael H., *Rationing Health Care*, New York: Halsted, 1975.

Davis, Karen, "Community Hospital Expenses and Revenues: Pre-Medicare Inflation," *Social Security Bulletin*, 35(October):3, 1972.

Davis, Karen, "Equal Treatment and Unequal Benefits: The Medicare Program," *Health and Society*, 53:449, 1975.

Davis, Karen, "Achievements and Problems of Medicaid," *Public Health Reports*, 91(4): 316, 1976.

Davis, Karen, Testimony before the Subcommittee on Health, Ways and Means Committee, U.S. House of Representatives, February, 1980.

Donabedian, Avedis, "An Examination of Some Directions in Health Care Policy," *American Journal of Public Health*, 63:243, 1973.

Durenberg, Sen. David F., "Health Incentives Refor.n Act" (S. 1968), *Congressional Record*, November 1, 1979.

Dyckman, Zackary U., *A Study of Physician Fees*, Washington, D.C.: Council on Wage and Price Stability, 1978.

Eckhardt, Rep. Bob, Hearings on Hospital Waste and Inefficiencies, Subcommittee on Oversight and Investigations, Interstate and Foreign Commerce Committee, Washington, D.C.: U.S. House of Representatives, March 21, 1980.

Eilers, Robert D., "National Health Insurance: What Kind and How Much (Parts 1 and 2)," *New England Journal of Medicine*, 284:881, 945, 1971.

Eilers, Robert D., and Moyerman, Sue S., Eds., *National Health Insurance: Conference Proceedings*, Homewood, Ill.: Irwin, 1971.

Ellwood, Paul M., Jr., "Health Maintenance Strategy," *Medical Care*, 9:291, 1971.

Ellwood, Paul M., Jr., "Alternatives to Regulation: Improving the Market," in *Controls on Health Care, Conference on Regulation in the Health Industry*, Washington, D.C.: National Academy of Sciences, 1974.

Ellwood, Paul M., Jr., and McClure, Walter, "Health Delivery Reform," Minneapolis: Interstudy, mimeo, November 17, 1976.

Enthoven, Alain C., "Consumer-Choice Health Plan," *New England Journal of Medicine*, 298:650–658, 709–720, 1978.

Falk, I. S., "Medical Care in the USA—1932–1972. Problems, Proposals and Programs from the Committee for National Health Insurance," *Health and Society*, 51:1, 1973.

Falk, Isador S., "Proposals for National Health Insurance in the U.S.A. Origins and Evolution, and Some Perceptions for the Future," *Milbank Memorial Fund Quarterly*, Spring: 161, 1977.

Fein, Rashi, "Some Health Policy Issues: One Economist's View," *Public Health Reports*, 90:387, 1975.

Feldman, Paul, "Efficiency, Distribution, and the Role of Government in a Market Economy," *Journal of Political Economy*, 79(3):508–526, 1971.

Feldstein, Paul J., *Health Associations and the Demand for Legislation: The Political Economy of Health*, Cambridge, Mass.: Ballinger, 1977.

Fennor, R., "The Internal Distribution of Influence: The House," in Truman, D., Ed., *The Congress and America's Future*, Englewood Cliffs, N.J.: Prentice-Hall, 1965.

Fennor, R., *Congressmen in Committees*, Boston: Little, Brown, 1973.

Fried, Charles, "Equality and Rights in Medical Care," *Hastings Center Report*, 6(February):29–34, 1976.

Fuchs, Victor R., *Who Shall Live?: Health, Economics, and Social Choice*, New York, Basic Books, 1974.

Hetherington, Robert W., Hopkins, Carl E., and Roemer, Milton I., *Health Insurance Plans: Promise and Performance*, New York: Wiley-Interscience, 1975.

Huitt, R., "The Internal Distribution of Influence: The Senate," in Truman, D., Ed., *The Congress and America's Future*, Englewood Cliffs, N.J.: Prentice-Hall, 1965.

Hyde, David R., and Wolff, Payson, "The American Medical Association: Power, Purpose, and Politics in Organized Medicine," *Yale Law Journal*, 63:938–1022, 1954.

Inglehart, John, "Health Report/Congress Expands Capacity to Contest Executive Policy," *National Journal Reports*, 7:730, 1975.

Institute of Medicine, *Medicare-Medicaid Reimbursement Policies*, Washington, D.C.: National Academy of Sciences, 1976.

Jonas, Steven, "Copayment and National Health Insurance in the United States: A Critique of Work by Newhouse, Phelps and Schwartz," *International Journal of Health Services*, 7(2), 1977.

Katz, Jay, and Capron, Alexander M., *Catastrophic Diseases: Who Decides What?* New York: Russell Sage Foundation, 1975.

Keeler, Emmett B., Morrow, Daniel T., and Newhouse, Joseph P., "The Demand for Supplementary Health Insurance, or Do Deductibles Matter?" *Journal of Political Economy*, 85(4):789, 1977.

Kennedy, Sen. Edward M., "Health Care for All Americans Act" (S. 1720) *Congressional Record*, September 6, 1979.

Leaf, Philip J., "The Medical Marketplace and Public Interest Law, Part 2," in Weisbrod, Burton, *Public Interest Law: An Economic and Institutional Analysis*, Berkeley: University of California Press, 1978.

Le Clair, M., "The Canadian Health Care System," in Andreopoulos, S., Ed., *National Health Insurance: Can We Learn From Canada?*, New York: Wiley, 1975.

Lindblom, Charles E., *The Intelligence of Democracy*, New York: Free Press, 1965.

Luft, Harold S., "How do Health Maintenance Organizations Achieve Their 'Savings'?" *New England Journal of Medicine*, 298:1336–1343, 1978.

Marmor, Theodore, and Thomas, D., "The Politics of Paying Physicians: The Determinants of Government Payment Methods in England, Sweden and the United States," *International Journal of Health Services*, 1:71–78, 1971.

"Martin, Rep. James G., "Medical Expense Tax Credit Act" (H.R. 3974), *Congressional Record*, May 7, 1979.

Martin, Rep. James G., "Medical Expense Protection Act" (H.R. 6405), *Congressional Record*, February 4, 1980.

Mayhew, D., *Congress: The Electoral Connection*, New Haven: Yale University Press, 1974.

McNeil, Richard, and Schlenker, Robert, "HMOs, Competition, and Government," Minneapolis: Interstudy, 1974.

Mechanic, David, "The Right to Treatment: Judicial Action and Social Change," in Mechanic, D., *Politics, Medicine, and Social Science*, New York: Wiley-Interscience, 1974.

Mitchell, Bridger M., and Phelps, Charles E., "Employer-Paid Group Health Insurance and the Costs of Mandated National Coverage," Santa Monica, Rand Corporation, 1974.

Mitchell, Bridger M., and Schwartz, William B., *The Financing of National Health Insurance*, Rand Publication R-1711–HEW, May 1976.

Newhouse, Joseph P., Phelps, Charles E., and Schwartz, William B., "Policy Options and the Impact of National Health Insurance," *New England Journal of Medicine,* **290**: 1345–1359, 1974.

Newhouse, Joseph P., and Acton, Jan P., "Compulsory Health Planning Laws and National Health Insurance," in Havighurst, C. C., *Regulating Health Facilities Construction,* Washington, D.C.: American Institute for Public Policy Research, 1974.

Office of Health Maintenance Organizations (OHMO), USPHS, *Projections for HMO Development, 1980–1990,* Washington, D.C.: USDHEW(PHS), 1980.

Pauly, Mark V., "The Welfare Economics of Community Rating," *Journal of Risk and Insurance,* September 1970.

Pauly, Mark V., *Medical Care at Public Expenses: A Study in Applied Welfare Economics,* New York: Praeger, 1971.

Phelps, Charles, *Demand for Health Insurance: A Theoretical and Empirical Investigation,* Santa Monica: Rand Corporation, 1973.

Phelps, Charles, "The Effects of Insurance on Demand for Medical Care," in Anderson, Ron, et al., Eds., *Equity in Health Services,* Cambridge, Mass.: Ballinger, 1975.

Phelps, Charles E., "Public Sector Medicine: History and Analysis," in *New Directions in Public Health Care,* San Francisco: Institute for Contemporary Studies, 1976.

Polsby, Nelson, "Strengthening Congress in National Policymaking," in Polsby, N., Ed., *Congressional Behavior,* New York: Random House, 1971.

Pressman, Jeffrey L., and Wildavsky, Aaron, *Implementations: How Great Expectations in Washington Are Dashed in Oakland, or, Why It's Amazing that Federal Programs Work at All. This Being a Saga of the Economic Development Administration as Told by Two Sympathetic Observers Who Seek to Build Morals on a Foundation of Ruined Hopes,* Berkeley: University of California Press, 1973.

Rafferty, John, "Enfranchisement and Rationing Effects of Medicare on Discretionary Hospital Use," *Health Services Research,* **10**:51–62, 1975.

Reinhardt, Uwe E., "Proposed Changes in the Organization of Health Care Delivery: An Overview and Critique," *Milbank Memorial Fund Quarterly,* **51**(Spring):169–222, 1973.

Rivlin, Alice M., *Social Policy: Alternate Strategies for the Federal Government,* Washington, D.C.: Brookings Institution, 1974.

Roemer, Milton I., et al., "Copayments for Ambulatory Care: Penny-Wise and Pound-Foolish," *Medical Care,* **13**:457, 1975.

Sade, R. M., "Medical Care as a Right: A Refutation," *New England Journal of Medicine,* **285**:1288, 1971.

Samuelson, Paul A., *Economics,* New York: McGraw-Hill, 1967.

Singer, Neil, *Public Microeconomics: an Introduction to Government Finance,* 2nd ed., Boston: Little, Brown, 1976.

Somers, Herman M., and Somers, Anne R., *Doctors, Patients and Health Insurance,* Washington, D.C.: Brookings Institution, 1961.

Somers, Herman M., and Somers, Anne R., *Medicare and the Hospitals: Issues and Prospects,* Washington, D.C.: Brookings Institution, 1968.

Stevens, Robert, and Stevens, Rosemary, *Welfare Medicine in America: A Case Study of Medicaid,* New York: Free Press, 1974.

Strickland, Stephen P., *U.S. Health Care: What's Wrong and What's Right,* New York: Universe, 1972.

Strickland, Stephen P., *Politics, Science, & Dread Disease: A Short History of United States Medica,* Cambridge: Harvard University Press, 1972.

Sun Valley Forum on National Health, "Medical Cure and Medical Care," *Milbank Memorial Fund Quarterly,* **50**(4, Part 2):entire issue, 1972.

Sunley, Emil M., Deputy Assistant Secretary of The Treasury, statement before the Health Subcommittee of The Committee on Ways and Means, U.S. House of Representatives, 1980.

Susser, Merwyn, "Ethical Components in the Definition of Health," *International Journal of Health Services,* 4:539, 1974.

Titmus, Richard M., *Social Policy: On Introduction,* New York: Pantheon Books, 1974.

Ullman, Rep. Al, "Health Cost Restraint Act" (H.R. 5740), *Congressional Record,* October 30, 1979.

USDHEW, "Patient Cost Sharing," Washington, D.C.: USDHEW, Assistant Secretary for Planning and Evaluation, mimeo, 1978.

USDHEW, "Financing National Health Insurance," Washington, D.C.: USDHEW, Assistant Secretary for Planning and Evaluation, mimeo, 1978a.

USDHEW, "Lead Agency Memorandum on a National Health Plan," Washington, D.C.: USDHEW, Assistant Secretary for Planning and Evaluation, mimeo, 1978b.

USDHEW, "Hospital Cost Containment—Fact Sheet," Washington, D.C.: USDHEW, Assistant Secretary for Planning and Evaluation, mimeo, 1979a.

USDHEW, "Fact Sheet on The National Health Plan," Washington, D.C.: USDHEW, Office of the Secretary, mimeo, 1979b.

U.S. Senate, Finance Committee, *Medicare and Medicaid: Problems, Issues, and Alternatives, Report of the Staff,* Washington, D.C.: Government Printing Office, 1970.

Waldman, Saul, *National Health Insurance Proposals,* USDHEW, Social Security Administration, Office of Research and Statistics, USDHEW Publication No. (SSA) 76–11920, Washington: U.S. Government Printing Office, 1976.

White, R., *Right to Health: The Evolution of an Idea,* Ames: University of Iowa Press, 1971.

Wildavsky, Aaron, *The Politics of the Budgetary Process,* Boston: Little, Brown, 1974.

Woodcock, Lennard, "Testimony re National Health Insurance," testimony before the Subcommittee on Health, House Committee on Interstate and Foreign Commerce, December 8, 1975.

Cumulative Index